Surgery
of the
Knee Joint

Surgery of the Knee Joint

EDITED BY

J.P. Jackson FRCS

Emeritus Consultant Orthopaedic Surgeon
Queens Medical Centre
Nottingham

and

W. Waugh MA, MChir, FRCS

Professor of Orthopaedic and Accident Surgery
Medical School
Queens Medical Centre
Nottingham

With illustrations by
G. Lythe BASMAA
Medical Illustrator
Queens Medical Centre
Nottingham

J. B. Lippincott Company
PHILADELPHIA

First published 1984
by Chapman and Hall Ltd
11 New Fetter Lane, London EC4P 4EE

© 1984 Chapman and Hall Ltd

Printed in Great Britain
at the University Press, Cambridge

ISBN 0–397–58291–9

Library of Congress Catalog Card Number 83–82568

Published and distributed in North America by
J.B. Lippincott Company, Philadelphia

A. Steindler	*There is no joint in the body upon which locomotion has placed a heavier burden, nor is there any so ready to resent abuse.*
	Constructing a joint so exposed to mechanical stresses with any assurance of safety has been a strain on nature's ingenuity.
King Henry V, Act IV, Scene I	*Canst thou, when thou command'st the beggar's knee, command the health of it?*
King Henry VIII, Act II, Scene II	*They have all new legs and lame ones: one would take it, that never saw 'em pace before.*
Pericles, Act IV, Scene II	*Therefore lets have fresh ones, what'ere we pay for them.*
P. Hammond	*The human knee is a joint, and not an entertainment.*
P. Ayres	*Let man's hands stay off the knees.*
Isaiah XXXV.3	*Strengthen ye the weak hands and confirm the feeble knees.*

Contents

CONTENTS

List of Contributors

P. M. Aichroth
MS, MB, BS, FRCS

Consultant Orthopaedic Surgeon at Westminster Hospital, Westminster Children's Hospital, Queen Mary's Hospital, Roehampton and Honorary Consultant to the Hospital for Sick Children, Great Ormond Street and Honorary Research Fellow to the Institute of Orthopaedics, London.

D. J. Dandy
MA, MB, BChir, FRCS

Consultant Orthopaedic Surgeon at Newmarket General Hospital and Addenbrookes Hospital, Cambridge.

J. W. Goodfellow
MB, BS, FRCS

Consultant Orthopaedic Surgeon at Nuffield Orthopaedic Centre and Clinical Lecturer to Oxford University Medical School, Oxford.

J. P. Jackson
MB, BS, FRCS

Emeritus Consultant Orthopaedic Surgeon to Harlow Wood Orthopaedic Hospital, Nottingham General Hospital and Nottingham University Hospital, and Clinical Teacher to Nottingham University Medical School, Nottingham.

F. Johnson
BSc, MASc, PhD,
MIEE, MBES

Formerly Lecturer in Bioengineering, Nottingham University Medical School, Nottingham. Now with Oxford Medical Systems.

J. K. Lloyd Jones
MA, MB, BChir, FRCP

Consultant in Rheumatology and Rehabilitation, Harlow Wood Orthopaedic Hospital and Mansfield District General Hospital, and Clinical Teacher to Nottingham University Medical School, Nottingham.

B. J. Preston
MB, BS, FRCS, FRCR,
FFR, DMRD

Consultant Diagnostic Radiologist, Nottingham University Group Hospitals, Nottingham.

Mrs M. Tew
MA

Statistician, Nottingham University Medical School, Nottingham.

E. L. Trickey
MB, BS, FRCS

Consultant Orthopaedic Surgeon at Royal National Orthopaedic Hospital and Edgware General Hospital, and Dean of Institute of Orthopaedics, London University, London.

W. Waugh
MA, MChir, MB, BChir,
FRCS

Professor of Orthopaedic and Accident Surgery, Nottingham University, Nottingham.

J. N. Wilson
ChirM, MB, BS, FRCS

Consultant Orthopaedic Surgeon at Royal National Orthopaedic Hospital (London) and National Hospital for Nervous Diseases (Queens Square), and Surgeon-in-Charge of Accident Unit, Royal National Orthopaedic Hospital (Stanmore), and Consultant Orthopaedic Surgeon to Garston Moor Medical Rehabilitation Centre.

Foreword

The timeliness of this book on arthritis of the knee is unquestionable. In the last decade, the diagnosis and treatment of knee disorders have been brought into a new era, principally by knee replacement and arthroscopy. Both are beautifully covered in the text.

Further, the book is outstanding because Peter Jackson and William Waugh have been a unique team – a partnership – for these many years. Their combined efforts have greatly improved our knowledge of the knee and they have published numerous papers on this joint. Their pioneering procedure of upper tibial osteotomy for degenerative arthritis, first reported in 1968, is a classic.

The material in this book is written by experts in the subject who have achieved international reputations in their respective fields. A complete review of all knee replacements available in the world today would require a two or three volume work. Rather, this book deals with selected topics based on the authors' personal experience and the evaluations are the result of intensive, controlled studies. Among the chapters are unexpected pearls, such as one on restoration of knee flexion. Another on the evaluation of results points out how easily we can be led down the primrose path of false assumptions and false deductions to false conclusions.

This is an extremely readable text. Although it may be presumptuous for an American to comment on the literary style of a book by English authors, the reader will appreciate that the sentence structure is uncomplicated and that, in essence, the book is written in 'plain English'. The language of the text is direct and to the point, devoid of meaningless superlatives and unnecessary additives. When one is so assailed today by needless technicalities and euphemisms, it is reassuring to see that the patient is fat, not 'obese' or 'overweight'; that he walks, not 'ambulates'.

Jackson and Waugh, the team, have thus put together their own experiences and the personal experiences of their chapter contributors. This makes a text which, as they emphasize in their preface, is basically a collection of essays or monographs. It is not just a summary of the literature, but a report of personal knowledge by the authors of each chapter. It is gratifying that the references cited are up-to-date in a book which has taken much time to prepare.

I recommend this book to all physicians interested in the knee joint. While admittedly written primarily for the orthopedic surgeon, it has great appeal for the clinical orthopedist, the internist, rheumatologist, family physician, and the accident surgeon – in short, for all who strive for medical understanding of the knee as an important functioning unit of the musculoskeletal system.

Mark B. Coventry
*Emeritus Professor
of Orthopedic
Surgery,
Mayo Clinic,
Rochester,
Minnesota, U S A*

Preface

During the past five or ten years, orthopaedic surgeons have become increasingly interested in the function of the knee joint and its disorders. In the 1950s there was little successful treatment which could be offered to sufferers from arthritis of the knee and knowledge of the management of athletic injuries was relatively limited. At this time, many considered meniscectomy to be a trivial procedure, although since then an awareness of the importance of the meniscus has gradually developed. The knee is certainly a complex mechanism, but greater understanding has altered the approach to the management and treatment of many of its disorders. Many papers are published and there are now a number of new books (as well as new editions of old favourites) available for the edification and instruction of orthopaedic surgeons.

What then have we to offer? First, our own long-standing interest in osteoarthritis and meniscectomy. Second, the collaboration of a group of colleagues who, although they would not make the claim themselves, have an international reputation for their knowledge of particular disorders of the knee. Although written primarily for orthopaedic surgeons, we hope that this book will also be of value to others interested in the knee joint (for example, rheumatologists, radiologists and bioengineers). The subject matter deals with topical and controversial problems which are relevant to orthopaedic practice in North America and other parts of the world as well as in the United Kingdom.

Many of the chapters have been produced by those who have worked with us at Harlow Wood Orthopaedic Hospital and in Nottingham. We have, however, also been fortunate that colleagues in other centres in the United Kingdom have written about aspects of the knee of which they have a special interest and experience. It is also a particular privilege to have a foreword written by Dr Mark Coventry of the Mayo Clinic, USA, whom we have known for many years.

Arthroscopic surgery, the management of ligamentous injuries and knee replacement are all subjects of current interest and development. These as well as other related topics, are fully discussed; but we have excluded fractures as outside the scope of this book.

We have, however, not attempted to produce a comprehensive text book but we would like each chapter to be regarded as an essay or monograph which expresses the author's individual opinion. Nonetheless, we intend that the book as a whole should give a coherent and up to date account of methods of diagnosis and management of the most important disorders which affect the knee joint.

We are grateful to other authors and publishers who have given permission for their illustrations to be reproduced, and who are acknowledged at the appropriate places in the text. Most of the diagrams have been drawn by Mr Geoffrey Lythe of the Audio-Visual Department in the Medical School at Nottingham. His experience, clarity of line and, above all, his ability to produce work of a high standard at short notice, have made life a lot easier for us.

Finally, we must thank our contributors, some of whom have put up with a good deal of pressure and badgering. Our publishing editor, Dr Barry Shurlock, and his staff have smoothed out path and imposed a literary house-style of a high standard.

Our two secretaries, Mrs E. Morris and Mrs D. Harrap, have been responsible for all the typing and retyping and have shown admirable patience in the face of the demand for better and better versions to send to our publishers.

J.P. Jackson
W. Waugh

PART ONE

Anatomy, Biomechanics and Diagnosis

CHAPTER 1

Surgical Anatomy

J. P. Jackson

1.1 Limb alignment

An accurate knowledge of what is normal in the anatomy of the knee is necessary in order that abnormalities can be properly assessed. The bones forming the joint have a definite relationship to each other and any departure from this produces alteration in function and leads to secondary changes, which may be progressive if uncorrected. Because of the arrangement of ligaments and muscles, the joint is essentially very stable, but the length of the bones involved leads to considerable magnification of any deforming forces and as a result it is more liable to injury than any other joint in the body.

1.1.1 CORONAL TIBIOFEMORAL ANGLE (CTF) (FIG. 1.1)

The anatomical axes of the femur and tibia are represented by lines drawn down the centre of the diaphyses. These will normally be set at an angle to each other which varies between 4–9° and is known as the coronal tibiofemoral angle (CTF). The higher values occur in the female as a result of the wider pelvis. Variations occur due to abnormalities caused by trauma, disease or dysplasia.

1.1.2 MECHANICAL AXIS (FIG. 1.1)

The mechanical axis is represented by a line joining the centre of the head of the femur to the centre of the ankle joint. Normally this will pass through the centre of the knee joint. In those knees in which there is a lateral deformity, the mechanical axis will be deviated to one or other side of the centre.

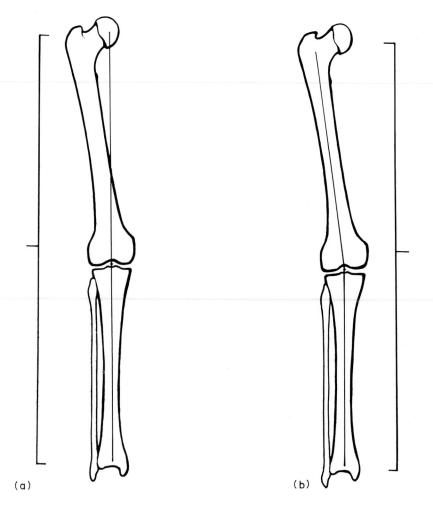

(a)   (b)

Fig. 1.1   The mechanical axis (*a*) and the coronal tibiofemoral angle (CTF) (*b*).

1.2   The articular surfaces

(a) Femur

The articulating part of the femur consists of two condyles. Posteriorly they are circular and parallel to each other. Anteriorly the two condyles flatten out and the medial inclines towards the lateral side, so that in effect it is the longer of the two condyles (Fig. 1.2). The patellar surface of the lateral condyle is normally rather more prominent than the medial. This prominence varies in size. It may be underdeveloped in patients who suffer from subluxation or habitual dislocation of the patella. On the peripheral surface of the medial

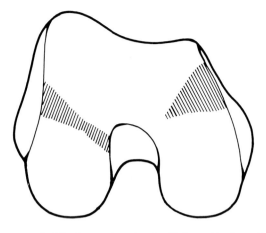

Fig. 1.2   The lower end of the femur showing the V-shaped indentation on the medial femoral condyle and the strip shape on the lateral condyle.

condyle there is a V-shaped indentation. On the lateral condyle the groove is strip-shaped. These indentations are situated at the anterior end of the part of the condyle that articulates with the tibia. Into these indentations the anterior horns of the appropriate meniscus fit when the knee is in full extension. If for some reason there is a fixed flexion deformity of the joint so that there is no contact between these areas and the menisci, then the articular cartilage undergoes degeneration (Tasker and Waugh, 1982). It has also been noted that it is eroded much earlier than the rest of the articular cartilage in inflammatory joint disease (Waugh *et al.*, 1980).

(b) Tibia

The upper surface of the tibia presents two rounded condyles, though the medial is rather more oval in shape (Fig. 1.3). It is also slightly concave from side to side and anteroposteriorly. The lateral condyle, which is more nearly circular, is concave from side to side but has a slight convex contour when viewed anteroposteriorly. It is this convexity which accounts for the fact that rare cases of osteochondritis dissecans occur at this site. Both condyles are covered by articular cartilage and this is further prolonged on to the posterior surface of the tibia towards the medial side.

(c) Patella

The patella articulates with the upper part of the articular surface of the femur to a varying degree, depending on the amount of flexion. It is a sesamoid bone developed in the quadriceps tendon and has the function of making the quadriceps muscle mechanically more efficient. It may also have a secondary role in protecting the front of the joint. There are two facets

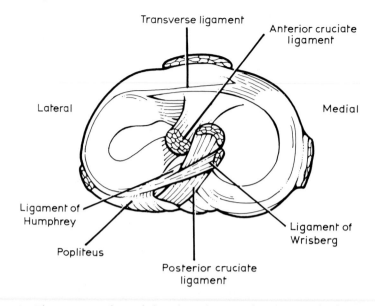

Fig. 1.3 The upper surface of the tibia, showing the menisci, the ligaments of Wrisberg and Humphrey embracing the posterior cruciate ligament. (After Heller and Langman, 1964.)

divided by a median ridge into lateral and medial. The size of these varies in relation to each other. Depending on the ratio between them, Wiberg (1941) classified them into three groups (Fig. 1.4). Reider *et al.* (1981), who investigated a series, found that in the first group (type I), of which the lateral and medial facets were approximately equal, there were 24% of cases. The second group (type II), which is the most common and in which the lateral facet is significantly larger than the medial, was found to be present in 57% of cases. In the third group (type III), in which the lateral condyle was considerably greater than the medial facet, which was almost vertical, there were 19%. Wiberg was of the opinion that chondromalacia was much more common in type III, though this has not subsequently been confirmed. On the medial side of the patella there is a small facet which comes into contact with the femoral condyle only in the last part of the flexion range (the occasional medial facet). It is very probable that the characteristic shape of the patella varies with the forces acting on it and it may be modified in those patients who suffer from congenital dislocation (Green and Waugh, 1968). The patella is further subdivided into an upper, middle and lower facet by transverse ridges running across the articular cartilage and roughly dividing the surface into three equal areas (Fig. 1.5). The lower articulates with the femur only in full extension. As flexion proceeds, the middle facet comes into contact at about 30°. Finally, at about 90° and beyond, the upper facet lies in contact with the femur.

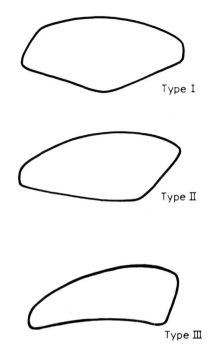

Type I

Type II

Type III

Fig. 1.4 Wiberg Classification of patellar shapes.

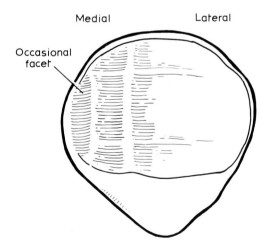

Medial   Lateral

Occasional
facet

Fig. 1.5 Posterior surface of the patella.

The height of the patella in relation to the tibia and femur is remarkably constant. In the normal position the length of the patella from the upper surface down to the tip of the lower pole is equal to the length of the patellar

7

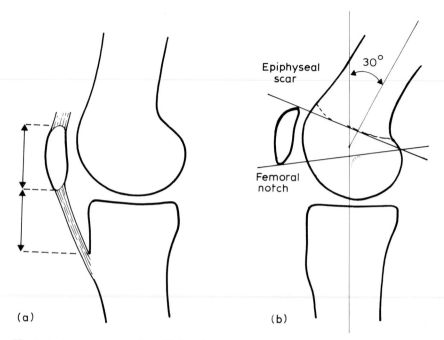

Fig. 1.6 Measurement of patella height: (*a*) The method of Insall; (*b*) Blumensaat's lines.

tendon (Insall and Salvati, 1971) (Fig. 1.6). This is most easily measured on a lateral radiograph. The patella is also said to lie between a line drawn through the epiphyseal scar and the line of the intercondylar notch when the knee is in 30° of flexion (Blumensaat's lines (Blumensaat, 1958)). This method is probably less accurate than that described by Insall and Salvati, 1971. The patella occupies a higher position in patients suffering from subluxation and recurrent dislocation of the patella. Insall *et al.* (1976) have suggested that variations in the ratio are also associated with chondromalacia.

(d) The Q-angle

This is the angle between the axis of pull of the quadriceps and the patellar tendon. In practice it is measured by drawing a line from the anterior superior iliac spine to the centre of the patella and then a further line from the centre of the patella to the tibial tuberosity (Fig. 1.7). Insall *et al.* (1976) found that these two lines met an an angle averaging 14°. He considered that anything above 20° was abnormal.

1.2.1. OSSIFICATION

The femoral epiphysis appears at about the ninth month and joins at the

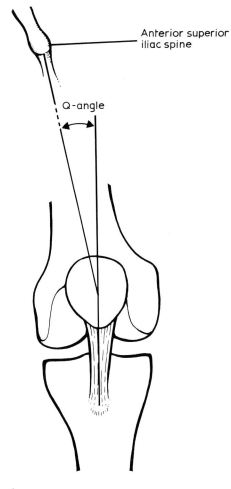

Anterior superior
iliac spine

Q-angle

Fig. 1.7 The Q-angle.

twentieth year. That at the upper end of the tibia appears before or shortly after birth and joins at age twenty. Both of these epiphyses, particularly that of the femur, may have rather unusual and irregular appearances during growth (Fig. 1.8). The changes are so variable that in order to decide whether or not they are pathological a radiograph of the opposite knee may be required. The variation may well be mistaken for osteochondritis dissecans. The centre for the patella appears in the second or third year but may be delayed to as long as the sixth. It is complete at puberty. The absence of the patellar centre may make the diagnosis of congenital dislocation of the patella extremely difficult (Green and Waugh, 1968). If it is dislocated there may well be even further delay in the appearance of the centre.

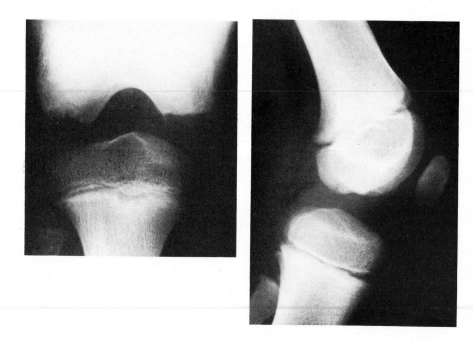

Fig. 1.8 Normal ossification of femoral condyles (aged 8) showing changes suggestive of osteochondritis dissecans.

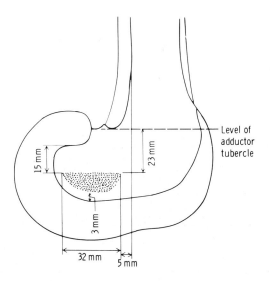

Fig. 1.9 Attachment of anterior cruciate ligament to medial side of the lateral femoral condyle. (After Girgis and Marshall, 1975.)

1.3   Ligaments

1.3.1   INTRODUCTION

These are an important factor in maintaining the stability of the knee. They are complementary to each other in that the cruciates in the centre of the joint cross each other. The collateral ligaments also cross; the medial running forwards and downwards and the lateral downwards and backwards. The crossed relationship means that all four ligaments simultaneously tighten as the joint screws home. This gives a very solid, stable joint.

(a) *The anterior cruciate ligament*

This ligament is attached above to the medial surface of the lateral femoral condyle, just anterior to the articular surface on the posterior part of the condyle. Its origin is crescentic in outline. The convexity is directed posteriorly and slightly upwards (Fig. 1.9). Below, it is attached to a depressed area in front of and between the tibial spines (Fig. 1.10). It gives a well-marked

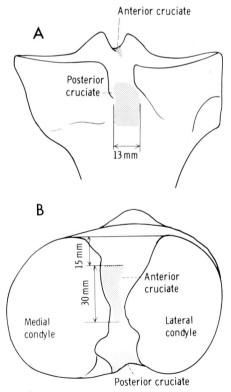

Fig. 1.10   Attachment of anterior and posterior cruciate ligaments to the tibia. (After Girgis and Marshall, 1975.)

slip which runs forward to join with the anterior horn of the lateral meniscus. It measures about 11 mm in width and is 38 mm long (Girgis and Marshall, 1975). There is some divergence of opinion as to when the ligament is tight and when it is relaxed. The probability is that in no part of the flexion cycle is it more than very slightly relaxed, although the fibres are not, in fact, under tension. Girgis and Marshall (1975) suggest that as the knee flexes the posterior attachments of the anterior cruciate ligament are brought closer together and it becomes looser. The anteromedial band, however, tends to remain tight (Figs 1.11 and 1.12). Kennedy *et al.* (1974) concluded that some fibres of the cruciate were taut in full extension, in 5° to 20° of flexion and again at around 70–90° of flexion. They thought that there was probably maximum relaxation at about 45°. The amount of rotation, however, also has an effect on the tension. As the tibia internally rotates during flexion this also has the effect of tightening the fibres. External rotation conversely tends to relax them.

(b) The posterior cruciate ligament

This is attached above to the lateral surface of the medial femoral condyle. This also has a crescentic origin but the convexity is downwards (Fig. 1.13).

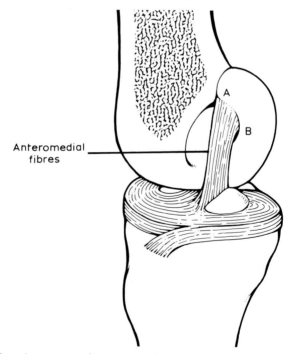

Fig. 1.11 Anterior cruciate ligament with knee in extension. (After Girgis and Marshall, 1975.)

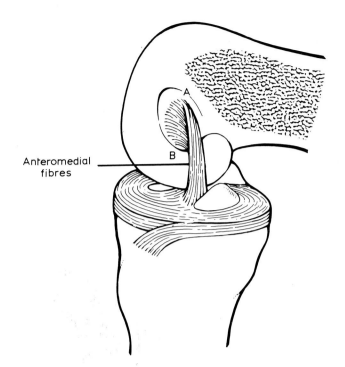

Anteromedial
fibres

A

B

Fig. 1.12 Anterior cruciate ligament with knee in flexion. (After Girgis and Marshall, 1975.)

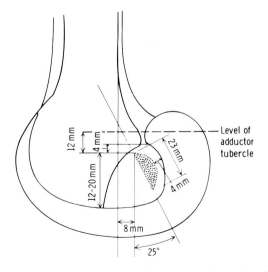

12 mm

4 mm

12-20 mm

8 mm

25°

23 mm

4 mm

Level of
adductor
tubercle

Fig. 1.13 Attachment of posterior cruciate ligament to lateral surface of medial femoral condyle. (After Girgis and Marshall, 1975.)

Below, it attaches to the groove between the tibial condyles, extending down between them on to the upper part of the tibial shaft (Fig. 1.11). Both the cruciate ligaments are extra-articular and are normally excluded from the knee joint by a covering of synovial membrane. As the knee flexes the more posterior femoral fibres of the posterior cruciate are carried downwards and forwards and relax, although the remainder of the ligament remains taut (Figs 1.14 and 1.15). At about 30° of flexion the bulk of the fibres are quite tight. The posterior cruciate ligament is of similar length to the anterior, measuring about 38 mm in length and 13 mm in width (Girgis and Marshall, 1975). It is, in fact, the strongest ligament in the knee and is of considerable importance in maintaining stability.

Both cruciate ligaments are multifascicular. The fibres tend to be spiral, though in some cases pass directly from tibia to femur. They are separated from their neighbours by loose connective tissue and tortuous blood vessels (Kennedy *et al.*, 1974). This suggests that they can undergo rotation as flexion and extension take place. Nerve fibres have been identified in the cruciate ligaments. Their destination may be the cerebellum and they may

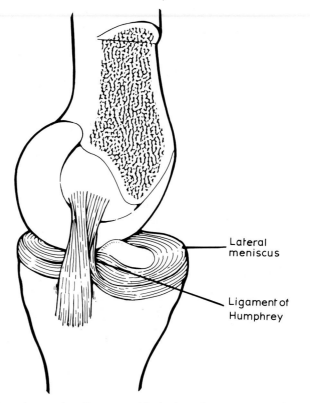

Lateral
meniscus

Ligament of
Humphrey

Fig. 1.14 Posterior cruciate ligament with the knee in extension. (After Girgis and Marshall, 1975.)

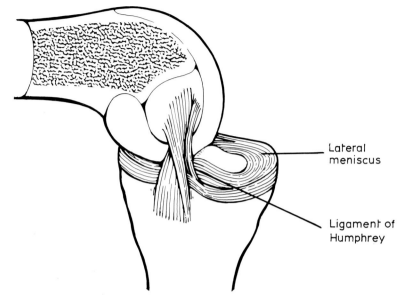

Fig. 1.15 Posterior cruciate ligament with the knee in flexion. (After Girgis and Marshall, 1975.)

participate in reflex subcortical activity (Kennedy *et al.*, 1974). The two ligaments wind on each other, as the tibia turns into internal rotation, and consequently tighten. They relax to some degree as they become unwound as external rotation takes place. This, of course, would indicate that they wind in flexion and unwind as the joint comes into extension.

1.3.2 THE MEDIAL SIDE OF THE KNEE

The structures on the medial side are difficult to isolate since they blend intimately with each other. This has led to varying descriptions of the anatomy. Warren and Marshall (1979) thought that they could best be considered in three layers.

(a) The first layer

This is the deep fascia which invests the sartorius and extends forward to envelop the patellar tendon. It then passes posteriorly in a sheet to the mid-line of the popliteal fossa, overlying the medial head of the gastrocnemius and the other structures in this fossa.

(b) The second layer

The superficial part of the medial collateral ligament is the most important

15

(Fig. 1.16). This ligament is composed of both parallel and oblique fibres. Those that are parallel towards the anterior part of the ligament measure about 11 cm in length. The origin above is from the medial epicondyle. The fibres extend downwards and forwards to be inserted on to the medial surface of the medial tibial condyle. These fibres are about 1.5 cm wide. Extending posteriorly from them and forming the oblique part of the superficial medial collateral ligament there are fibres that sweep backwards and blend with the capsule of the joint, which forms the third layer. They envelop the medial condyle of the femur. This area also has a contribution from the semi-membranosus sheath and its tendon. It forms the so-called posteromedial corner (Fig. 1.17(a)). In full extension this part of the ligamentous support is tight and helps to give stability to the knee joint. When the knee is flexed it forms a lax pouch. As the knee flexes, the anterior or parallel fibres of the superficial ligament pass posteriorly, moving over the deep part of the collateral ligament. Movement between these two components of the collateral ligament is facilitated by a small bursa, which from time to time may become inflamed. The position of this bursa is variable in relation to the joint line and it may be either actually over or, not infrequently, just above or below it. The lower part of the superficial collateral ligament is covered by the insertion of the anserine muscles (sartorius, gracilis and semitendinosus) (Fig. 1.16). The tendons of these muscles are also separated by a small bursa from the collateral ligament, which may undergo inflammatory change and be a source of pain.

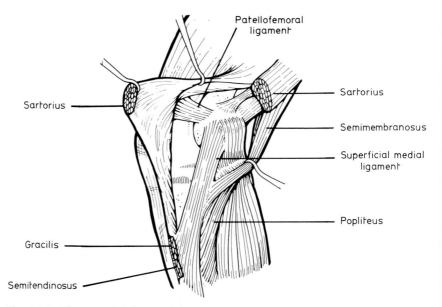

Fig. 1.16 The superficial part of the medial collateral ligament. (After Warren and Marshall, 1979.)

(c) The third layer

This is the true capsule of the knee. Anteriorly it is quite thin and passes forward to cover the fat pad below and to invest the suprapatellar pouch above. As it passes posteriorly it becomes thickened just deep to the superficial collateral ligament, forming the deep collateral ligament (Fig. 1.17(b)).

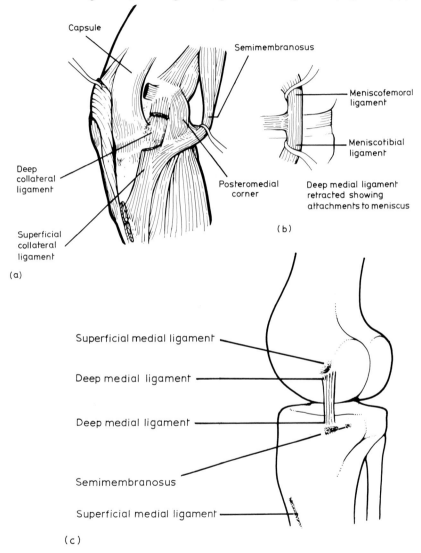

Fig. 1.17 (a) Deep part of the medial collateral ligament with areas of attachment of superficial collateral ligament and semimembranosus; (b) superficial part cut away to show deep part of collateral ligament; (c) attachments of deep part to medial meniscus. (After Warren and Marshall, 1979.)

17

The fibres are attached above, to the area immediately below the epicondyle. They then pass downwards to obtain attachment to the meniscus as the meniscofemoral ligament (Fig. 1.17(c)). Below the meniscus, the fibres pass downwards to obtain a further attachment to the tibia just below the joint line, and may be referred to as the coronary or meniscotibial ligament. The fibres of this ligament are short but will allow movement of the meniscus forwards and backwards to the limit of the length of the fibres as the knee flexes and extends. Should it rupture, not only is control of the meniscus lost, but rotatory instability of the joint can result. Posteriorly this ligament, which is a continuation of the capsule, blends with the superficial ligament and contributes to the posteromedial corner.

1.3.3 THE LATERAL SIDE OF THE JOINT

There is a layer of investing fascia which extends anteriorly from the tibial tendon backwards to the mid-line of the popliteal fossa where it joins the fascia investing the medial side. Posteriorly, it covers over the head of the gastrocnemius and the contents of the popliteal fossa. On the lateral aspect of the knee and the thigh it is thickened and forms the iliotibial band.

(a) Iliotibial band

This strong band of fascia takes origin above from the anterior superior iliac spine and an area of 2–3 cm posteriorly along the crest of the ilium. It passes down the lateral surface of the thigh and is inserted into Gerdy's tubercle on the lateral condyle of the tibia. These lower fibres act as an accessory collateral ligament of the knee. The upper part is fairly thin, but as it passes down the thigh towards the lower third it becomes thick and well demarcated. There is no attachment between the lateral femoral condyle and Gerdy's tubercle. The intermuscular septum, through which the fascia gains attachment to the linea aspera, maintains the iliotibial band under some tension. If it is severed in the middle of the thigh the upper fibres retract upwards and the lower ones downwards. The upper part is under the control of two muscles, the tensor fasciae femoris above and in front, and the gluteus maximus above and behind. These two muscles pass downwards to be attached obliquely into it. As a result it can be moved slightly forwards and backwards during movements of the knee and the hip. Kaplan (1958) was of the opinion that contraction of these muscles did not produce active movement at the knee. He reported that stimulation of the tensor fasciae femoris in anaesthetized patients did not move the joint. Blaimont et al. (1971) were, however, able to produce some effect on the knee joint by faradic stimulation. Later still, Paré et al. (1981) found that proximal traction of the fascia lata on the lateral aspect of the thigh and as high as the level of the tensor produced tension in the tract as far distally as the lateral tibial tuberosity. Furthermore, they found activity of the posterolateral fibres of the tensor at heel strike.

They concluded that muscular action through the fascia lata could compensate for anterior cruciate instability in the Ellison transplant procedure, though they were not sure that the force applied was great enough to be effective.

The iliotibial band is often sacrificed, particularly for operations in stabilizing the knee. Its loss, however, by itself does not appear to produce instability provided the lateral collateral ligament and the biceps tendon remain intact. If one or both of these structures has been damaged, giving rise to instability, then removal of the iliotibial tract may well accentuate the problem.

(b) Lateral collateral ligament

The lateral collateral ligament runs from the lateral epicondyle of the femur downwards and backwards to the styloid process of the fibula (Fig. 1.18). It is a rounded cord-like structure which has no attachment to the lateral meniscus. In full extension it is taut but as soon as the knee flexes it relaxes. The biceps femoris muscle exerts continual tension on the ligament by means of tendinous fibres which loop around it (Marshall *et al.*, 1972) (Fig. 1.18). By this means as some slack occurs with rotation of the tibia during flexion and extension the collateral ligament is kept under continual tension. This helps to maintain the stability of the joint.

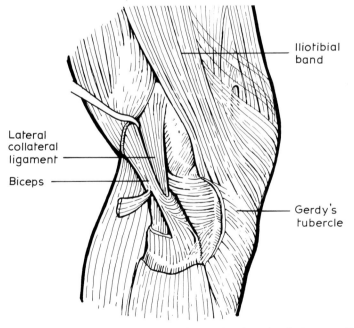

Fig. 1.18 Attachment of biceps femoris to fibular head, with relation to collateral ligament. (After Marshall *et al.*, 1972.)

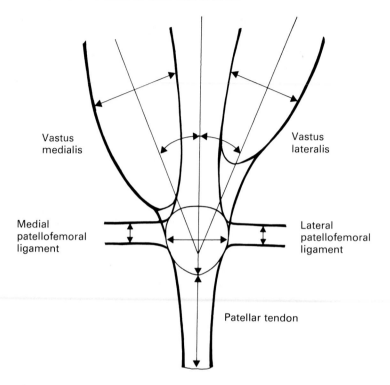

Fig. 1.19 Diagrammatic attachments of the patella.

The capsule of the joint is similar to that on the medial side. In front, the fibres invest both the fat pad below and the suprapatellar bursa above. It passes posteriorly and blends with the capsule of fibres from the medial side. In the posterior intercondylar area the capsule is thickened to form the oblique popliteal ligament.

1.3.4 PATELLAR LIGAMENTS

In addition to the attachments of the quadriceps muscles and tibial tendon, further ligamentous attachments are inconstantly found on each side of the patella (Fig. 1.19). A patellofemoral ligament passes from the medial side of the bone and is attached to the medial femoral epicondyle, but was found in only about six out of twenty specimens dissected by Reider *et al.* (1981). On the lateral side a similar ligament runs to the lateral epicondyle. This is rather more frequently present and was found in over half the dissected specimens. These ligaments vary in thickness and are about 1 cm broad. Two further small bands extend from the lower part of the patella and pass obliquely down diverging from the patellar tendon to obtain attachment to the anterior aspect of the tibia. They are probably not of any great importance but occasionally when a lateral angulation develops they can be felt passing over the femoral condyles as the joint flexes and extends. Patients with lateral deformity may complain of pain and discomfort as these bands pass over lipping on the femoral condyles.

The patella, as has already been suggested, has a shape which reflects the forces acting on it. Since it is a sesamoid bone, this is very largely, therefore, the effect of the quadriceps pull. During flexion and extension it takes a rather oblique path on the front of the femur. In full flexion it lies to the lateral side of the midline, but is more central in extension. If the oblique fibres of the vastus medialis fail, more particularly due to injury, then subluxation or dislocation may occur. When present the medial patellofemoral ligament must also be ruptured when the bone dislocates. At one time it was suggested that loss of the patella led to improved efficiency of the knee (Brooke, 1937; Hey-Groves, 1937; Watson-Jones, 1945). Later work, however, has shown that this is not so and that its loss leads to impairment of the mechanical efficiency (Haxton, 1945). Since more power is required over the last 15° to extend the knee, weakness of the quadriceps may produce a lag of extension. Patellar tendon advancement, as recommended by Kaufer (1971), may be sufficient to overcome the lag by improving the mechanical efficiency.

1.4 Musculature

1.4.1 THE EXTENSION MECHANISM

The four component muscles of the quadriceps contribute in varying degrees of power to the extension of the knee joint (Reider *et al.* 1981) (Fig. 1.20).

(a) Rectus femoris

This, the most central part, narrows at the lower end to form a wide aponeurosis, about 5–8 cm across. The fibres then sweep over the anterior surface of the patella. Almost all the fibres of the rectus femoris continue onwards across the front of the patella into the patellar tendon.

(b) Vastus lateralis

This has a more direct attachment to the patella. The lower fibres approach the patella at about 12–15° in the coronal plane. It becomes tendinous 2–3 cm from the upper border of the patella. Almost all the fibres are directly inserted into the patella, though some do continue onwards in the lateral retinaculum. A small proportion of its fibres pass laterally giving a contribution to the iliotibial band. They are thus better placed mechanically to produce lateral rotation of the tibia on the femur when the joint is flexed.

21

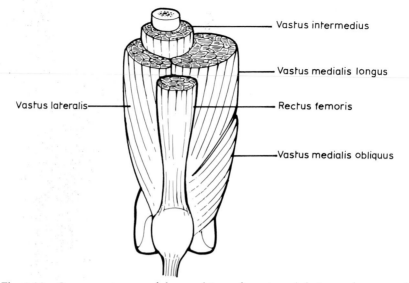

Vastus intermedius

Vastus medialis longus

Vastus lateralis

Rectus femoris

Vastus medialis obliquus

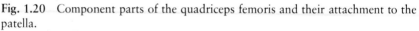

Fig. 1.20 Component parts of the quadriceps femoris and their attachment to the patella.

(c) Vastus medialis

This is functionally two muscles. The longer and more vertical fibres form an angle with the shaft of the femur of 15–18°. The lower ones are more oblique and approach the superomedial border of the patella at about 50–55°. These two muscles, which may be referred to as the vastus medialis longus and the vastus medialis obliquus, have different nerve trunks. In some limbs there is an actual fascial separation (Reider *et al.*, 1981). The muscle becomes aponeurotic only a few millimetres from the patella and inserts directly into it. Some fibres contribute to the medial retinaculum.

(d) Vastus intermedius

This is the smallest of four components of the quadriceps and inserts almost directly into the superior border of the patella. It does not continue beyond this.

1.4.2 FUNCTION

The primary function of the quadriceps is to extend the knee, but the rather prominent fibres of the vastus medialis obliquus at the lower end do not, in fact, contribute to this action. Their only function is to prevent the patella subluxating laterally. It has been stated that without the vastus medialis the last 15° of extension cannot be achieved (Nicoll, 1943). This was questioned by Brewerton (1955) and later by Lieb and Perry (1968). Brewerton showed that if the vastus medialis action was decreased by infiltration of the oblique muscle's nerve supply with local anaesthetic there was no evidence of loss of power of extension. Lieb and Perry attached weights to the vastus medialis oblique tendon in the line of a pull and showed that, however large the load, no extension was produced. They also demonstrated that the quadriceps muscle requires 60% more force for the last 15° of extension than it does throughout the remainder of its excursion. The vastus intermedius and the rectus femoris are the most efficient of the muscles producing extension due to their mechanical positioning. The external rotation of the tibia, which occurs as the joint moves into full extension, the so-called screw home movement, is partly dictated by the shape of the bones but also by the cruciate ligaments. As indicated above, the vastus lateralis does have some external rotation power. It contributes this in the last part of extension. Since it is necessary to use more force during the last 5° to 15° of extension, it follows that this part of the range is most easily lost in those limbs in which there is a decrease in the total power of the muscles (Kaufer, 1971). As a result, patients with a knee damaged by injury or disease may have difficulty in obtaining the last part of extension. Flexion contractures may then develop.

1.4.3 THE KNEE FLEXORS

These are a diverse group of muscles, all of which have other functions. A detailed description of these will be found in books of anatomy but the following points are of particular interest in relation to the knee joint.

(a) Biceps femoris

The biceps femoris has already been referred to in the description of the lateral side of the knee, indicating that its insertion produces a pull on the collateral ligament and by exerting tension helps as a lateral stabiliser of the knee. The superficial fibres form a broad band which continues down the lateral side of the leg. Marshall *et al.* (1972) were of the opinion that these fibres formed a strong flexion lever and in addition produced external rotation. They also pointed out that there was a strong fascial connection between these fibres and the iliotibial band, so that they helped to keep it under tension when the knee was semiflexed, thus providing further stability of the joint.

(b) Semitendinosus

The semitendinosus is characterized by the length of its tendon of insertion which starts just below the middle of the thigh, curves around the medial tibial condyle and then passes over the medial collateral ligament, from which it is separated by a bursa, to take part in the anserine insertion.

The semimembranosus tendon reinforces the posteromedial corner of the

23

capsule. Other fibrous extensions which pass downwards are rather better placed mechanically to assist in medial rotation of the tibia when the joint is semiflexed.

1.5 Menisci

Although for many years there has been doubt about the exact function of these two bodies (MacConaill, 1932), their anatomy has been well described (Fig. 1.3).

1.5.1 MEDIAL MENISCUS

This is semicircular in shape. The posterior horn is much broader than the anterior part. Anteriorly it is attached just in front of the anterior cruciate ligament between the two condyles of the tibia. Some fibres continue across the front of the joint to join the anterior horn of the lateral meniscus. They form the transverse ligament. Posteriorly it is attached to the intercondyloid fossa just in front of the posterior cruciate ligament and underlying the posterior horn fibres of the lateral meniscus. Around the periphery of the joint it is loosely attached to the capsule. This is thickened in the middle third where it forms the meniscofemoral and meniscotibial ligaments (the deep medial collateral ligament), which limit the movement of the meniscus.

1.5.2 LATERAL MENISCUS

This forms two-thirds of a circle. It is broader throughout its length than the medial meniscus. The anterior horn is attached behind the anterior cruciate ligament, blending with it. The posterior horn has an attachment just behind the intercondyloid eminence of the tibia. In most cases the meniscus gives off a small ligament from the posterior horn, which is fixed to the lateral aspect of the medial femoral condyle. This ligament may pass either in front of or behind the posterior cruciate ligament. Lying in front it is usually referred to as the ligament of Humphrey (Fig. 1.21) and behind as the ligament of Wrisberg. These ligaments help to control the meniscus during movement of the knee. During flexion the ligament tightens and pulls the posterior horn of the meniscus forwards and medially to fit into the tibio-femoral space and increase congruity. The popliteus tendon passes under the lateral collateral ligament and grooves the lateral meniscus at the junction of the middle and posterior thirds. It is separated from the meniscus as it passes over it by a synovial sheath. As the muscle passes posteriorly, some of its fibres are attached to the posterior horn of the lateral meniscus (Fig. 1.21). These fibres help to control the movement of the meniscus in conjunction with the ligaments of Wrisberg and Humphrey (Last, 1950). Their action is to pull the posterior horn backwards. It has been shown that the greatest activity of this

Popliteus tendon

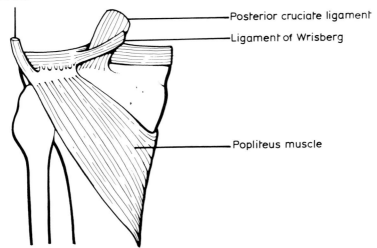

Posterior cruciate ligament

Ligament of Wrisberg

Popliteus muscle

Fig. 1.21 Posterior attachments of the lateral meniscus.

muscle is when the knee is in about 90° of flexion, producing internal rotation of the tibia (Heller and Langman, 1964).

The majority of the fibres of the menisci are disposed in a circumferential direction (Fig. 1.22). There are some radially disposed fibres in the mid-zone and also on exposed surfaces, particularly the tibial aspect. The tensile strength of the menisci increases with age in a way similar to that of articular cartilage (Bullough *et al.*, 1970). This very possibly accounts for the more frequent occurrence of longitudinal tears in younger and middle-aged

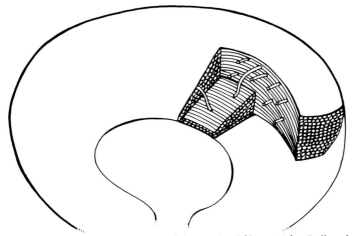

Fig. 1.22 Diagrammatic representation of the meniscal fibres. (After Bullough *et al.*, 1970.)

25

patients rather than in later life. Seedhom *et al.* (1974) have estimated that the medial meniscus carries 57% of the total load through the knee, the lateral some 69%. The vascular supply of the menisci is only to the outer third. The inner two-thirds rely for nutrition on synovial fluid. The blood supply is probably rather better in the attached area of the horns as there is no direct pressure in these parts. Similarly, the inner two-thirds of the menisci do not have any sensory innervation. In consequence, pain which is provoked by a tear of a meniscus must be due to damage to the outer third or to the ligamentous attachment being stretched.

1.6 Arterial supply (Fig. 1.23)

The knee joint is extremely well supplied with blood which comes from the superior, middle and inferior geniculate vessels of the popliteal artery. The vessels anastomose in front, above, behind and below the patella. From above they also receive a small contribution from the highest geniculate and below

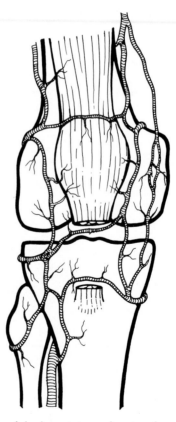

Fig. 1.23 Arterial supply of the knee joint – showing the anterior anastomosis.

from the recurrent anterior tibial vessel. The rich vascularization of the joint, which occurs as a result of all these vessels, probably explains the frequency of haemarthrosis (Scapinelli, 1967; 1968). In haemophilia the knee is the site of bleeding more often than any other articulation. The blood supply to the posterior aspect of the knee joint is from all the geniculate vessels, but they are irregular in size and position. Anteriorly they come together to form a well-marked anastomosis which lies around the patella. Above, the highest geniculate joins the lateral superior geniculate vessel in an anastomosis which lies anterior to the quadriceps aponeurosis just above the patella. On the medial side there is a contribution from the medial superior geniculate.

Below the lower pole of the patella and running posterior to the tibial tendon, there is an anastomosis between the medial and lateral inferior geniculate vessels, which receives reinforcement from the anterior tibial recurrent on the lateral side.

There is a junction between the two arches on either side to complete the anastomotic ring around the patella.

The interosseous vessels are grouped into two systems, the first represented by the mid-patellar vessels which enter the bone by foramina in the middle third of the anterior surface. The vessels pass upwards and penetrate to the chondro–osseous junction.

The second system from the infrapatellar arch penetrates the patella at the lower pole and passing upwards supplies the lowest third of the bone and communicates with the mid-patellar system. These vessels may be interrupted by fractures across the lower part of the patella so that necrosis results. Similarly, lateral marginal and superior third fractures may give rise to necrosis because of isolation of bone fragments, and resulting slow union.

Whilst all the vessels give some blood supply to the inner part of the knee joint, the cruciate ligaments are largely supplied by the middle geniculate. This vessel passes forwards into the upper end of the anterior cruciate ligament and runs distally. At arthroscopy quite a large branch can be seen lying on the anterior surface of the ligament. This artery ends in the tibial plateau and has little or no anastomosis with any other vessel and is in effect an end artery. This is of relevance in injuries to the anterior cruciate when the distal part may be cut off from its blood supply so that healing does not occur. The posterior cruciate ligament has some supply from the popliteal artery directly but also from the inferior geniculate vessels through its base.

1.7 The synovium

The synovial cavity of the knee is the largest in the body. Above, it forms a long pouch (the suprapatellar pouch) which extends upwards for two finger breadths above the patella. The synovium extends down behind the quadriceps aponeurosis and peripherally covers the surfaces of the femoral condyles to form the lateral and medial gutters. Distally, it extends to the attachment of the menisci. Below them, it covers the small area of capsule and the sides of the tibial plateau up to the articular cartilage; an area which may be affected by inflammatory arthritis and cause early erosions.

Centrally the synovium covers the fat pads and extends into the inter-condylar fossa as the patellar (or infrapatellar) fold. If this fold is large, it may form an obstacle to the passage of an arthroscope from one tibiofemoral compartment to the other. The anterior and posterior cruciates are covered by the membrane and it also lines the cul-de-sac at the back of the lateral meniscus for the tendon of the popliteus muscle.

In embryonic life the suprapatellar pouch is separated from the tibio-femoral compartments by an infolding of the synovium at the level of the upper pole of the patella. This may persist in its entirety with only a small centrally-placed opening with crescentic folds on either side. These are referred to as the medial and lateral suprapatellar plicae. They may be traumatized or inflamed and give rise to symptoms.

Another fold which may persist runs distally from the medial suprapatellar fold to the membrane covering the fat pad and is known as the medial patellar plica or shelf (Fig. 1.24). These folds may be found in 20% of normal knees (Hardaker *et al.*, 1980).

1.8 Bursae

There are numerous bursal sacs around the knee joint, all of which may be affected by inflammation, producing pain and, not infrequently, cystic

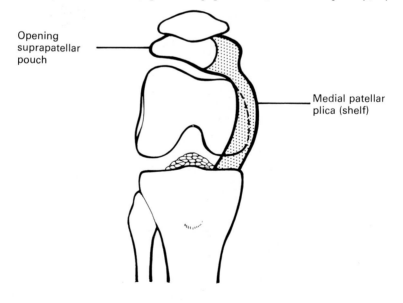

Opening suprapatellar pouch

Medial patellar plica (shelf)

Fig. 1.24   Medial patellar plica (shelf). (After Hardaker *et al.*, 1980.)

swelling. Those that most commonly give rise to symptoms lie in the front of the knee where they are more liable to pressure. The prepatellar bursa lies over the lower part of the patella and its tendon. It becomes inflamed in such people as miners, who not only work on their knees but also apply a sheering stress to the bursa as they shovel and turn at the same time. It is recognized as the 'beat knee' which initially is due to bleeding into the bursa (Sharrard, 1965) and is later followed by inflammation and serous effusion. The infrapatellar bursa lies between the patellar tendon and the upper part of the tibia. When it is inflamed it may be seen bulging on either side of the patellar tendon. There is also a small pretibial bursa overlying the tibial tuberosity.

The semimembranosus bursa lies beneath the tendon of that muscle and over the medial head of the gastrocnemius. It may present as a cystic swelling on the posteromedial aspect of the knee. The anserine bursa lies beneath the insertion of the anserine muscles and over the superficial surface of the lower part of the tibial collateral ligament. There is a small bicipital bursa which may enlarge and appear over the head of the fibula but beneath the biceps tendon. It may in this position simulate enlargement of the fibular head.

A small bursa lies underneath the superficial tibial collateral ligament and over the deep part. In this position it facilitates movement between the two components of the collateral ligament. It may lie at any point beneath the superficial collateral ligament from the femur above, across the joint line down on to the tibial surface. When inflamed, if it is near the joint line, it may well simulate a meniscal tear.

1.9 Movements of the knee

1.9.1 FLEXION–EXTENSION

Flexion–extension of the joint is accompanied by the so-called screw-home movement. This movement, which is involuntary, occurs entirely as a result of the bony configuration and the ligamentous attachments of the joint. It is a rotational movement of the tibia on the femur. The tibia rotates laterally over the last 30° of extension. As the knee passes from full flexion towards extension the femoral condyles, which are parallel posteriorly, roll on the tibial condyles. During this phase the menisci, particularly the medial, are held back and exert a stabilizing effect on the knee. Their function in this movement is to act as a wedge which fills the space between the tibial and femoral condyles, moving to accommodate the changing tibiofemoral space. This movement continues until the knee is in about 30° of flexion. At this point the screw-home movement begins. It is guided by the anterior cruciate, which by now is quite taut, and forces the tibia into external rotation. The amount of rotation that occurs reaches a maximum at about 10° of flexion and thereafter the degree of rotation decreases until full extension has been reached. At this point the joint is locked home. The axis of rotation is about the medial tibial spine (Shaw and Murray, 1974). It is noteworthy that if the anterior cruciate ligament is sectioned then irregular screw-home movement patterns can be shown to occur. At the start of the screw-home movement the initial rolling of the femoral condyles on the tibia converts to a sliding motion as the flat part of the femoral condyles comes in contact with the tibia. The medial condyle, being bigger, has to move backwards more rapidly and further than does the lateral. At the end of the screw-home movement the ligaments are tight. The superficial part of the medial collateral, which has an oblique path, can only become tight in full extension when the tibia has finally rotated outwards as far as it can go. As extension takes place the cruciate ligaments become wound on each other so that they are almost completely tight in full extension, as indeed is the posterior cruciate.

As the knee proceeds in the opposite direction from extension to flexion it initially has to be unlocked. This movement is activated by the popliteus muscle (Last, 1950). Electromyographic studies (Mann and Hagy, 1977) show that the popliteus contracts at the start of flexion. Not only does it flex the knee but it also initiates internal rotation. During flexion the popliteus muscle stabilizes the tibia in internal rotation and also pulls the lateral meniscus posteriorly. This protects the meniscus from the lateral femoral condyle and adjusts it to the tibiofemoral space. This movement is partly aided by the passive pull of the meniscofemoral ligament.

The lateral femoral condyle moves posteriorly about 1 cm during flexion, a range which is possible because of the potential laxity of the lateral collateral ligament. The lateral meniscus has to move a similar amount to accommodate the condylar movement. On account of this active movement carried out by the popliteus muscle, the posterior horn of the lateral meniscus is less often damaged than the medial. The latter is pushed posteriorly by the femoral condyle but only moves a few millimetres. Its excursion is controlled by the meniscotibial and meniscofemoral ligaments.

Medial rotation of the tibia is carried out, once the movement has been initiated, by the medial hamstrings (sartorius, gracilis, semitendinosus and semimembranosus). These muscles also contribute to the power of flexion. Perry et al. (1975) have shown that much of the flexion power of the anserine muscles is converted to internal rotator power by the Slocum procedure. This is due partly to the more proximal insertion, but also by lengthening the medial rotator arm, utilizing the flare of the medial tibial condyle.

Lateral rotation of the tibia is carried out by the biceps and to a lesser extent by the vastus lateralis, the fibres of which are in part inserted with the iliotibial tract. This tract itself does not exert any active force on the knee, although its fibres do have a passive stabilizing effect on the lateral side. The role of the popliteus muscle in producing internal rotation has already been mentioned.

During extension of the knee the mechanical advantage of the quadriceps is

30

increased by the presence of the patella. The muscle fibres are carried anteriorly and the patella also holds the tibia forward and in consequence exercises an anterior stabilizing effect. This can best be seen when testing for posterior subluxation in a knee in which the posterior cruciate ligament has been torn. As the knee flexes and comes to rest with the back of the heel on the couch, the tibia immediately subluxes backwards once the quadriceps ceases to function. During movements of the knee the patella moves laterally as the joint flexes. The lowest part of the patella is in contact with the femoral surface of the joint in full extension. As the joint flexes so the area in contact moves from the lower pole of the patella through the middle facet up to the superior facet. The odd small facet on the medial side of the patella only comes into contact with the femur when the joint is almost in full flexion (Goodfellow et al., 1976).

1.9.2 ROTATION

As has already been stated, rotation of the tibia takes place during the screw home movement. During locomotion a range of rotation is necessary to conform to the changing position of the hips and feet. This range varies from 0° when the knee is in full extension up to about 20° as the joint approaches full flexion (Markolf et al., 1976). Clinically, it is difficult to measure the range of flexion with any exactitude.

1.9.3 LATERAL MOVEMENT

Other movements which take place at the knee are abduction and adduction and a small amount of anteroposterior movement. These have also been measured by Markolf et al. (1976). Like rotation, the range of abduction and adduction increases with flexion. In full extension, it is only about 2° but increases up to 8° in full flexion. Anteroposterior movement is small in the intact knee and is of the order of 3 mm at 45°, decreasing as the knee approaches 90° of flexion.

References

Blaimont P, Burnotte J, Ballion JM, Duby P. Contribution biomécanique à l'étude des conditions d'équilibre dans le genou normal et pathologique. Application au traitement de l'arthrose varisante. *Acta Orthop Belg* 1971;**37**:573–92.

Blumensaat C. Cited by Andersen. Congenital deformities of the knee joint in dislocation of the patella and achondroplasia. *Acta Orthop Scand* 1958;**28**:27–50.

Brewerton DA. The function of the vastus medialis muscle. *Am Phys Med* 1955;**2**:164–8.

Brooke R. The treatment of fractured patella by excision. A study of morphology and function. *Br J Surg* 1937;**24**:733–47.

Bullough PG, Munera L, Murphy J, Weinstein AM. The strength of the menisci of the knee as it relates to their fine structure. *J Bone Joint Surg* [Br] 1970; **52–B**:564–70.

Girgis FG, Marshall JL. The cruciate ligaments of the knee joint. Anatomical, functional and experimental analysis. *Clin Orthop Rel Res* 1975;**106**:216–31.

Goodfellow J, Hungerford DS, Zindel M. Patello-femoral joint mechanics and pathology. *J Bone Joint Surg [Br]* 1976;**58–B**:287–90.

Green JP, Waugh W. Congenital lateral dislocation of the patella. *J Bone Joint Surg [Br]* 1968;**50–B**:285–9.

Hardaker WT, Whipple TL, Bassett FH. Diagnosis and treatment of the plica syndrome of the knee. *J Bone Joint Surg [Am]* 1980;**62–A**:221–5.

Haxton H. The function of the patella and the effects of its excision. *Surg Gynecol Obstet* 1945;**80**:389–95.

Heller L, Langman J. The menisco-femoral ligaments of the human knee. *J Bone Joint Surg [Br]* 1964;**46–B**:307–13.

Hey-Groves EW. A note on the extension apparatus of the knee joint. *Br J Surg* 1937;**24**:747–8.

Insall J, Falvo KA, Wise DW. Chondromalacia patellae. A prospective study. *J Bone Joint Surg [Am]* 1976;**58–A**:1–8.

Insall J, Salvati E. Patellar position in the normal knee joint. *Radiology* 1971;**101**:101–4.

Kaplan EB. The ilio-tibial tract. *J Bone Joint Surg [Am]* 1958;**40–A**:817–31.

Kaufer H. Mechanical function of the patella. *J Bone Joint Surg [Am]* 1971;**53–A**:1551–60.

Kennedy JC, Weinberg HW, Wilson AS. The anatomy and function of the anterior cruciate ligament. *J Bone Joint Surg [Am]* 1974;**56–A**:223–35.

Last RJ. The popliteus muscle and the lateral meniscus. *J Bone Joint Surg [Br]* 1950;**32–B**:93–9.

Lieb FJ, Perry J. Quadriceps function. *J Bone Joint Surg [Am]* 1968;**50–A**:1535–48.

MacConaill MA. The function of intra-articular fibro-cartilage with special reference to the knee and inferior radio-ulnar joints. *J Anat* 1932;**LXVI**:210–27.

Mann RA, Hagy JL. The popliteus muscle. *J Bone Joint Surg [Am]* 1977;**59–A**:924–7.

Markolf KL, Mensch JS, Amstutz HC. Stiffness and laxity of the knee. The contribution of the supporting structures. *J Bone Joint Surg [Am]* 1976;**58–A**:583–94.

Marshall JL, Girgis FG, Zelko RR. The biceps femoris tendon and its functional significance. *J Bone Joint Surg [Am]* 1972;**54–A**:1444–50.

Nicoll EA. Principles of exercise therapy. *Br Med J* 1943;**1**:747–50.

Paré EB, Stern JT, Schwartz JM. Functional differentiation within the tensor fasciae latae. *J Bone Joint Surg [Am]* 1981;**63–A**:1457–71.

Perry J, Antonelli D, Ford W. Analysis of knee joint forces during flexed knee stance. *J Bone Joint Surg [Am]* 1975;**57–A**:961–7.

Reider B, Marshall JL, Koslin B, Ring B, Girgis FG. The anterior aspect of the knee joint. *J Bone Joint Surg [Am]* 1981;**63–A**:351–6.

Scapinelli R. Blood supply of the human patella. *J Bone Joint Surg [Br]* 1967;**49–B**:563–70.

Scapinelli R. Studies on the vasculature of the human knee joint. *Acta Anat* 1968;**70**:305–31.

Seedhom BB, Dowson D, Wright V. *The loadbearing function of the menisci. A preliminary study. The knee joint.* Amsterdam: Excerpta Medica, 1974:37–42.

Sharrard W J W. Pressure effects on the knee in kneeling miners. *Ann R Coll Surg (Eng)* 1965;**36**:309–24.

Shaw J A, Murray D G. The longitudinal axis of the knee and the role of the cruciate ligaments in controlling transverse rotation. *J Bone Joint Surg [Am]* 1974;**56–A**:1603–9.

Tasker T, Waugh W. Articular changes associated with internal derangement of the knee. *J Bone Joint Surg [Br]* 1982;**64–B**:486–8.

Warren F L, Marshall J L. The supporting structures and layers on the medial side of the knee. *J Bone Joint Surg [Am]* 1979;**61–A**:56.

Watson–Jones R. Excision of patella. *Br Med J* 1945;**2**:195–6.

Waugh W, Newton G, Tew M. Articular changes associated with a flexion deformity in rheumatoid and osteoarthritic knees. *J Bone Joint Surg [Br]* 1980;**62–B**:180–3.

Wiberg G. Roentgenographic and anatomic studies on the femoro-patellar joint with special reference to chondromalacic patellae. *Acta Orthop Scand* 1941;**12**:319–410.

CHAPTER 2

Biomechanics

Frank Johnson

2.1 Introduction

This chapter provides an overall view of the biomechanics of the knee. The diversity of the subject will be emphasized, and special reference will be made to those aspects relevant to trauma and chronic arthritis.

The material presented covers: first, the properties of material in the structures of the knee; and second, the mechanics, function and movement of the entire knee joint.

A note on *the units used* in this chapter may be helpful. The SI unit of force is the newton (N), roughly one-tenth of a kilogram. Pressure is expressed in force per unit area or Newtons per square metre. The unit of pressure is the pascal (Pa), and this is also used for stress. The pascal is so low that a prefix is used in most instances. Thus kPa is a thousand and MPa a million pascals. The moduli of elasticity have the dimensions of stress over strain. Strain is extension per unit length, and thus dimensionless; the moduli therefore have the same dimensions as that of stress, but are usually quoted in mega-newtons per square metre ($MN\ m^{-2}$). In Table 2.1 giga newtons per square metre ($GN\ m^{-2}$) are used. Friction is a force per unit force, and thus is dimensionless. Torque is force times distance and is given in newton metres (Nm).

Table 2.1 Properties of materials used in endoprostheses

Material	Ultimate tensile strength $MN\ m^{-2}$	Young's Modulus $GN\ m^{-2}$
Stainless steel	500–1500	200
Aluminium oxide ceramic	270	350
High molecular weight polyethylene	43	0.5
Polyacetal – Delrin	70	3
Polymethylmethacrylate	25	2
Cortical bone	80–160	20

Data taken from Weightman (1977a).

2.2 Properties of materials

2.2.1 BASIC CONCEPTS

There are a number of mechanical engineering terms and methods which should be understood.

The study of the behaviour of a material under load includes the relation between deformation of the material and the applied stress. In simplest terms this will be of the form shown in Fig. 2.1. The stiffness of the material will be related to slope of the curve. If the plot is of applied load against extension of the material, then the slope of the graph is the longitudinal elasticity, or Young's modulus of the material. Other elastic constants in common use are the torsion modulus and the bulk modulus, which respectively define the response to shear stress and compression stress.

All biological materials exhibit a number of deviations from the ideal curves of Fig. 2.1. Most important are anisotropy, hysteresis and viscosity.

(a) Anisotropy

The moduli will be different in different directions of stress. In addition, the ultimate compression or tensile strength may depend upon direction of testing. This is illustrated for samples of cortical bone in Fig. 2.2.

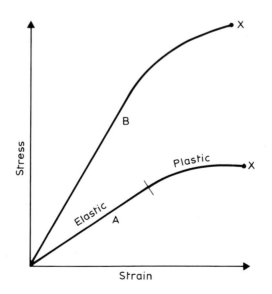

Fig. 2.1 Generalized stress–strain curves. Material B is stiffer than A. Both exhibit a linear, elastic region followed by a region of plastic deformation until fracture at X.

(b) Hysteresis

The deformation observed when the load increases may be different from that seen when the load is decreasing on the same specimen. The separation between the two curves (Fig. 2.3) provides an estimate of the amount of energy dissipated by the process.

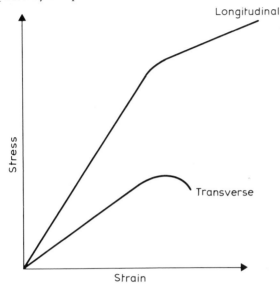

Fig. 2.2 Anisotropy in cortical bone. The longitudinal sample is stiffer and takes a higher stress at fracture than the transverse sample.

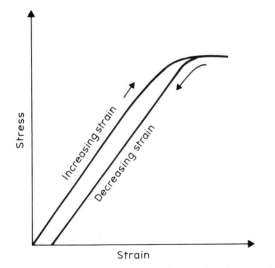

Fig. 2.3 Hysteresis. Deformation of materials into the plastic region is not usually reversible, and some residual strain will remain on removal of the stress.

(c) Viscosity

Measurements made at different rates of application of strain demonstrate a range of results. In general, materials with interstitial fluid (as in the menisci and articular cartilage) will be stiffer for higher rates of loading. The slower phenomenon of creep is also seen. The apparent modulus of articular cartilage may reduce from 12 MN m^{-2} to 7 MN m^{-2} after 30 minutes of load (Hayes and Mokros, 1971).

In any simple material testing these deviations need to be considered, and even more difficulty is caused by boundary problems. Consider the testing of cartilage under compression. Since natural cartilage is supported by bone, the response to gross compression is greatly modified and tests which assume infinite thickness of material clearly do not apply.

A method of theoretical analysis which has received considerable attention in recent years is finite element analysis. This attempts to divide the structure into a large number of discrete regions, or elements. The characteristics of each element may be specified separately, and the overall response of the structure is obtained by summation. The method can be used in three dimensions and will in principle cope with all of the anomalies mentioned above. The restriction lies in the size of computer available, and the results of any analysis can only be as good as the data and boundary conditions put into the computation. An example of the application of finite element analysis to the knee may be found in O'Connor *et al.* (1982).

2.2.2 BONE

For trabecular bone the stiffness has been shown to be correlated with volume fraction of bone and contiguity of trabeculae (Pugh *et al.*, 1973). Changes in stiffness in specimens that had early signs of arthritis in the cartilage were higher than that in specimens from below normal cartilage (Pugh *et al.*, 1974). This relationship between the two changes does not, however, confirm the genesis of osteoarthritis.

The anisotropic distribution of strength of bone has been investigated by Brehens (1974) who showed highest strength (load to yield point) in the region subject to load at 45° of flexion, and also on the medial side of the knee. The importance of fluid movement in bone has been demonstrated by Hayes and Swenson (1981) who showed that marrow flow contributed to the apparent stiffness of bone samples.

Cortical bone stiffness has been measured to be about twenty times that of cancellous bone (Evans, 1973). The development of a stiff subcortical layer of bone in osteoarthritis has been proposed by Hayes and Swenson (1981) in their finite element model of the knee.

Fatigue experiments on cortical bone (Carter *et al.*, 1981) have shown that samples from the mid-diaphysis of the femur have a fatigue strength of about

7 MPa at 10^7 cycles. Stresses up to 40 MPa have been reported by Hayes and Swenson (1981) and at these levels it was considered that fatigue fractures would occur after one day of activity. Bone remodelling may thus be considered to be essential to the stability of the skeletal system, and fatigue damage accumulation may be related to loss of ability for repair, rather than any pathological changes.

2.2.3 ARTICULAR CARTILAGE

The structure of articular cartilage reveals much about its function and behaviour. The tissue consists of collagen fibres in a dense matrix with considerable interstitial fluid.

The movement under load of the interstitial fluid is responsible for the properties of the cartilage. Because the behaviour of cartilage is determined by fluid flow within the tissue, McCutchen (1959) advocates the term 'poroelastic' to distinguish the effect from simple viscoelasticity. He points out that under compression pore, fluid flow occurs within (and out of) the cartilage. This flow is opposed by viscous forces in the fluid, and an appreciable time is required for equilibration. A poroelastic tissue creeps at different speeds during compression and, because the behaviour is determined by fluid flow, the response to strain is dependent upon the sample size. The behaviour is non-linear and time-dependent, and these factors bedevil simple measurement of the mechanical properties of the tissue. Elementary estimates may be obtained by taking cartilage–bone plugs from a large joint and obtaining slices of cartilage. Experiments with intact joints have been performed by Linn and Radin (1968). They arrived at the much lower result for linear modulus of 2.2 MN m⁻².

The process of stress relaxation follows from redistribution of strain within the material. Mow *et al.* (1980) illustrated this behaviour with the data shown in Fig. 2.4.

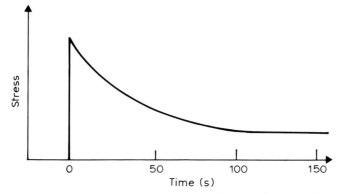

Fig. 2.4 Stress relaxation is demonstrated in the reduction of stress with time following applications of a fixed strain.

Friction between cartilage surfaces has also attracted attention. Malcolm (1976) reported a comprehensive series of tests using axisymmetric samples of bovine articular cartilage under cyclic dynamic loading. He demonstrated a minimum mean friction coefficient of 0.0026 at 500 KPa normal stress, rising to a maximum of 0.0038 at 2 MPa normal stress. Loads in the human knee are of the order of 2.5 MPa. The coefficients of friction may be compared with figures of 0.05 to 0.1 for plastic and metal (Fung, 1981).

The possible reasons for the efficacy of cartilage in reducing friction have been discussed by Fung (1981). Four theories are salient. McCutchen (1959) proposed that the slow squeezing out of fluid under load is effective, provided that the point of application of load is moved during load bearing. MacConaill (1932) suggested that the viscosity of synovial fluid is high at low shear rates. This may ensure a thin lubrication layer at all times, since the shear rate at the boundary tends to zero. Dowson (1967) mentioned the deformation of cartilage as a contributory to redistribution of load under stress, and Radin *et al.* (1970) speculated on the existence of a lubricating molecular species which forms a boundary layer in the cartilage.

Whatever the resolution of this problem, Fung (1981) showed that in disease the coefficient of friction increased to the range 0.01–0.1. He did not, however, state the condition of his 'osteoarthritic' sample, and the reason for the increase has not been determined.

2.2.4 SYNOVIAL FLUID

Ogston (1970) attributes the viscosity of synovial fluid to the presence of hyaluronic acid. He explains the action of this polysaccharide with reference to its high molecular weight of 10 million. Each molecule occupies a sphere of $1 \mu m^3$ and 1 g of the substance would occupy $5 \times 10^{-3} m^3$. Thus, in a solution of 2.4 mg ml^{-1} (the concentration present in human synovial fluid) there has to be 90% overlap of the molecules. This entanglement implies that considerable energy will be absorbed when movement of the fluid is attempted, and the material therefore appears to have high viscosity.

At high rates of shear the molecules do not have time to move apart, and the fluid exhibits a high elasticity. The elastic and viscous components of the behaviour are measured as the real and imaginary components of the bulk shear modulus.

Using an oscillating cuvette rheometer, Balazs (1968, see Fung, 1981) determined the range of values for these two components for synovial fluid taken from two groups of normal subjects and a group of patients with osteoarthritis. Figure 2.5 illustrates these data. It may be seen that the changeover from a predominantly viscous action to a predominantly elastic behaviour occurs rapidly. Age of the sample influences both the point at which the changeover takes place, and also the absolute value of the moduli. The comparison with normal rates of walking and running are indicated in

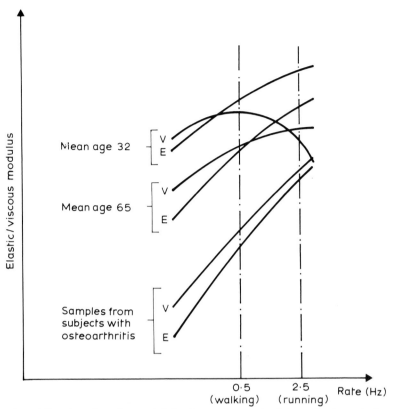

Fig. 2.5 The viscosity of synovial fluid may be resolved into elastic and viscous components. These vary with rate of application of shear strain, age and disease. (After Fung, 1981.)

Fig. 2.5, and this suggests that the synovial fluid contributes a significant elastic, or shock-absorbing, role at physiological rates of movement.

Disease seriously effects the constitution and function of the synovial fluid. The data on samples with osteoarthritis showed an average of only half of the hyaluronic acid concentration, and the moduli were almost an order of magnitude lower than those of the same age group. There is also no cross-over of the two moduli at higher speed, indicating a further reduction in the energy and absorbing capacity of the fluid in the aged.

2.2.5 MENISCI AND JOINT CAPSULE

Histological study of the menisci using polarized light has shown the arrangement of fibres to be mainly circumferential anteriorly with a division into two parts in the posterior oblique ligament. Some of the superior fibres have attachments to the joint capsule, and there is some evidence for the

39

suggestion of an element of muscular control (Last, 1950). Attachment of the posterior meniscofemoral ligament to the femur will modify the length, and hence the load bearing properties of both menisci.

Oretorp *et al.* (1978) considered that the collagenous fibres of the medial and posteromedial knee capsule, the meniscus and the lateral collateral ligament are all anatomically integrated and therefore act as a mechanical unit. The mechanics of these structures are interrelated, and it is not sensible to isolate the role played by each part.

Much mechanical work on the menisci has been carried out using an inferential technique. This is illustrated in Fig. 2.6. In order to determine the load-bearing characteristics of the meniscus, the response of the entire system is first determined. The meniscal component is removed, and the response again found. By subtraction, it is argued, the load carried by the meniscus may be between 10 and 95% of the total load. This wide range of possibilities

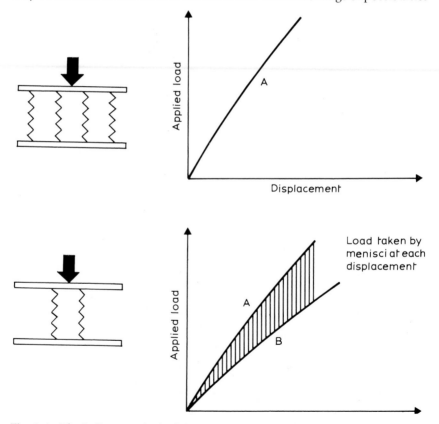

Fig. 2.6 The indirect method of determining meniscal load. A is the stress–strain curve for the entire knee. B is the curve for the knee without the menisci. The vertical separation between the two curves is taken to represent the load taken by the menisci. The meniscal proportion of the load is a constant fraction of the whole.

40

reflects the dependence upon the load used and method of loading. As Fig. 2.7 shows, the proportion of load taken by the meniscus depends upon the point of the curve used. Walker and Erkman (1975) used a load of 1500 N. This is a reasonable limit for a test rig, but the loads in the natural knee may reach twice this value.

Speed of application of load is also critical. All the tissue components of the knee exhibit viscoelastic response to some degree. Walker and Erkman did not observe any change up to 2 seconds. Jaspers *et al.* (1978) have examined porcine knees loaded at rates approaching that seen in walking, and demonstrated quite different results. Since the cross-over point in Fig. 2.5 occurs around this speed, it appears imperative to control rate during any measurement.

The most important function of the meniscus is to distribute the load over a wider area. Walker and Erkman (1975) estimate an increase from 200 mm² to 600 mm² between no-menisci and menisci present at 1500 N. This observation has two consequences. First, the pressure on any part of the articular cartilage is reduced in the same proportion. Secondly, the cartilage underneath the menisci is loaded uniformly and consistently during use.

The fibres of the menisci are highly anisotropic. Bullough and Walker (1976) determined tensile strengths of around 1 MPa in a direction parallel to the fibres for normal menisci. Tests on the tissues of the joint capsule show similar strength.

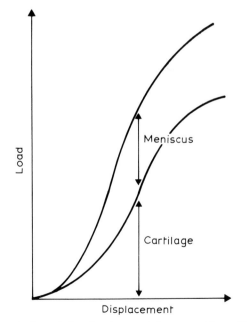

Fig. 2.7 A more typical result for the tissues of the normal knee. The proportion of load taken by the menisci depends upon the imposed load.

41

The menisci contribute to the stability of the knee and the apparent extent of this contribution is determined to some degree by the method of testing. The unconstrained rig of Goodfellow and O'Connor (1978) and used by Biden (1981) has demonstrated that the ligaments and muscles, and not the menisci, contribute most to torsional stability of the knee. If this were not the case, then a knee replacement of the Oxford design (Goodfellow and O'Connor, 1978) would not provide torsional stability until the meniscal bearings met the tibial eminence.

2.2.6 LIGAMENTS AND TENDONS

These are parallel-fibred collagenous structures to which all the foregoing comments about testing and mechanical properties apply. The stress–strain relationship for slow strain rates are of the form shown in Fig. 2.8. A segment of laxity is followed by a state of high stiffness for a static test. The ultimate tensile stress of human tendon (C in Fig. 2.8) is in the range 50–1000 MPa, at strains between 10 and 15%.

Ligaments exhibit stress relaxation. If strain is applied and then held constant, the load will decrease with time, as illustrated in Fig. 2.4. Repeated loading and unloading cycles, with time between each cycle for recovery, will not follow the same course (Fig. 2.9). The difference between cycles decreases, and the asymptote is the point at which preconditioning has been achieved.

The response to deformation of any tissue depends upon the internal structure. Fung (1981) has examined the behaviour in terms of change in internal energy and change in entropy. He shows from thermodynamics that:

Stress = (Increase in specific internal energy − decrease in specific entropy).

Materials such as metal respond to stress by a change of internal energy and will cool when stretched. Collagen or muscle, on the other hand, assume a more ordered formation under stress, and the change in entropy results in a rise in temperature.

2.2.7 ENDOPROSTHESES

Extensive work has been done on the properties of materials of plastic, metallic and ceramic components of endoprostheses for the knee. Fixation has also received considerable attention, and much thought has been given to the use of prostheses for ligament repair.

In this section it is not intended to review the functional mechanics of joint replacement. Instead a brief summary will be give of salient details about tribology, wear and mechanical testing. An excellent review of these subjects may be found in Weightman (1977a;b).

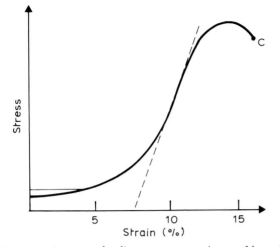

Fig. 2.8 Stress–strain curve for ligamentous specimens. Note that point C, the rupture point, occurs at strains of the order of 15%.

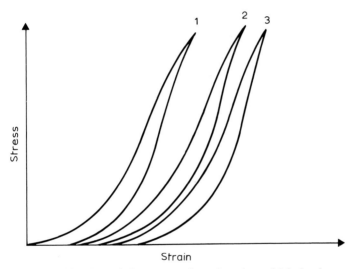

Fig. 2.9 Repeated loading of a ligament will produce data which slowly approach an asymptote.

The mechanical properties of materials used in knee joint replacement are summarized in Table 2.1. For the majority of designs for knee joint replacement it is considered that the strength and durability of the metallic components far exceeds that required. Some concern has been expressed about the strength at critical sites within a small surface replacement; for example, the internal corners of the femoral components of an Oxford Meniscal Knee (Fig. 2.10) (O'Connor, 1981).

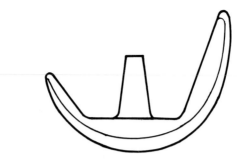

Fig. 2.10 Cross-section of a femoral component of the Oxford Knee prosthesis.

The load sharing between an intramedullary stem and the surrounding bone depends upon the difference between the Young's Moduli. For all the steels mentioned in Table 2.1, cortical bone is at least five times less stiff, and effective transfer of load throughout the length of a stem will depend upon the behaviour of the bone cement.

The plastic components of knee replacements have received most attention, both from the point of view of wear and creep as well as the problems of fixation. To illustrate the last point, the fracture *in situ* illustrated in Fig. 2.11 was attributable to failure of the support of the component.

Wear between two sliding surfaces is assumed to follow the relation:

Volume of wear = k × load sliding distance

(where k is a property of the materials used, and will vary with the temperature, lubrication and roughness of the surfaces.)

The behaviour of metal–plastic interfaces exhibits unusual properties when the roughness of the metallic surface is considered. Dowson (1982) has shown from simulator studies that the wear rate falls with decreasing roughness of the metal component down to a finish of ± 1 μm. Below this value of roughness the rate of wear begins to rise again. Values for k of 10–20 × 10^{-10} have been obtained for metal–plastic combinations in normal use.

The survival time of knee joint replacement is such that wear is not the limiting factor. The detritus from wear, however, may be absorbed by macrophages and cause local tissue reaction. The study of patterns of wear in recovered implants provides confirmation of the distribution of load predicted by gait analysis. Figure 2.12 indicates the regions of wear by a holographic method used by Lalor *et al.* (1979). Gait analysis on this patient before revision indicated that the load on the medial side was 83% of the total (Johnson *et al.*, 1981).

The problems of fixation have been reviewed by Swanson (1977). He showed that the polymethylmethacrylate–bone interface withstands compressive loads only. The forces in the knee involve loads in all three orthogonal directions and torsion about all three orthogonal axes. Transmission of

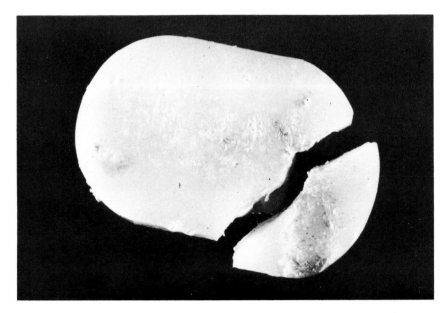

Fig. 2.11 A fractured tibial component, after four years implantation in a 75 kg man.

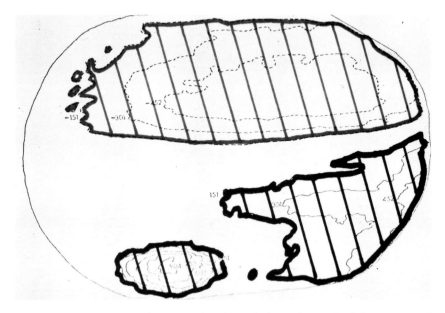

Fig. 2.12 Contour map of wear produced by a holographic method (by courtesy of Lalor *et al*, 1979).

loads other than compression is therefore achieved by soft tissue stress and accommodated by the shape of the fixation surface.

The femoral fixation is either by an intramedullary stem, or by close fitting of a concave prosthesis surface over a wide area of cut bone surface. Transmission of torsional and shear forces in the second case is easy to ensure. Reliance upon a stem requires consideration to be given to resist torsion, either by fluting the stem or using multiple stems.

Fixation to the tibial surface is more difficult owing to its flatter shape. Dovetailed keyways or stems of a greater or lesser degree have been used for tibial fixation. Promotion of bone ingrowth has been proposed. Swanson (1977) reviewed five papers which indicated that 'shear strengths at least equal to and probably greater than those obtained with methylmethacrylate can be expected' for bone ingrowth. Such equivocal results do not establish the case for bone ingrowth fixation in the knee, and problems of torsion still remain.

2.3   Function and measurement

The second half of this chapter will consider the function of the knee as a whole. Methods of measurement will be discussed, and the relevance of mechanical assessment will be examined.

2.3.1   METHODS OF MEASUREMENT

(a) Measurement of position and movement

Range of movement of the knee in clinical examination may be estimated by using simple goniometers. The addition of longer, extensible, arms and the use of carefully found landmarks can improve the precision. Best results attainable on normal knees are $\pm 1.0°$ in the coronal plane, and $\pm 2°$ in the sagittal plane (Lawrence, 1980).

Radiographs may be used to give a more precise measurement of knee angles provided no distortion or deformity is present. A flexion deformity of the knee confounds measurement of alignment, particularly if rotation is present, as Fig. 2.13 shows. Alignment to the radiograph machine may be improved by biplanar screening, but this is expensive and cannot always be achieved.

Measurement of patterns of movement of the knee can be made with a variety of electrogoniometers and other systems. Paul (1978) reviews the techniques available to record the movement of the knee during normal activities. Cinephotography was the first system to be used, but involves tedious manual analysis. More recently there has been development of fully-automated methods using polarized light (Mitchelson, 1978; Grieve, 1969) or television (Winter et al., 1972). By using cameras in more than one plane it

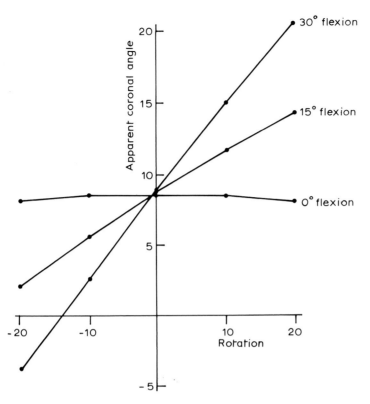

Fig. 2.13 Error in apparent coronal tibiofemoral angle caused by flexion deformity and misalignment with X-ray beam.

is possible to obtain three-dimensional movement data. The direct method of Mitchelson (Coda 3, made by Movement Techniques Ltd) provides such data with a precision of better than 0.5 mm.

Using apparatus of this latter kind, it is conceivable that rotations of the knee about all three axes may be recorded. Three-axis electrogoniometers such as those used by Godfrey and Falconer (1980) can also be used to give this information. Data from normal walking are shown in Fig. 2.14.

(b) Measurement of load

The direct measurement of load in any part of the knee is notoriously difficult. The stratagem of a strain-gauged implant, which has been used successfully in the hip by Rydell (1966) and English and Kilvington (1978), is not easily applied to the knee as there are no conveniently cantilevered structures for strain measurement. Loads in the ligament and muscle structures are equally difficult to assess because of the inaccessibility and the duplication of loading across several structures.

47

Because of the importance of estimating the stresses in the knee's structures for implant design, much effort has been expended into indirect methods of measurement. The mechanical principle of all indirect methods is simple. Figure 2.15 illustrates a much amplified model of a person 'frozen' in the middle of stance phase. The entire body load is carried by one knee, and contact at the floor is made at one point.

If it is assumed that static equilibrium has been attained and that measurement has been obtained of the vertical and horizontal force reactions at the floor, the position of the tibia in space and the dimension of the knee, then, for the purpose of the analysis, the force diagram of Fig. 2.16 may be constructed. This amputates the body at the level of the tibial plateaux and replaces its action by a single vertical load equal to body weight, plus quadriceps force. The item of interest is the load in the knee. The outline of how this is found is simply by taking moments about the centre

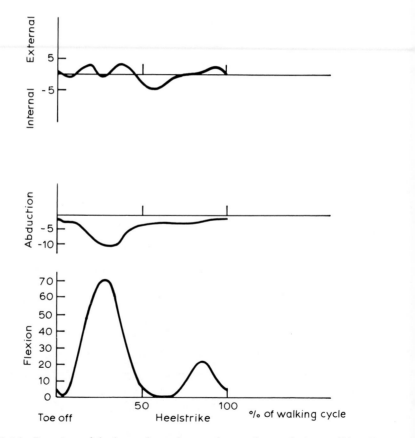

Fig. 2.14 Rotation of the knee about three orthogonal axes during walking. Data from Godfrey and Falconer (1980).

48

of the knee:

$$Md = yl\sin\varnothing + xl\cos\varnothing$$
$$\therefore M = (y\sin\varnothing + x\cos\varnothing)\, e/d \tag{2.1}$$

and the total joint force is:

$$F = M + B \tag{2.2}$$

where M = muscle force; B = reaction between joint surfaces; x and y are the reactions at the floor.

In these equations, all the anatomical, force and angle data are known. The estimates for M and F follow. It should be noted that Equation (2.1) reduces to:

$M = xl/d$ if the tibia is vertical, and further reduces to $M = 0$ if the horizontal reaction at the floor is zero. Thus, if the person is upright and not moving, no muscle force is predicted. This emphasizes a major assumption of the model: that minimal muscle action is assumed, and no account is taken of the possible antagonal action.

The elementary analysis also depends upon knowing the distance d, the separation between the point of contact of the joint surfaces and the line of

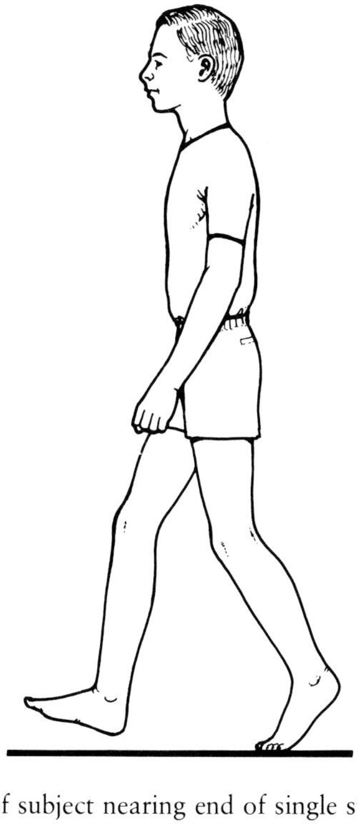

Fig. 2.15 Lateral view of subject nearing end of single stance phase.

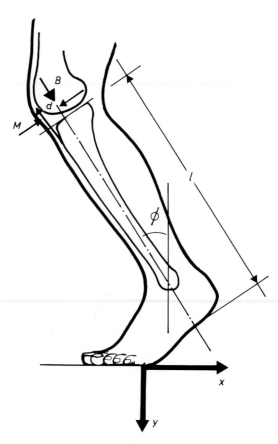

Fig. 2.16 Free-body diagram to show forces on lower limb at the position of Fig. 2.15.

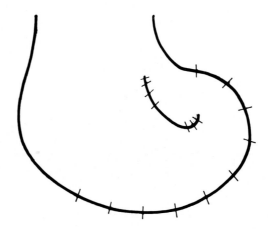

Fig. 2.17 The centre of rotation of the tibia on the femur according to Fick (1910).

action of the patellar tendon. This introduces the problems of measuring the kinematics of the knee joint, and is the subject of the next section.

2.3.2 KINEMATICS OF THE KNEE

Since Fick (1910) described the involutes which are shown in Fig. 2.17, much time has been spend upon computing the 'centres of rotation' of the knee. The method of Reuleaux (1900) is deceptively simple, and for two bodies moving in one plane will produce results of value. Figure 2.18 demonstrates the method.

The danger in applying the method to the knee lies in the assumption of monoplanar motion (Soudan and Van Audekercke, 1979). Fig. 2.14 illustrates that rotation occurs about all three axes. If the tibia rotates with respect to the femur by as little as 5°, then the apparent centre of rotation can move by up to 2 cm and if some sliding occurs, the centre of rotation lies at infinity.

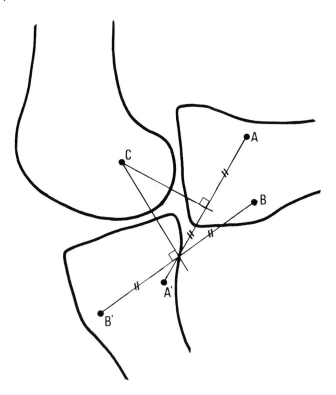

Fig. 2.18 Illustrating the construction of Reuleaux (1900) to determine the apparent centre of rotation as the tibia moves from position AB to position A'B'. The perpendicular bisectors of the lines AA' and BB' intersect at C, the required centre of rotation.

Whilst the centre of rotation has some meaning for the knee, it is better to determine the instantaneous axis of rotation, which is a moving line in three-dimensional space about which the knee rotates. Careful interpretation is required before use of this in prosthesis design. The use of screw axes as an example of a more rigorous analysis of movement has been demonstrated by Biden (1981).

Studies of the kinematics of the knee have provided a valuable means to measure the contribution of structures to constraint of motion and hence distribution of load. Goodfellow and O'Connor (1978) have demonstrated the efficacy of the cross-linked four-bar mechanisms, formed by both the cruciate and the collateral ligaments, in producing the rolling–sliding action of the knee.

By modelling the action of the cruciates, Fig. 2.19, it is possible to construct the ideal shape of the femoral articular surfaces for congruence throughout the range of motion. Laxity in flexion follows from loss of congruence, as indicated by tracing of the anatomical joint shape. The locus of movement of the medial and lateral condyles are different and Biden (1981) has produced a most detailed analysis of joint kinematics using the cross-linked model.

2.3.3 KINETICS OF THE KNEE

Estimation of loads in the structures of the knee is of considerable interest. Fairbank (1948) was the first to demonstrate the role of the menisci as something more than a filler to prevent the posterior capsule being trapped during movement! The problem of meniscal loading has been examined in detail above. Use of unconstrained rigs of many forms have added to our understanding of the function of the components of the joint, although the assessment of contact areas under load remains a complex problem. Maquet (1976) used radio-opaque dye and compressive forces of 2200 N to show the relationship between contact area and knee position to be of the form shown in Fig. 2.20. His measurement suffers, of course, from the rigid restraint

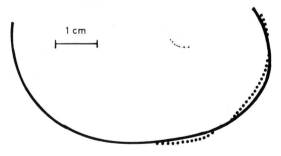

Fig. 2.19 The profile of the medial femoral condyle (solid line), and the profile calculated from the action of the cruciate ligaments. (By courtesy of Biden, 1981.)

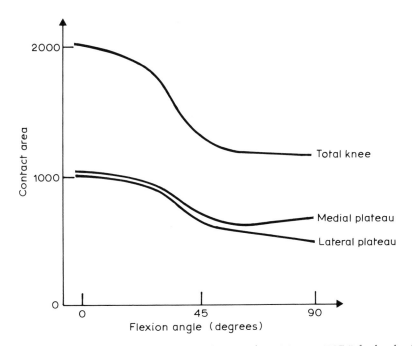

Fig. 2.20 Contact area against flexion angle. Data from Maquet (1976) for loads of 2200 N.

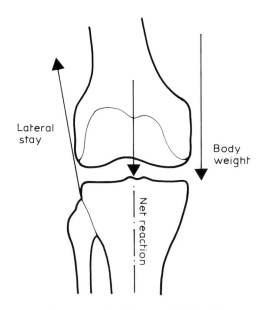

Fig. 2.21 The system of forces used by Maquet (1976) in his static analysis of loads in the knee.

imposed upon the joint, so the question remains whether without this restraint the loads might have been distributed differently.

The relationship between distribution of load and alignment of the knee is important, both for the operation of tibial osteotomy and the total replacement of the joint. Maquet (1976) has proposed that the resultant load should pass through the centre of the knee. In his analysis, he balances the action of the iliotibial band against the mass of the body acting vertically through the centre of gravity (Fig. 2.21). He then applies his analysis to compute the correction necessary in cases of osteoarthritis. This analysis is essentially static, and does not provide any explanation of the horizontal reaction at the floor seen during walking.

It is possible to analyse the forces in the knee without making any assumption about ligament loads, iliotibial band contribution, or distribution of load between the compartments of the joint. Using a simplification of the methods published by Morrison (1969), Johnson *et al.* (1981) examined results of this type of analysis for knees with a wide range of deformities in the coronal plane. Figures 2.22 and 2.23 summarize their conclusions for share of load between medial and lateral compartments and the loads in the medial and lateral ligament or muscle structures.

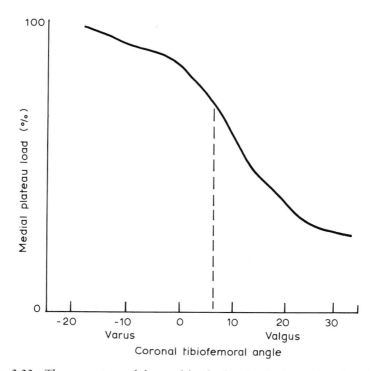

Fig. 2.22 The percentage of the total load taken by the knee plotted against the coronal tibiofemoral angle. (From Johnson *et al.*, 1981.)

Analyses of this kind are based upon complex and difficult laboratory work. The gait of disabled patients is not noted for its reproducibility, and large numbers of observations have to be collated in order to derive meaningful statistics. The results demonstrate that the loads are predominantly carried on the medial compartment of the knee for joints with tibiofemoral angles in the normal range. The average load in the collateral ligaments or muscle structures at these angles is less than $0.05 \times$ body weight. This does not mean that no higher stress can exist in the iliotibial band; the analysis used only predicts the minimum force required for stability.

This points to a possible reconciliation between these results and the theoretical analysis of Maquet (1976); his data suggest that a higher load may be present, and this could be accommodated in the dynamic model and result in a reduction of the load in the medial compartment.

The importance of alignment is demonstrated in Fig. 2.19. A change of 2° in the coronal tibiofemoral angle will result in a 5° alteration in the distribution of load between the medial and lateral compartments of the knee. The preponderance of load carried on the medial side of the knee suggests that wear of a symmetrical prosthesis will occur on that side. This hypothesis has been confirmed by the pattern of wear seen in recovered implants. Fig 2.24

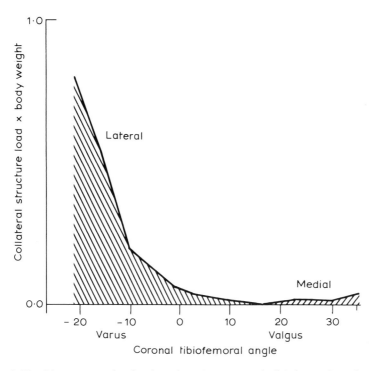

Fig. 2.23 Ligamentous loads plotted against coronal tibiofemoral angle. (From Johnson *et al.*, 1981.)

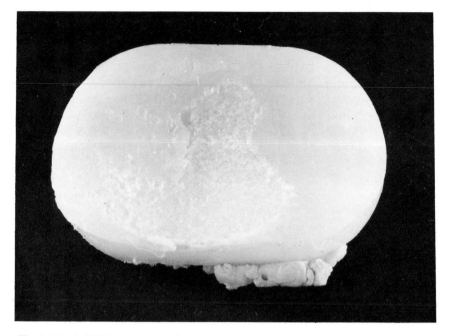

Fig. 2.24 A tibial component of a Freeman–Swanson knee joint, recovered after four years in use.

shows moderate wear in a Freeman–Swanson tibial component after four years use in the body. This joint was removed because of loosening. The presence of such asymmetric loads, together with a fixation method unable to withstand eccentric stress, will inevitably tend to loosen the plastic component.

Debate continues over the use of static analyses to predict the dynamic loading of the knee in normal activities. Minns (1981) provides a concise review of previous analyses. He investigated the effect of anatomical variations on medial and lateral compartment forces. In addition to variation of the tibiofemoral angle, he examined the changes caused by subluxation, altered plateau widths, patellar tendon angles and modification of the tibial attachment of the patellar tendon. Anatomical data were gathered from radiography of patients and a static analysis was performed. This indicated that the loads carried by the knee were critically dependent upon the anatomy. The amount of subluxation and the relative displacements of the femoral condyles were shown to affect the distribution of load, and these factors resulted in a final distribution of 60% medial plateau load for a 7° coronal tibiofemoral valgus angle.

The use of analysis of gait as a 'patient evaluation tool' has received critical comment from Brand and Crowninshield (1981). They survey 150 years of 'gait analysis' and dismiss any prospect of its use as an aid to diagnosis. They also conclude that there is no technique of analysis in current use which provides any information which would assist in the discrimination between disease processes.

The role of gait analysis as an aid to patient evaluation then has to be assessed on the basis of its contribution as a numerical tool. To perform this function the method should provide data which is not directly observable and which is accurate and reproducible. It is not enough merely to increase the precision of information as this may not of itself be of value in overall assessment (Corston et al., 1981).

To consider the analysis of gait in this narrow way precludes a fair judgement of its benefit to biomechanical understanding of the function of the knee. Knowledge of the average distribution of forces, however variable the underlying data may be, provides a useful source of criteria for the design of a suitable endoprosthesis. Comprehensive biomechanical assessment of the knee includes much more than measurement of walking ability.

Ligament laxity has been measured *in vitro* using a variety of standardized tests. Shoemaker and Markolf (1982) have examined the rotatory stability of the knee. Lowe (1977) used a similar mechanical rig to test varus–valgus

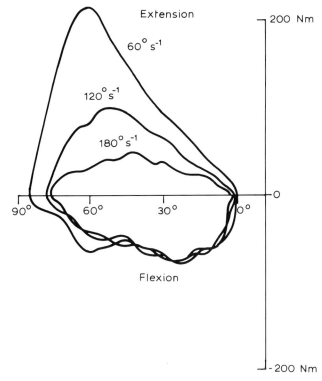

Fig. 2.25 Results from an isokinetic dynamometer meaurement of function at the knee. The difference in power developed at each speed is shown.

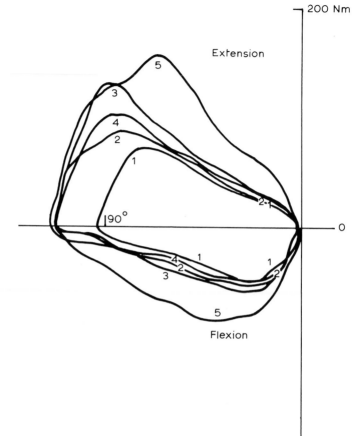

Fig. 2.26 A series of dynamometer tests over five days to show the variability of the results. The overall trend is towards increasing performance.

laxity and provide information about collateral ligament state. Shoemaker and Markolf (1982) described measurement of cruciate stability. The importance of muscle forces in these tests is recognized by carefully controlling the position of the hip, knee and ankle joints. The contribution of the muscle action to protection of the knee ligaments was shown to be up to 100%. The forces required to rupture ligaments under conditions of maximal muscle action approached those which could produce tibial fractures.

Recognition of the importance of muscle protection of the joint has led to development of testing and training machines which may be used to evaluate extensor and flexor action around the knee. Static measurement of muscle force provides some information just as static exercise can be beneficial to a degree. Muscle action, however, is known to be related to the speed of movement. Fig. 2.25 shows data from an isokinetic dynamometer test at three speeds, from 60° s⁻¹ to 180° s⁻¹. This figure illustrates that maximal torque is produced at around 60° of flexion and that quadriceps torque is related to speed of contraction, falling to less than half the peak value at 180° s⁻¹. The flexor effort is much more feeble, and not so markedly dependent upon speed.

The instrument used to produce Fig. 2.25 provides an interesting example of the problem of biomechanical muscle testing. Isokinetic activity has been shown to be an effective exercise, which by definition produces change in performance. Results from sequential tests on one subject shown in Fig. 2.26 illustrate an improvement and consolidation of performance over several days.

This problem makes the interpretation of results of any measurements which involve active participation of the subject difficult. Laboratory tests of muscle function and gait analysis all depend to some degree upon subject co-operation. In using standardized tests to assess disability it is important to be able to relate the results of the tests to the amount of disability the patient suffers in daily living.

Recordings of daily activity have been attempted for many years (Seedhom et al., 1973), and Johnson et al. (1982) reported a method which specifically examines the range of movement at the knee during normal daily activities. Bilateral recordings of knee angle and heel contact are made continuously for periods of up to 18 hours. Such data may be compared with the results of standardized clinical evaluations (Tew and Waugh, 1980; Waugh, 1982), as well as used to provide information for the study of wear and loosening in prosthetic joints.

Data about the change in activity following a knee-joint replacement may be of value in estimating the benefit of the treatment. This introduces philosophical and economic considerations which lie beyond the scope of biomechanics (Taylor, 1976), but which are nonetheless the concern of both engineer and surgeon. This chapter has attempted to give a brief review of relevant biomechanics, and to provide sufficient pointers for further reading.

References

Biden E. The mechanics of synovial joints. DPhil. (Oxford) 1981.

Brand R A, Crowninshield R D. Comment on criteria for patient evaluation tools. *J Biomech* 1981;14:655.

Brehens J C, Walker P S, Shoji H. Variations in strength and structure of cancellous bone at the knee. *J Biomech* 1974;7:2–1–207.

Bullough P G, Walker P S. The distribution of load through the knee joint and its possible significance to the observed patterns of articular cartilage breakdown. *Bull Hosp Joint Dis* 1976;37:110–23.

Carter D R, Caler W E, Spengler D M, Frankel V H. Uniaxial fatigue of human cortical bone. The influence of tissue physical characteristics. *J Biomech* 1981;14:461–70.

Corston R N, Johnson F, Godwin-Austen R B. The assessment of drug treatment of spastic gait. *J Neurol Neurosurg* 1981;44:1035–9.

Dowson D. Modes of lubrication of human joints. *Proc Inst Mech Eng* 1967;**181**:45–54.

Dowson D. Personal communication 1982.

English T A, Kilvington M. A direct telemetric method for measuring load. In: Harris J D, Copeland K. eds. *Orthopaedic engineering*. London: Biological Engineering Society, 1978.

Evans F G. *Mechanical properties of bone*. Springfield: Charles C. Thomas, 1973.

Fairbank T J. Knee joint changes after meniscectomy. *J Bone Joint Surg* 1948;**308–B**:663–70.

Ficks R. *Handbuch der Anatomie und mechanik der Gelenke*. Jena: Fischer, 1910.

Fung Y C. *Biomechanics*. Berlin: Springer-Verlag, 1981.

Godfrey C M, Falconer K A. Reliability of the C.A.R.S. – U.B.C. Electrogoniometer In: *Proceedings of human locomotion I*. London, Ontario: Canadian Society of Biomechanics, 1980.

Goodfellow J, O'Connor J. The mechanics of the knee and prosthesis design. *J Bone Joint Surg [Br]* 1978;**60**:358–69.

Grieve D W. A device called POLGON for the measurement of the orientation of parts of the body relative to a fixed external axis. *J Physiol* 1969;**201**:70.

Hayes W C, Mockros L F. Visco-elastic properties of human articular cartilage. *J Appl Physiol* 1971;**31**:562–8.

Hayes W C, Swenson L W. Finite element stress analysis of the human knee. *In*: Ghista D N, Roaf R, eds. *Orthopaedic mechanics: procedures and devices*. New York: Academic Press, 1981:29–78.

Jaspers P, Lange A, Huiskes R, von Rens ThJB. The mechanical function of the meniscus, experiments on cadaveric pig knee-joints. *Proc Europ Soc Biomech* 1978:151–6.

Johnson F, Oborne J, Allen M, Waugh W. Continuous assessment of knee function and patient mobility. *J Bio Med Eng* 1982;**4**:2–8.

Johnson F, Scarrow P, Waugh W. Assessment of loads in the knee joint. *Med Biol Eng* 1981;**19**:237–43.

Lalor M J, Groves D, Atkinson J T. Holographic studies of wear in implant materials and devices. In: Von Bally G, ed. *Holography in medicine*. New York: Springer-Verlag, 1979.

Last R. The popliteus muscle and the lateral meniscus. With a note on the attachment of the medial meniscus. *J Bone Joint Surg [Br]* 1950;**32–B**:93–9.

Lawrence M R. The role of goniometry and radiography in the assessment of tibio-femoral alignment and knee joint stability. B Med Sci Thesis (Nottingham) 1980.

Linn F C, Radin E L. Lubrication of animal joints III. The effect of certain chemical alterations of the cartilage and lubricant. *Arth Rheum* 1968;**11**:674–82.

Lowe P J, Saunders G A B. Knee analyser: an objective method of evaluating mediolateral stability in the knee. *Med Biol Eng* 1977;**15**:548–52.

MacConaill M A. Function of intra-articular fibro-cartilages, with special reference to knee and inferior radio-ulnar joints. *J Anat* 1932;**66**:210–27.

McCutchen C W. Mechanism of animal joints. *Nature* 1959;**184**:1284–5.

Malcolm L L. Frictional and deformational responses of articular cartilage interface to static and dynamic loading. PhD Thesis University of California (San Diego) 1976.

Maquet P. *Biomechanics of the knee*. Berlin: Springer-Verlag, 1976.

Minns R J. Forces at the knee joint. Anatomical considerations. *J Biomech* 1981;**14**:633–43.

Mitchelson D L. The clinical assessment of gait using the polarised light goniometer. In: Harris J D, Copeland K, eds. *Orthopaedic Engineering* London: Biological Engineering Society, 1978;74–179.

Morrison J B. Function of the knee joint in various activities. *Biomed Eng* 1969;**4**:573–9.

Mow V C, Kidel S C, Lai W M, Armstrong C G. Stress-relaxation of articular cartilage in compression – theory and experiments. *Trans Am Soc Mech Eng* 1980;**102**:73–84.

O'Connor J. The strength of the femoral components of the Oxford Knee. Personal communication, 1981.

O'Connor J, Goodfellow J, Perry N. Fixation of the tibial components of the Oxford Knee. *Orthop Clin North Am* 1982;**13**:65–87.

Ogston A G. In: Balazs E A, ed. *Chemistry and molecular biology of the intercellular matrix*. New York: Academic Press, 1970:1231–40.

Oretorp N, Alm M, Ekstrom H, Gillquis J. Immediate effects of meniscectomy on knee-joint – effects of tensile load on knee joint ligaments in dogs. *Acta Orthop Scand* 1978;49:414.

Paul J P. Gait analysis. In: Harris J D, Copeland K, eds. *Orthopaedic engineering*. London: Biological Engineering Society, 1978:145–55.

Pugh J W, Radin E L, Rose R M. Quantitative studies of human subchondral cancellous bone – its relationship to state of its overlying cartilage. *J Bone Joint Surg [Am]* 1974;56–A:313–21.

Pugh J W, Rose R M, Radin E L. Structural model for mechanical behaviour of trabecular bone. *J Biomech* 1973;61:657–70.

Radin E L, Swann D A, Weisser P A. Separation of a hyaluronate-free lubricating fraction from synovial fluid. *Nature* 1970;228:377.

Reuleaux E. *Theoretische Kinematic: Grundzeige Theories des Madrinemesen*. Brauschwaig: F. Kieveg und Sohn 1900.

Rydell N W. Forces acting on the femoral head prosthesis. *Acta Orthop Scand* 1966;Suppl 88.

Seedhom B B, Longton E B, Dowson D, Wright V. Biomechanics background in the design of a total replacement knee prosthesis. *Acta Orthop Belg* 1973;39:164–80.

Shoemaker S S, Markolf K L. *In vivo* rotatory stability of the knee. *J Bone Joint Surg [Am]* 1982;64–A:208–16.

Soudan K, Van Audekercke Rd. Methods, difficulties and inaccuracies in the study of human joint kinematics and pathokinematics by the instant axis concept. Example: the knee joint. *J Biomech* 1979;12:27–33.

Swanson S A V. Mechanical aspects of fixation. In: Swanson S A V, Freeman M A R. eds. *The scientific basis of joint replacement*. London: Pitman Medical, 1977:1–27.

Taylor D G. The costs of arthritis and the benefits of joint replacement surgery. *Proc R Soc* 1976;B192:145–52.

Tew M, Waugh W. Guide to recording information about knee replacements. University of Nottingham, 1980.

Walker P S, Erkman M H. The role of the menisci in force transmission across the knee. *Clin Orthop Rel Res* 1975;109:184–93.

Waugh W. Assessment of knee function. *Acta Orthop Belg* 1982;48:36–44.

Weightman B. Properties of materials. In: Swanson S A V, Freeman M A R, eds, *Scientific basis of joint replacement*. London: Pitman Medical, 1977a.

Weightman B. Friction, lubrication and wear. In: Swanson S A V, Freeman M A R, eds. *Scientific basis of joint replacement*. London: Pitman Medical, 1977b:46–85.

Winter D A, Hobson D A, Greenlow R K. TV – computer analysis of kinematics of human gait. *Comput Biomed Res* 1972;5:489–509.

61

CHAPTER 3

Radiography

B. J. Preston

3.1 Routine radiography

Conventional radiographs are invariably requested when a patient seeks medical attention for knee symptoms. The radiological examination is a most important and useful ancillary investigation, but its aim is to confirm a clinical diagnosis obtained by a careful history and examination, and to detect such lesions as tumours, infections and arthropathies. In many common conditions such as a torn meniscus, chondromalacia patellae and early osteoarthritis, the radiographs will be normal.

Radiographs of both knees, the hips, other joints and the spine are likely to be needed in any full examination. Pain from the hip can be referred to the knee and this seems particularly so in slipped upper femoral epiphyses. It is not unusual in this condition for there to have been two or three radiological examinations of the knee prior to the correct diagnosis being made.

In describing radiographic techniques precise angles are often quoted for the position of the bony structures relative to one another but such accuracy is difficult to obtain consistently, often due to the build of the patient and the disease present. Radiography is devised to solve a clinical problem and not just to obtain perfect pictures.

Finally, the information required should be obtained by using the minimum number of exposures and the gonadal dose reduced by appropriate shielding.

Anteroposterior and lateral views are essential and almost invariably an axial view (skyline) view of the patella should be included. If this view is omitted, fractures of the patella and abnormalities of the patellofemoral joint will be missed. Intercondylar, oblique, stress and standing films may all be necessary.

3.1.1 ANTEROPOSTERIOR VIEW

This is obtained with the knee fully extended and should show the lower femur with the overlying patella, the femorotibial joint space, the upper tibia and fibula, and the surrounding soft tissues. Slight flexion of the knee will cause superimposition of the femur and tibia and the joint space will not be depicted.

Routine radiographs do not accurately show the extent of a depression of a tibial plateau and this has been stated to be due to the superior surface of the tibia sloping posteroinferiorly. Moore and Harvey (1974) indicated that the accurate measurement of depression of a tibial plateau fracture could be obtained by directing the X-ray beam at right angles to the superior tibial surface. They found that reproducible and comparable radiographs could be obtained by directing the X-ray beam 15° caudally. Slight magnification of any anterior depression is encountered when using this tibial plateau view and in any unusual knee the appropriate tube angulation will have to be worked out from the lateral view.

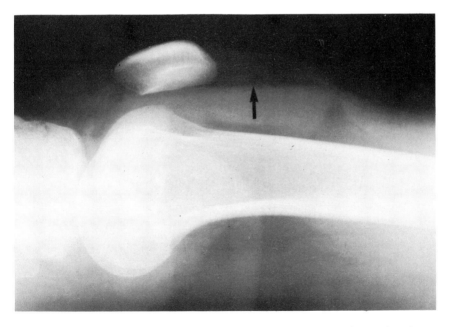

Fig. 3.1 Lipohaemarthrosis: the suprapatellar effusion has separated into a fatty layer anteriorly which appears relatively radiolucent compared with the blood posteriorly producing an interface (arrowed).

3.1.2 LATERAL VIEW

Different techniques are used to obtain a lateral film of the knee in the uninjured patient and patients with a suspected fracture.

The lateral film on the uninjured patient is obtained by turning the patient onto the side of the leg being examined. The knee is flexed between 20° to 35° and a vertical X-ray beam is employed. The lateral femoral condyle is nearest the film and can be recognized on the film as its overall size is slightly smaller and its cortex is thinner and sharper than the medial femoral condyle. If there has been a recent injury, the patient lies on his back and the X-ray cassette is placed vertically by the side of the knee and the X-ray beam is horizontal. Because of this, fluid levels such as a lipohaemarthrosis (Fig. 3.1) will be detected. A lipohaemarthrosis usually accompanies a fracture and occasionally it can indicate that there is a minor fracture which may not have been recognized. The fluid level is produced by the fatty components of the blood rising to the upper layers of the effusion and appears as a more radiolucent area.

Some surgeons use a lateral view of the knee in maximal extension to assess and measure the degree of flexion contracture (see p. 290).

3.1.3 INTERCONDYLAR (TUNNEL) VIEW

This view reveals the intercondylar notch and brings the more posterior part of the subchondral cortex of the femoral condyles into profile. It is useful for detecting loose bodies and osteochondritis dissecans. It can be obtained as either an anteroposterior (patient supine) or posteroanterior (patient prone) projection. In the anteroposterior view a curved cassette is placed behind the knee and in both views the knee is flexed. The X-ray beam is directed perpendicularly through the knee to the centre of the film.

If a more posterior view of the notch is required to be visualized then further cephalad angulation of the tube is required (Fig. 3.2).

3.1.4 OBLIQUE VIEWS

Oblique views are usually taken by internally or externally rotating the leg through 45°. The patient may be either supine or prone such that anteroposterior or posteroanterior views are obtained. Oblique views are of value to demonstrate osteochondral fragments of the femoral condyles (Fig. 3.3). They may also be of help in further visualization of the patella and tibial condyles.

3.1.5 STRESS VIEWS

The status of the medial and lateral collateral, and anterior and posterior cruciate ligaments is important in both the injured patient and those with

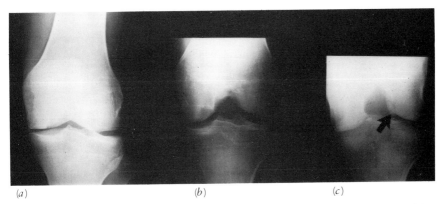

(a)   (b)   (c)

Fig. 3.2 Intercondylar view: (a) the anteroposterior and (b) the routine intercondylar view, show the osteochondral defect of the medial femoral condyle but not the loose body. (c) An intercondylar view with 40° cephalad angulation reveals the loose body (arrowed).

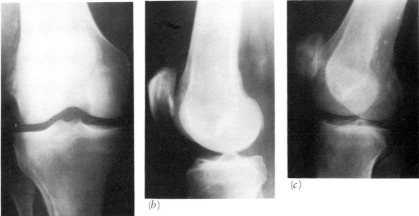

(a)   (b)   (c)

Fig. 3.3 Oblique view: (a) and (b) are the routine anteroposterior and lateral views and the osteochondral fracture of the lateral femoral condyle is difficult to identify but is easily demonstrated in (c), the oblique view.

other disease processes. Clinical examination of the ligaments can be supplemented with radiographic techniques which demonstrate abnormal movement of the tibia on the femur. The abnormalities can be recorded using spot films or an image intensifier and video recorder.

3.1.6 STANDING FILMS

Routine radiographs of the knee give considerable information about the morphology and pathology of the bones. However, films taken with the

65

patient bearing weight give more information about the state of the articular cartilage.

Standing anteroposterior and lateral films will give considerably more information in diseases of the femorotibial joint. Angular deformity and joint space narrowing (Fig. 3.4) may become more obvious on these films. The patient's whole weight is placed on the affected limb when possible. This is difficult in some patients who are extremely unsteady and thus a supporting stand for them to hold is necessary. The target film distance should be 90 cm.

Narrowing of the medial and lateral femorotibial articulations has been graded by Ahlbäck (1968) into three groups:

(1) The joint space is narrower than half the width of the articular space in (i) the other articulation of the same knee or (ii) the same articulation of the other knee.

(2) There is a reduction in the space in a weight-bearing as compared to non-weight-bearing position, and/or

(3) The space is narrower than 3 mm.

Leach *et al.* (1970) found that normal knees had a joint space from 5–11 mm wide but found many painful knees with a joint space of 4 mm. Narrowing of the space on one side may lead to opening up of the opposite side of the joint on bearing weight.

3.1.7 AXIAL (SKYLINE) VIEW OF THE PATELLA

There are numerous radiographic techniques for assessing the patellofemoral joint and the patella.

In patients with a suspected fracture, the simplest method is required. It is usually done by gently flexing the knee sufficiently (usually 30°) so that the X-ray tube can be placed along the tibia and the beam directed parallel to the posterior surface of the patella and striking the X-ray plate at right angles which is placed on the anterior aspect of the thigh. Flexion of the knee should be done under medical supervision, and after the anteroposterior and lateral films, and possibly oblique views have been looked at.

The advantages and disadvantages of the various techniques for assessing the patellofemoral joint in such conditions as osteoarthritis, chondromalacia patellae and subluxation are summarized in Table 3.1. The ideal is to obtain a view of the joint with the patella in the upper part of the intercondylar sulcus, where most subluxations and dislocations occur and with the X-ray beam striking the film as near as possible at right angles so that minimal distortion occurs.

In addition to the above method described for trauma, we also use the technique described by Laurin *et al.* (1979). For the Laurin view the knee is flexed 20° and the X-ray beam is directed along the anterior aspect of the tibia and parallel to the longitudinal axis of the patella. The X-ray film is pressed

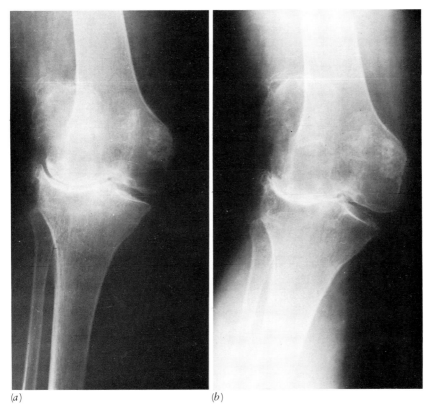

(a)   (b)

Fig. 3.4 (a) This radiograph has been taken with the patient supine and (b) with the patient standing. The standing films shows the joint space narrowing in the lateral compartment and the valgus angulation.

against the anterior aspect of the thigh and held at 90° to the tibia and hence at right angles to the X-ray beam. The film is best obtained with the patient seated with his feet at the edge of the table so that the X-ray tube can be lowered below the level of the table. Both patellofemoral joints are X-rayed simultaneously. Laurin has suggested certain measurements on the image of the structures obtained by this view which will be of help in confirming or excluding a clinical diagnosis.

(a) Lateral patellofemoral angle

The angle is obtained by drawing a line joining the apices of the femoral condyles and another line joining the limits of the lateral patellar facet (Fig. 3.5). Laurin found that this angle was open laterally in 97% of normal patients and the lines were parallel in 3%. In patients with subluxation of the patella, the lines were parallel in 60% and open medially in 40%.

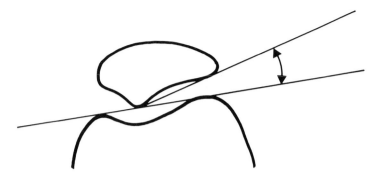

Fig. 3.5 Lateral patellofemoral angle: this is obtained by lines passing through the most superior points of the femoral condyles and through the limits of the lateral patellar facet.

Table 3.1

Name	Diagram	Advantages	Disadvantages
Furmaier		No image distortion	Difficult due to large size of X-ray tubes
		Patella in position where pathology occurs	
Laurin		Patella in position where pathology occurs	Technically difficult especially in obese individuals
		No image distortion	
Merchant		Radiographically easy	Some distortion
Settegast		No special equipment required	Patella is deep in the intercondylar groove and not in the position where dislocations and subluxations occur
		Easy positioning for the radiographer	
		Patella not distorted	The view cannot be taken if knee is painful and swollen as it requires acute flexion

Name	Diagram	Advantages	Disadvantages
Hughston		No special equipment required	Image is distorted as the X-ray beam does not strike the film at right angles
		Relatively easy positioning for the radiographer	
Knutsson		Minimal image distortion	Difficult due to large size of X-ray tubes
		Patella in position where pathology presents	
Ficat		A 'dynamic' visualisation of the joint	Three exposures
			Difficult to obtain a good image on the film at 90°

(b) Patellofemoral index

This index is the ratio between the thickness of the medial and lateral patellofemoral spaces. The medial patellofemoral interspace is the shortest distance between the lateral limits of the medial patellar facet and the medial femoral condyle and the lateral patellofemoral interspace is the shortest distance between the lateral patellar facet and the lateral femoral condyle. In normal individuals this index was 1.6 or less and more than 1.6 in 97% of patients with chondromalacia patellae.

3.2   Normal radiographic variations

Normal structures may vary in their appearances and in some cases simulate disease. Structures around the knee joint are no exception to this and a knowledge of these variations may prevent an incorrect diagnosis, unnecessary tests and even biopsy.

Cortical irregularity of the lower femur (Fig. 3.6) is one of the commonest variations which may lead to an incorrect diagnosis of osteosarcoma. This irregularity is often very slight and there may be fine bony spicules perpendicular to the shaft. A distinguishing feature from osteosarcoma is the absence of associated soft-tissue swelling. The pathological nature of the cortical irregularity on the medial aspect of the lower femur has been found to

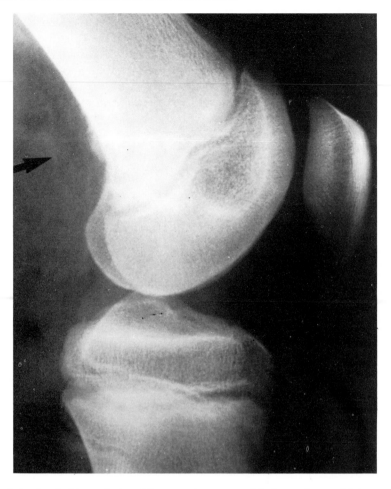

Fig. 3.6 Cortical irregularity of the posterior aspect of the lower femur: this is normal radiological variation which can be mistaken for an osteosarcoma.

be a fibrous lesion similar to the benign fibrous cortical defect (Brower *et al.*, 1971; Prentice, 1974). Occasionally quite considerable new bone formation is seen on the posterior aspect of the femur and this is thought to be due to either avulsion injury (Bufkin, 1971) or to a fibrous lesion.

Benign fibrous cortical defects are often seen as an incidental finding on radiographs of the knee in adolescence. Usually they can be recognized immediately but if they are only visualized 'en face' they can be mistaken for a more serious lesion.

Irregularities in normal ossifications of the lower femoral epiphysis have been described by Caffey *et al.* (1958). Confusing appearances are fragmentation and radiolucencies in the ossific nucleus (Fig. 3.7). Marginal irregularities of the femoral condyles may be mistaken for osteochondritis dissecans.

In the mature skeleton, small indentations may be present in the condyles on the lateral view. The indent on the lateral femoral condyle is approximately at its mid-point while that on the medial femoral condyle is approximately at the junction of the anterior and middle thirds.

The patella usually ossifies from a single centre which is normally radiographically visible at the age of 2–3 years but may be delayed as long as six years. Occasionally there may be two, three or more centres so that the patella may be bipartite, tripartite or multipartite. These accessory centres of ossification are usually sited on the superolateral aspect of the patella. In the

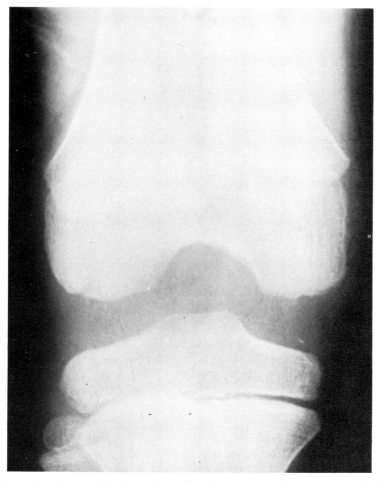

Fig. 3.7 Irregularity of the lower femoral epiphysis: a normal appearance which can be mistaken for osteochondritis dissecans.

growing period the bone may appear speckled and linear radiolucencies may be present which can be mistaken for fractures.

The ossification centre for the tibial tubercle may also be fragmented and this can be a normal variation. Scalloping of the anterior aspect of the upper tibia may be present before the development of the ossification centre for the tibial tubercle and this can be mistaken for pressure erosion.

3.2.1 SOFT TISSUES

Most radiographs of the knees are looked at with the bones in mind and frequently little attention is paid to the soft tissues. Subtle signs of an effusion can be overlooked and yet an effusion may be the first radiographic manifestation of a joint disorder.

The most reliable sign of an effusion is an increase in width of the suprapatellar pouch as seen on the lateral film (Hall, 1975). The part of the pouch which is easily visualized and can be measured, is just proximal to the patella where it is outlined by fat anteriorly (the anterior suprapatellar fat pad) and posteriorly (the prefemoral fat pad) (Fig. 3.8). The radio-opaque line produced by the synovium is normally less than 5 mm in width and if more than 10 mm, this invariably indicates an effusion (Fig. 3.9). When the distance measures between 5 and 10 mm, this probably means a small effusion is

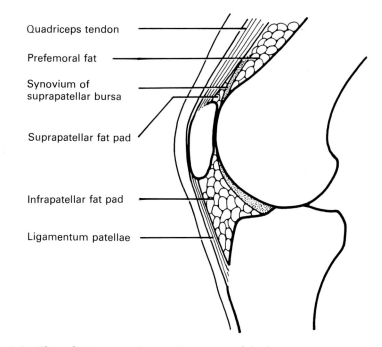

Fig. 3.8 The soft tissues on the anterior aspect of the knee.

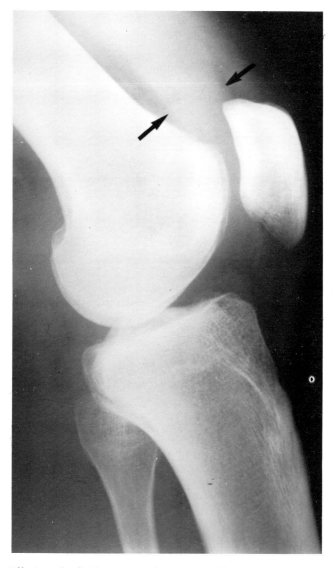

Fig. 3.9 Effusion: the fluid is seen in the suprapatellar region between the anterior suprapatellar and prefemoral fat pads (arrowed).

present but the accuracy is less than when it is 10 mm or more. Hall (1975) states that this sign of an effusion is best seen on radiographs of the knee which are not too overexposed and are taken with the knee in minimal flexion with the tube angle 5° towards the head.

Other signs of an effusion seen on the lateral film are: anterior displacement of the patella; distension of the posterior capsule; bulging of the infrapatellar ligament and posterior displacement of the ossified fabella.

On the anteroposterior film of a knee, fluid in the suprapatellar pouch can be detected by observing a curved radiolucent line medial and/or lateral to the distal femoral shaft (Harris and Hecht, 1970).

The extrasynovial fat pads on the posterior aspect of the knee have been described by Weston (1977). They have the configuration of a '3', conforming with the outline of the femoral and lateral tibial condyles. The posterior cruciate ligament may be outlined by fat lying on its posterior aspect. Behind this fat is the oblique ligament of Winslow and it is seen as a vertical density with a further layer of fat lying posteriorly separating it from the gastrocnemius muscle (Fig. 3.10). These extrasynovial fat pads can be displaced posteriorly by an effusion. In rheumatoid arthritis, where a synovial mass is produced by oedema, effusion and synovial hypertrophy, the '3' pattern may be replaced by an irregular margin.

3.2.2 PATELLA ALTA AND BAJA

Three main methods of measuring patellar height have been employed and they are those of Blumensaat (1938), Insall and Salvati (1971) and Blackburne and Peel (1977). Blumensaat's technique entails taking a lateral

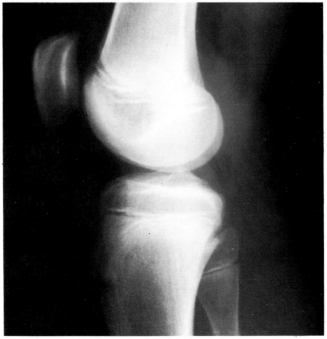
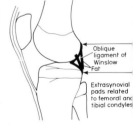

Oblique ligament of Winslow
Fat
Extrasynovial pads related to femoral and tibial condyles

Fig. 3.10 Radiograph and line diagram of soft tissues on the posterior aspect of the knee.

radiograph with the knee flexed exactly to 30° and in the normal knee the lower pole of the patella should lie between a line projected forward from the intercondylar notch and the line of the epiphyseal scar. It is easy to draw the line along the intercondylar notch but it is difficult to obtain routine radiographs flexed precisely to 30° and the method has been found to be inaccurate by Insall and Salvati (1971). Because of these disadvantages they used the ratio between the length of the patella to that of the patellar tendon as measured on a lateral radiograph of the flexed knee. The length of the patella is taken as the greatest diameter and the length of the patellar tendon is measured on its posterior surface, from its origin on the lower pole of the patella, to its insertion into the tibial tuberosity (Fig. 3.11). The advantages of the method are that it can be carried out on routine radiographs provided the knee was flexed between 20–70 degrees and, because a ratio was employed, photographic enlargement could be ignored, and direct measurements made on the film.

The ratio was found to be 1.0 in normal patients and the normal variation does not exceed 20%. Lancourt and Cristini (1975) found this to be 0.8 in patients with dislocations, 0.86 in those with chondromalcia and 1.2 in those with apophysitis of the tibial tubercle.

Blackburne and Peel (1977) criticized Insall's method since it depended on the tibial tubercle being a standard distance below the tibial plateau and

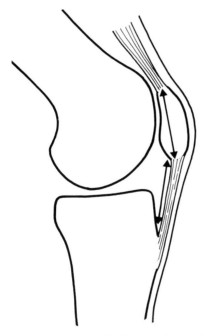

Fig. 3.11 Diagram showing the method of measuring the lengths of the patella and ligamentum patellae. After Insall and Salvati (1971).

this is not so; it was also difficult to measure the length of the patellar tendon particularly in Osgood–Schlatter's and Sinding–Larsen–Johannson's disease. They proposed an alternative method on a lateral radiograph of the knee flexed to at least 30° (Fig. 3.12). A line is projected forward along the tibial plateau and two measurements are made. The first measurement called 'A' is the shortest distance from the distal end of the articular surface of the patella to the line along the tibial plateau and the second is called 'B' and is the length of the articular surface of the patella. The ratio A/B is calculated and they defined the normal as 0.8 and in patella alta it is greater than 1.0.

3.3 Tomography

Tomography, also known as planigraphy or stratigraphy, is a technique whereby structures in a particular plane are more easily visualized and those in a different plane are blurred. It is of value in knee radiography to determine the presence of a lesion (Fig. 3.13) and to determine its nature and extent by better visualization of its radiographic detail, for example, in osteomyelitis, neoplasms and fractures. The extent of depression of bony fragments of tibial plateau fractures can be well demonstrated by tomography.

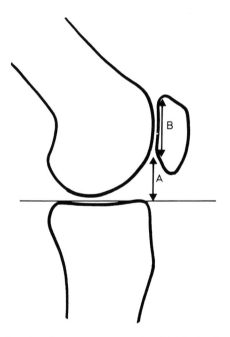

Fig. 3.12 Diagram showing the measurements A, which is the shortest distance from the distal end of the articular surface of the patella to the line along the tibial plateau, and B, which is the length of the articular surface of the patella. After Blackburne and Peel (1977).

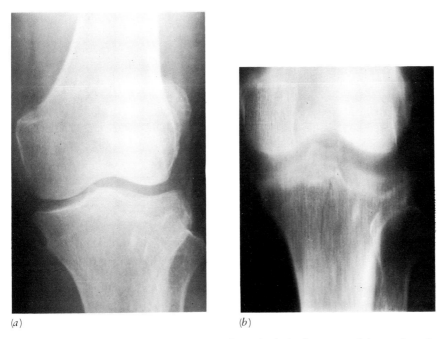

(a)   (b)

Fig. 3.13 (a) An anteroposterior radiograph in which the fracture and depression of the lateral tibial plateau is poorly demonstrated, but they are well demonstrated in (b) a tomogram.

3.4 Xeroradiography

Xeroradiography is a dry imaging process based on the photoconductor selenium and an image produced is based on a blue–white scale when it is viewed by reflected light. The patient has to be exposed to conventional X-rays in order to produce the image which can be obtained in either a positive or negative mode. In a positive xeroradiograph the radiolucent structures, such as soft tissues, appear white and radio-opaque structures, such as bone, appear blue. In negative xeroradiographs radio-opaque structures, such as trabecular and cortical bone, appear white, and radiolucent structures appear blue. Positive xeroradiographs are useful for the visualization of the soft tissues.

Xeroradiography is not usually a first choice examination but is employed as a second-line technique. One of the main advantages of xeroradiography is that it can record many tissues of different densities so that bone and soft tissues are equally visualized on a single film. This is useful in soft-tissue and bone tumours, and arthropathies. In cases of suspected Osgood–Schlatter's disease, xeroradiography could be satisfactorily employed as a first-line technique if the equipment is available as these will show both the soft-tissue

77

and bony abnormalities on the single view. The radiological findings in Osgood–Schlatter's disease are well described by Scotti *et al.* (1979) and they emphasize the role of xeroradiography. They also point out that if the routine (positive) radiograph is overexposed, making evaluation of the soft tissues difficult, then a negative image should be obtained which will help in their visualization.

3.5 Angiography

Angiography is not frequently requested in orthopaedic radiological practice because its role in the management of bone and soft-tissue tumours is limited. Angiography has been used to determine whether a tumour is either benign or malignant and to delineate its soft-tissue extent. It is now widely accepted that the method is not reliable enough to identify the nature of a lesion which must depend on the histological examination. Nowadays the soft-tissue and intraosseous extent of a tumour can be demonstrated by other techniques, such as computed tomography and nuclear magnetic resonance.

Angiography is, however, valuable for the assessment of arteriovenous malformations and these can occasionally be present around the knee joint. The extent of the lesion and in particular any synovial component can be delineated (Fig. 3.14).

More recently, selective arterial-embolization techniques have been used in the management of tumours and arteriovenous malformations and these are applicable to lesions around the knee.

3.6 Diagnostic ultrasound

Diagnostic ultrasonography is a useful technique for assessing soft-tissue swellings around the knee joint and particularly those of the popliteal space. The space-occupying lesions which may be encountered are synovial cysts, aneurysms, abscesses and soft-tissue tumours.

Sound is mechanical energy which travels in waves by compression of surrounding matter. Ultrasound is defined as sound higher than the human audible range; the upper limit of this being 20 kHz (1 Hz = 1 cycle per second). In diagnostic ultrasonic practice, frequencies of 1.5 to 10.0 MHz (1 MHz = 1 million cycles per second) are employed.

Medical ultrasound techniques depend on the detection of echoes from interfaces between tissues of different accoustic impedance.

An ultrasound machine consists basically of a transducer which both transmits a pulsed sound and receives the returned echoes. The returned echoes are converted into electrical pulses and are then displayed as either an A (amplitude) scan or B (brightness) scan on an oscilloscope. B-scans give a pictorial representation of the echoes so that a two-dimensional image of a section of the body is produced. Most B-scans nowadays use a 'grey scale'

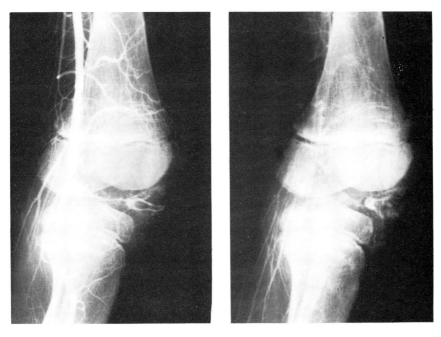

Fig. 3.14 Arterial and capillary phases showing a haemangioma of the synovium which is receiving most of its blood supply from the lateral inferior geniculate artery (reproduced by courtesy of Dr P.G. Small).

where various intensities of echoes are represented by shades of grey on the oscilloscope screen and recorded on polaroid film. New technology has introduced 'real time' ultrasonography in which dynamic events are recorded.

Soft-tissue masses which are investigated by ultrasonography will be shown to be either cystic, solid or complex. The definition of the images is inferior to those of computerized tomography but they will be obtained with minimal discomfort and risk to the patient. Ultrasound plays little part with visualization of bony structures.

In orthopaedic practice, ultrasonography will have most use in the diagnosis and detection of the complications of popliteal cysts. Popliteal cysts occur frequently in patients with rheumatoid arthritis but have also been recorded in osteoarthritis, Reiter's disease, Sjörgren's syndrome and tears of the medial meniscus (Gristina and Wilson, 1964). Genovese *et al.* (1972) found that clinical examination could only detect such cysts in 40% of patients. Ultrasonography has been found able to detect popliteal cysts in over 90% cases (Meire *et al.*, 1974). These authors found that ultrasonography was also useful to assess the progress of the lesions and measuring response of the cyst to treatment. They did note that ultrasonography failed to detect a cyst which was leaking.

Complications of these cysts are rupture into the calf (Tait *et al.*, 1965) and compression of the popliteal vein (Swett *et al.*, 1975), both of these may simulate deep vein thrombosis. A popliteal cyst will be demonstrated as an echogenic-free mass sometimes with small internal echoes (Fig. 3.15). It will distort the tissue planes and may extend into the calf for a variable distance. Oedema due to deep-vein thrombosis or any other cause will produce separation but not distortion of the tissue planes and no localized echogenic-free mass.

Ultrasonography has been applied to the assessment of the rheumatoid knee (Cooperberg *et al.*, 1978). Suprapatellar effusions and synovial thickening could be detected in addition to popliteal cysts.

3.7 Arthrography

Arthrography of the knee is now a procedure which is performed in many centres. The first arthrograms reported in the early part of the 20th century used negative-contrast media such as air, oxygen or carbon dioxide. Later, in the 1930s, positive-contrast media were used but such substances were relatively toxic.

The introduction of safe contrast media and good fluoroscopic equipment has lead to the increasing use of double-contrast techniques which are very accurate. The investigation has been developed and popularized by Andren and Wehlin (1960); Freiberger *et al.* (1966); Butt and McIntyre (1969); Ricklin *et al.* (1971) and Stoker (1980).

Single-contrast techniques are still employed and Tegtmeyer *et al.* (1979) have shown them to be as accurate as the double-contrast procedure. Most radiologists will use a single-contrast technique for the detection of popliteal cysts.

3.7.1 INDICATIONS

The usual indication for an arthrogram is to detect abnormalities of the menisci. It can also be used to evaluate the articular cartilage, ligaments and synovium.

3.7.2 TECHNIQUE

The various techniques of performing a double-contrast arthrogram are essentially similar in their basic approach and there are only minor variations.

Before beginning the procedure, plain films are taken (anteroposterior, lateral, skyline view of the patella and intercondylar views). It is important to look for bony fragments, loose bodies and evidence of an effusion.

Arthrography is carried out in sterile conditions with the patient lying supine on the screening table with the knee supported on a small foam pad. A

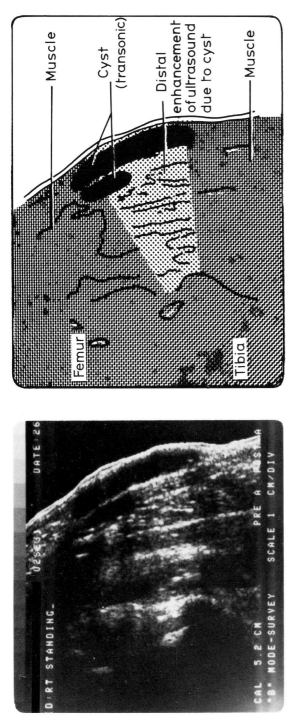

Fig. 3.15 Ultrasound examination of the posterior structures of the knee: a popliteal cyst is shown as a superficial transonic region. In this patient the cyst could only be demonstrated when the patient was standing (reproduced by courtesy of Dr P.G. Small).

short bevelled 20 gauge (5 cm) needle is inserted into the joint between the patella and femoral condyles at the mid-patellar level. This is usually done on the lateral side of the knee, although the medial approach can be employed. Any effusion must be aspirated. Frequently the needle can be felt to enter the joint, but if there is any doubt, a test injection of a small amount of gas should be given. If the joint is satisfactorily punctured, it will distend on the opposite side to the needle; but if there is still doubt, the image-intensifier can be employed. Either air, carbon dioxide or a combination of air and carbon dioxide can be used as the gas. The advantage of air is that it is 'readily available', whilst its disadvantage is that it is slowly absorbed and that some remains in the joint for several days afterwards.

Whatever gas is employed it is important to distend the joint. Approximately 50 ml are usually required in an adult although larger amounts may be necessary if an effusion is present. It is not necessary to distend the joint so much that it is painful.

The positive-contrast medium usually employed is Conray 280 and 3–5 ml are injected. More recently Hexabrix and Niopam have been introduced and Iohexol is to be shortly available in this country. Niopam and Iohexol are non-ionic contrast media and are less hypertonic than other conventional media. Thus the rate at which they induce synovial fluid into the joint is slower and thus the time in which the films can be taken is prolonged. The author is at present using Niopam 300.

Other contrast media such as Dimer X (Roebuck, 1977) and metrizamide (Johansen et al., 1977) have been used. However, Dimer X is no longer manufactured and metrizamide is generally considered to be too expensive for the slight advantage that it provides.

Hall (1974) advocated the use of 0.3 mg adrenaline (0.3 ml 1:1000 adrenaline solution) in order to delay the absorption of the positive-contrast.

After the injection of all the contrast media, the needle is removed and the knee is gently exercised with the patient still on the table. The patient is then turned on to his front with a pad under the thigh. A canvas band is placed around the lower thigh and attached to the side of the table and this is used in order to help apply a valgus or varus stress to open up the joint space. Joint distraction, in addition to the valgus or varus stress, is also required to show the meniscus.

It is customary to examine the medial meniscus first (unless the main abnormality is thought to be on the lateral side of the knee) and twelve spot-films are taken of each meniscus with at least four of these on the posterior horn. The leg is orientated so that each part of the meniscus comes into profile and the final positioning is determined with the help of the image intensifier. The films are marked to indicate that part of the meniscus which is visualized and usually a simple numbering system is employed. The films are scrutinized and, if necessary, a second series can be obtained.

The cruciate ligaments can be demonstrated by either vertical or horizontal beam methods. The vertical beam method is usually performed after the menisci have been demonstrated. The patient is turned on to the side under investigation with the knee flexed 60–80°. Lateral films are obtained, first with the leg at rest and then, to show the anterior cruciate ligament, the tibia is pulled or pushed forward (anterior drawer manoeuvre). The posterior cruciate ligament can be similarly demonstrated by using a posterior drawer manoeuvre.

The horizontal beam method described by Pavlov and Freiberger (1978) is usually done immediately after the injection of the contrast. The patient sits with his legs hanging over the edge of the table with a firm pad between the calf and the edge of the table. A chair is placed against the front of the foot which prevents extension at the knee and helps displace the tibia anteriorly. A lateral film of the knee is then taken using a horizontal X-ray beam.

Frontal views of the cruciate ligament have been described by Roebuck (1977) but they are not widely used.

When all the films on the image intensifier have been obtained then further anteroposterior, lateral with a horizontal beam, and skyline views of the patella are taken.

3.7.3 NORMAL FINDINGS

The knee joint consists of patellofemoral and femorotibial compartments and the synovium covering the cruciate ligaments and the infrapatellar fold separates the femorotibial joint into the medial and lateral compartments. The suprapatellar pouch extends for several centimetres above the patella and it may contain synovial folds. Occasionally there is a normal communication between the knee joint and the superior tibiofibular joint.

The medial meniscus is C-shaped with a larger posterior horn than anterior horn. The size of the mid-portion is usually between that of the anterior and posterior horns but can occasionally be smaller than the anterior horn. In cross-section, the meniscus is triangular with smooth superior and inferior margins which are approximately equal in length. The base of the meniscus is attached to the joint capsule and deep fibres of the medial collateral ligament, but a small recess may be present posterosuperiorly. The lateral meniscus is slightly larger than the medial meniscus and its size is more uniform from its anterior to posterior horn. Part of the popliteus tendon sheath is seen at the outer aspect of the posterior portion of the lateral meniscus (and the popliteus tendon is usually seen lying in its lateral wall). The posterior horn of the lateral meniscus is attached to the capsule by superior and inferior bands. Defects are present in these bands and that in the superior one is situated anteriorly and in the inferior one posteriorly.

The cruciate ligaments are intracapsular but are extrasynovial and can be demonstrated because they are surrounded by synovium anteriorly and on their sides. The anterior cruciate ligament has to be distinguished from the infrapatellar synovial fold (the ligamentum mucosum) which is situated more anteriorly. On lateral views, the anterior and posterior cruciate ligaments are seen to cross in the intercondylar region.

The articular cartilage is represented as the radiolucent band between the subchondral cortex and the positive contrast; its width is approximately 2–4 mm. The thickness of normal articular cartilage of both femoral condyles has been measured by Hall and Wyshak (1980) on arthrograms. They found that the articular cartilage was greater on the medial femoral condyle than the lateral condyle and there was also a correlation with the patient's weight such that it was thicker in heavier people.

3.7.4 ABNORMAL FINDINGS

(a) Meniscal tears

The main radiographic sign of a tear in a meniscus is a radiolucent defect within the meniscus with irregular edges coated with positive contrast. This finding depends on there being some displacement of the fragments. Occasionally positive contrast is seen extending into the meniscus; this is when a tear is short and closed or when stress has not been applied to open up the gap.

Tears of the menisci are of two types, vertical and horizontal. Vertical tears are either along the long axis of the meniscus or running transversely to the long axis. Long vertical tears which allow displacement of the central fragment are 'bucket-handle' tears (Fig. 3.16). Transverse tears are easy to miss because the tear is perpendicular to the X-ray beam and the meniscus on either side is normal. However, transverse tears are frequently associated with small longitudinal tears extending along the long axis of the meniscus, which are easier to detect. Such a combined tear is a 'parrot-beak' tear. A radial tear should be suspected if a meniscus remains adherent to the condylar surface in spite of adequate stress manoeuvres. Peripheral detachment is another type of vertical tear which may be complete or incomplete. In the medial meniscus the tear takes place through the outermost part of the meniscus or the meniscocapsular junction. Peripheral detachment of the lateral meniscus will cause rupture of one or both bands on either side of the popliteus tendon sheaths. If the detachment is total and both are torn this is usually obvious, but if only one is ruptured this is more difficult to detect, which may lead to a false negative result.

Horizontal tears are the other main type of tear detectable (Fig. 3.17). They usually occur in a meniscus that has undergone degenerative changes and are seen in the older patient.

Complex tears, consisting of a combination of vertical and horizontal tears may also occur (Fig. 3.18).

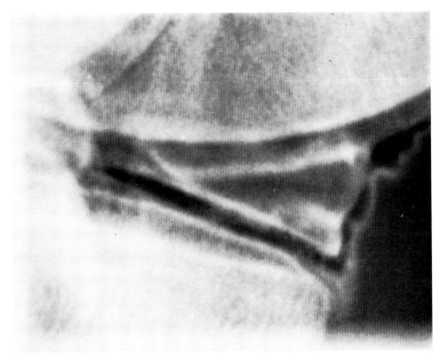

Fig. 3.16 Double-contrast arthrogram showing a vertical tear near the periphery of the posterior part of the medial meniscus.

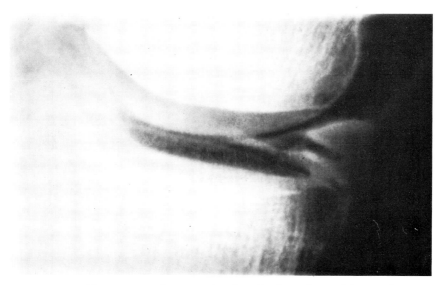

Fig. 3.17 Double-contrast arthrogram showing a horizontal tear of the anterior part of the medial meniscus.

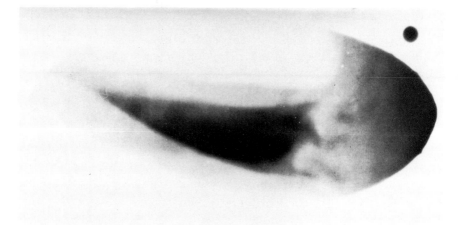

Fig. 3.18 A complex tear of a degenerate medial meniscus.

(b) The discoid meniscus

A discoid meniscus is usually found in the lateral side and is extremely rare on the medial side. Arthrographically a discoid meniscus appears larger than normal, extending towards the intercondylar notch and usually with parallel surfaces and a rectangular, rather than triangular, cross-section.

Any discoid meniscus must be carefully examined for tears and Stoker (1980) emphasizes that this may be difficult because the patient may resist normal stressing and there may be difficulty in bringing the meniscus into profile.

(c) After meniscectomy

An arthrographic study of the knee after meniscectomy has been reported by Debnam and Staples (1974). In approximately 25% of patients, multiple lesions were found. The main abnormalities detected were tears of the meniscus on the opposite side or tears in the remnant, distortion of the anterior cruciate ligament and ulceration of the articular cartilage of the femoral condyles in the region of the removed meniscus.

(d) Arthrography in children

Arthrography in children is of value particularly to confirm or exclude a meniscal tear or to detect a discoid meniscus. The technique employed is similar to that in adults, but general anaesthesia is required in very young children and the amounts of gas and contrast used are slightly less.

(e) Cruciate ligament tears

The cruciate ligaments can be demonstrated by either horizontal or vertical beam methods. An accuracy of over 90% using both techniques is claimed by Pavlov *et al.* (1979a). A completely torn ligament will show as an absent or acutely angulated contrast band whilst a partial tear will show a decreased slope. This is considerably better than earlier reports (Butt and McIntyre, 1969), where the accuracy was approximately 50%.

(f) Chondromalacia patellae (see Chapter 9)

Chondromalacia patellae is a frequently diagnosed condition in children and young adults who complain of pain on the anteromedial aspect of the knee which increases with activity. Invariably, plain radiographs of the affected knee appear normal. The early arthrographic findings of chondromalacia are swelling of the cartilage, increased absorption of contrast into the cartilage and occasionally fissures are identified. At a later stage, thinning of the cartilage may be recorded. Many experienced arthrographers (Dalinka, 1980; Stoker, 1980) state that arthrography is not helpful in the management of patients with this condition. The diagnosis is made on clinical grounds and if further assessment is required then arthroscopy is the method of choice. Arthrography can be of value for excluding associated meniscal lesions.

(g) Osteochondritis dissecans, chondral and osteochondral fractures

Arthrography can be used for assessing the overlying articular cartilage in these conditions (Fig. 3.19) and for detecting associated lesions such as loose bodies and meniscal tears.

(h) Loose bodies

Radio-opaque loose bodies are detected on initial plain films. Radiolucent loose bodies are difficult to identify on double-contrast studies because of many of the confusing shadows and even gas bubbles. A loose body is most likely to be a fragment of articular cartilage but portions of menisci, cruciate ligaments, pigmented villonodular synovitis fat and synovial tissue may all present as a loose body (Dalinka, 1980).

(i) Rheumatoid arthritis

Arthrography in patients with rheumatoid arthritis will reveal changes in the synovium, articular cartilage and menisci. The joint has an increased capacity and multiple filling defects due to hypertrophy of the synovium and fibrin bodies are recorded. Changes in the articular cartilage which may be noted

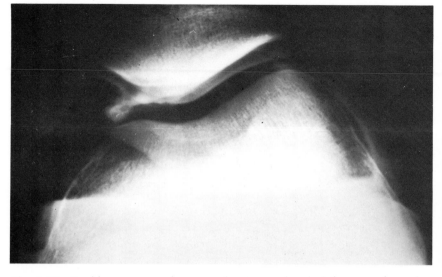

Fig. 3.19 Double-contrast arthrogram showing a chondral fragment from the articular surface of the patella.

are increased absorption of the contrast media, irregularity, thinning and disappearance, and those of the menisci, degeneration, tears and disappearance. Lymphatic filling is also occasionally recorded. Large popliteal cysts may be a feature of rheumatoid arthritis but they also occur in other connective tissue disorders, or without any predisposing cause (Dalinka, 1980). These cysts may cause tenderness in the calf and interfere with venous blood flow causing oedema (Fig. 3.20). Rupture of a cyst may cause symptoms mimicking deep-vein thrombosis. Arthrography can be used to confirm this diagnosis and should be done as a radiological emergency. The complicated double-contrast technique is not necessary. A single-contrast examination is employed injecting 15–20 ml of Conray 280 or Niopam 300. The knee is passively flexed and extended several times then a lateral film is obtained. If the cyst and rupture are not identified then the patient is encouraged to walk for 15–20 minutes and then a further film is obtained. A ruptured or dissecting cyst is identified by contrast between the muscle bundles and it will have an irregular edge (Fig. 3.21).

3.7.5 COMPARISON OF ARTHROGRAPHY AND ARTHROSCOPY

Inevitably there is a debate as to whether arthrography or arthroscopy is the method of choice to assess internal derangements of the knee. This debate is fully discussed by Stoker (1980), Ireland *et al.* (1980), Gillies and Seligson (1979), and De Haven and Collins (1975). When comparing arthrography and arthroscopy, it is reasonable to quote the results of operators in each

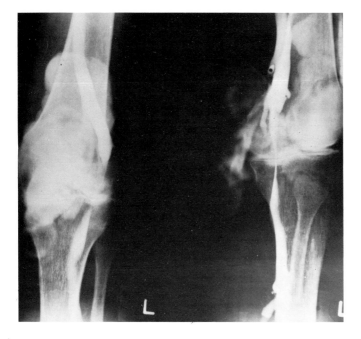

Fig. 3.20 Combined venography and arthrography: an enlarged popliteal bursa is seen compressing and displacing the popliteal vein.

procedure. However, when making a decision to request such an investigation, the experience of the persons undertaking the examination has to be considered.

Arthrography is performed by the radiologist as an out-patient procedure where as arthroscopy is done by the orthopaedic surgeon in the operating theatre usually under general anaesthesia. Arthrography is extremely accurate in detecting meniscal tears but is of less value in recording cruciate ligament tears, articular and synovial abnormalities.

An overall accuracy of 99.5% in detecting meniscal tears by arthrography has been achieved in one radiological unit (Nicholas *et al.*, 1970), but this high figure can be explained by the unique experience of the radiologist in charge of that unit. Other series reveal a diagnostic accuracy varying from 78% (De Haven and Collins, 1975), 83% (Gillies and Seligson, 1979) and 86% (Ireland *et al.*, 1980). Arthrography can demonstrate the whole of the medial meniscus. The posterior horn of the lateral meniscus is more difficult to visualize by arthrography because of its greater mobility and less secure peripheral attachments due to the intervening sheath of the popliteus tendon. Arthroscopy can produce similar results to arthrography in the detection of meniscal tears and an accuracy of 84% is recorded (Ireland *et al.*, 1980); in this paper the combined accuracy of both examinations was 98%.

Arthrography is less accurate in diagnosing chondromalacia patellae with rates of 55% compared with 99.5% for arthroscopy (Thijn, 1982).

3.7.6 ARTHROGRAPHY IN TOTAL KNEE REPLACEMENT

Arthrography for the detection of loosening and infection is not widely practised. However, it can provide additional information and can be combined with aspiration of the knee joint. The technique has been described by Ghelman and Dunn (1976) and they have incorporated the subtraction technique, which is a photographic method whereby densities on the preliminary and post-injection films are removed so that the injected contrast is

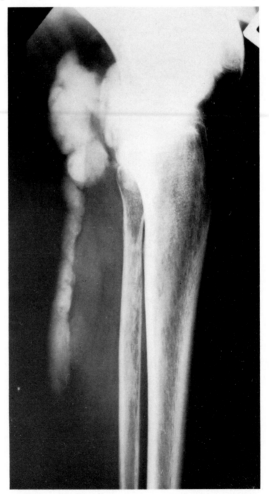

Fig. 3.21 Arthrogram showing extravasation of contrast into the muscles of the calf from a popliteal cyst indicating rupture of a cyst.

more easily seen. Contrast in the bone-cement interface of any of the prosthetic components indicates loosening (Ghelman *et al.*, 1978). It was also stated that arthrography is useful for assessing the tibial component, but of less value for the femoral component because the bone–cement interface is obscured on the anteroposterior view. Ghelman *et al.* (1978) concluded that loosening of the femoral component is better assessed by scintigraphy.

Abscess cavities may be demonstrated and if a cutaneous sinus is present, sinography can determine its extent and detect communication with the joint.

3.8 Bone scintigraphy

Bone scintigraphy is now done using technetium-99m phosphate compounds which have superseded other agents such as strontium-85, strontium-87 and fluorine-18. A variety of ^{99m}Tc-labelled compounds have been developed since their introduction by Subramanian *et al.* (1971). There are two types: condensed phosphates (inorganic compounds) and phosphonates (organic compounds). The development of these compounds has centred around the idea of improving the signal-to-noise ratio (the ratio between the bone (target) and blood, and soft tissues (non-target)) which should be as large as possible. The complex most frequently used is methylene diphosphonate (MDP). The usual adult dose is 444 MBq with blood pictures being obtained almost immediately and the bone scans after a period of at least three hours.

A gamma-camera is usually the instrument for recording the distribution of the radioisotope in the skeleton and the image is displayed on radiographic or polaroid film.

3.8.1 INDICATIONS

The common indications for bone scanning are the assessment of metastases, myeloma, lymphoma, primary bone tumours, osteomyelitis and benign bone lesions such as Paget's disease, fibrous dysplasia and bone tumours. These general indications apply to lesions around the knee, but in addition more specific conditions related to the knee such as osteonecrosis of the adult knee, partial transient osteoporosis, painful prostheses and arthropathies can also be usefully investigated by means of scintigraphy.

3.8.2 NORMAL SCAN

The appearance of a scan will depend on the age of the patient and the distribution of the radioisotope is not uniform. In the knee region of an adult, an almost symmetrical slight increased activity is noted which is proportional to the bony mass of the condylar structures. Slightly more activity may be seen in the region of the medial femoral condyle as this is slightly larger than the lateral femoral condyle. In the child, intense activity is seen in the epiphyseal–metaphyseal regions but this activity decreases with age until fusion occurs. In an infant, the growth complexes will appear as a rounded region of increased activity; this is because of the greatly increased uptake of the isotope and the natural posture so that the growth plate is superimposed on the epiphysis and metaphysis. When the child begins to walk the epiphyseal plate is visualized as a broad linear transverse area of preferential uptake.

3.8.3 ABNORMAL SCANS: GENERAL COMMENTS

The majority of bone lesions around the knee joint for which a bone scan is requested will manifest as a region of increased uptake. One of the commonest sites of osteosarcoma is around the knee joint and in such lesions increased activity is usually recorded on both the blood-pool and bone scan images. Various bone scan patterns have been noted with particular tumours (Murray, 1980). An osteosarcoma will show distortion of the bony outline and patchiness of uptake; however, the scan is unlikely to provide such good diagnostic information as the plain films. Bone scanning is an extremely sensitive technique for detecting lesions before they can be seen in routine radiographs. Thus the main purpose of carrying out a bone scan in patients with primary malignant bone tumours is to detect the presence of skeletal metastases. A study by Goldstein *et al.* (1980), on patients with an osteosarcoma who were receiving adjuvant chemotherapy, showed 16% developed skeletal metastases prior to pulmonary metastases.

The majority of benign bone tumours such as osteochondromata and chondromata will not show any significant increased activity on the blood-pool pictures and only slightly increased activity on the bone scan. One benign bone tumour which will cause increased activity on the blood pool and intense activity on the bone scan is an osteoid osteoma. This is important because these tumours may not always be identified on plain films.

The detection by radiographs of the bony changes of acute osteomyelitis is considerably delayed and they are not manifest until 10–14 days after the onset of the disease in the adult and 7–10 days in the child. Scans using ^{99m}Tc-compounds may be positive 24 hours after the onset of the disease and increased activity is recorded on both the blood-pool and the bone images. Cellulitis will show activity only on the blood-pool image and so can be distinguished from osteomyelitis. Occasionally false negative images will be obtained in osteomyelitis and even more rarely, regions of decreased activity (cold-spot) may be recorded (Jones and Cady, 1981).

Gallium 67-citrate can be used either as an alternative or in combination with ^{99m}Tc compounds to detect and evaluate activity of osteomyelitis. Lisbona and Rosenthall (1977) have suggested that subtle focal lesions adjacent to the growth place are often seen better on gallium scans.

3.8.4 ABNORMAL SCANS: SPECIFIC CONDITIONS

(a) Osteoarthritis of the knee

Scintigraphy is said to be the most sensitive method for detecting osteo-arthritis in the various compartments of the knee (Thomas *et al.* 1975). These authors have shown that bone scanning detected osteoarthritic changes in the lateral compartment of the femorotibial joint more frequently than clinical examination, plain film radiography and arthrography. This may be of value when tibial osteotomy is being considered for a particular knee joint.

Frontal and lateral views, and occasionally oblique views, are necessary to evaluate any one joint. Lateral views of the knees should be taken because increased activity in the overlying patella and patellofemoral compartment may be interpreted as lateral femorotibial compartmental disease.

A bone scan is also considered to be the most sensitive imaging technique for detecting active disease in rheumatoid arthritis and related arthropathies (Weissberg *et al.*, 1978).

(b) Osteonecrosis in the adult knee

Osteonecrosis in the adult knee may be secondary to such conditions as steroid therapy and sickle-cell anaemia but occasionally it may be a primary or idiopathic lesion. In this latter entity which was first described by Ahlbäck *et al.* (1968), the patient experiences pain over the medial femoral condyle followed by the development of a subchondral radiolucent lesion and an increased uptake of radioisotope in the appropriate region (Fig. 3.22). This condition is probably underdiagnosed because it is not widely known and routine radiography may not always detect a lesion. Lotke *et al.* (1977) described a series of 12 patients who had the clinical syndrome of osteone-crosis with a positive bone scan but no corresponding lesion on plain radiographs. The bone scans showed a high uptake of the radionuclide over the most distal portion of the femur in the affected condyle and sometimes there was a moderately increased uptake in the whole condyle radiating from a central nidus. In their series the medial femoral condyle was involved in 11 cases and the lateral femoral condyle in one case.

(c) Transient regional osteoporosis

This is a group of conditions which are manifested radiologically by self-limiting and reversible periarticular osteoporosis. There are two main diseases, transient osteoporosis of the hip and regional migratory osteo-porosis. The latter condition is also known as transient painful osteoporosis of the lower extremity (Langloh *et al.*, 1973) and recently Lequesne *et al.* (1977) have described a variation of this syndrome in which only part of an articulation is involved and they called it partial transient osteoporosis. They

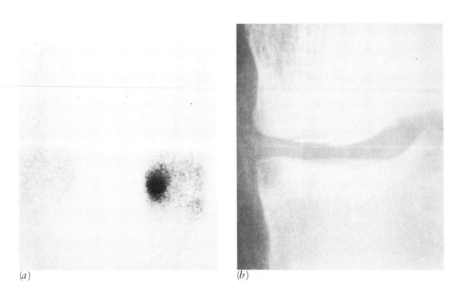

(a)   (b)

Fig. 3.22 Osteonecrosis of the medial femoral condyle: this was first detected by an area of increased activity on the bone scan (*a*) and then later by a radiolucent line near the articular surface (*b*).

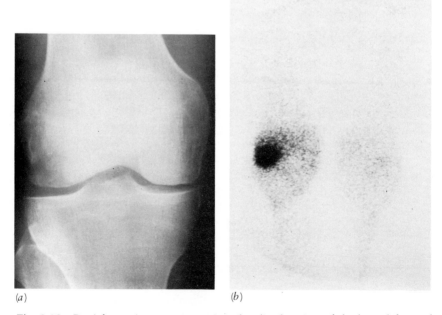

(a)   (b)

Fig. 3.23 Partial transient osteoporosis: a localized region of the lateral femoral condyle is recorded on the plain films (*a*) and the radionuclide scan (*b*) shows a corresponding area of increased activity.

subdivided this into two types: radial, where one or two rays of a foot or hand are involved, and zonal, where a portion of the bone in the joint is involved.

The knee, foot and ankle are most frequently involved in regional migratory osteoporosis. Radiographs show evidence of osteoporosis in a periarticular distribution and there may be associated soft tissue swelling. In partial transient osteoporosis the initial radiographs show a localized osteoporosis limited to a part of the articulation.

Scintigraphy shows increased uptake in the region of the osteoporotic bone (Fig. 3.23) and it can detect such an abnormality before plain film radiography. The migratory nature of the syndrome means that other joints are subsequently involved and thus bone scintigraphy is of particular value in predicting which joints are to be affected.

(d) Arthropathies

Initially joint images were obtained using ^{131}I-labelled albumin and ^{99m}Tc pertechnetate but now ^{99m}Tc-labelled phosphate compounds are used. The radionuclide scan has been found by Weissberg *et al.* (1978) to be a sensitive indicator of activity of disease in rheumatoid arthritis and its variants, and could detect disease in some patients with equivocal clinical examination and normal radiographs. They also found that in rheumatoid arthritis the pattern of activity was a symmetrical peripheral joint process whilst those of the rheumatoid variants showed asymmetrical peripheral joint involvement and more central involvement.

3.8.4 COMPLICATIONS OF KNEE REPLACEMENT

Pain after knee replacement is a common clinical problem. The routine radiographs are certainly the most useful ancillary investigation for detecting such complications as loosening, infection, instability, fractures of the metal components and stress fractures of the bone.

Bone scintigraphy using ^{99m}Tc phosphate compounds has been found to be a useful additional procedure for the detection of infection when taken in conjunction with the clinical and routine radiographic findings (Hunter *et al.*, 1980; Ghelman *et al.*, 1978). In addition to anterior and posterior scans of both knees a lateral scan is necessary (Ghelman *et al.*, 1978). The lateral scan is of value as increased activity in the distal femoral region on the anteroposterior images suggests a loosened femoral component but it could also be due to patellofemoral arthritis and this can be resolved by the lateral image. Arthritis of the patellofemoral joint will produce increased activity anteriorly whereas loosening or infection of the femoral component will create increased activity in the line of the femur.

Mild to moderate increased activity, particularly around the tibial component, may be present for several years after operation in the absence of any significant clinical abnormality. Abnormal increased activity will occur in infection, loosening, heterotopic bone formation and fractures.

95

Gallium-67 citrate is an isotope used for detecting neoplastic and inflammatory lesions. In the orthopaedic setting it is used mainly for diagnosing infective lesions. The increased concentration of ^{67}Ga at any site of infection is due to the isotope carried by the serum proteins and leucocytes.

Combined ^{67}Ga and ^{99m}Tc-labelled phosphate compound scans have been advocated for detecting infections in total joint replacement (Reing et al., 1979; Rosenthall et al., 1979). However, enhanced accumulation of ^{67}Ga citrate is not synonymous with infection and it has been recorded in non-inflamatory lesions. Rosenthall et al. (1979) have shown that if abnormal uptake in both the ^{67}Ga and ^{99m}Tc scans and the regions of increased uptake in the individual scans do not correspond (incongruent pattern) then infection is highly likely. An abnormal ^{67}Ga scan with congruent (matching) areas of increased uptake with the ^{99m}Tc phosphate scan is non-specific and no conclusion can be drawn.

More recently a new scintigraphic method using 'indium-labelled autologous' leucocytes has been employed to detect infection of a prosthesis. Rovekamp et al. (1981) investigated five patients with total hip replacement and in two of these patients the scans were positive and infection was confirmed at operation. Toghill and Waugh (1982) are using this technique to detect infection in knee prostheses as well as hip replacements.

3.9   Computerized tomography

Computerized axial tomography (CT) scanning is a relatively new method of radiological imaging. It was first developed by Sir Godfrey Hounsfield for brain scans and since then body scanners have been developed.

A synopsis of the technological advances from the first generation brain scanners to the highly sophisticated fourth generation body scanners is given by Genant et al. (1980).

All systems consist essentially of a scanning gantry, X-ray generator, a data-processing system and viewing and storage systems. There have now been four generations of scanners with the first generation scanners used for brain work and subsequent generations for both brain and body scanning. The latest scanners employ a 360° rotatory motion of the X-ray tube which is focused on a fixed stationary ring of detectors. The X-ray tube emits a very narrow collimated beam and the photons which are not absorbed by the patient fall on the detectors and are converted to scintillations. The scintillations can be quantified, recorded digitally and fed into the computer and an image is reconstructed. The image is displayed on a monitor usually using a grey, but occasionally a colour, scale. In a grey scale the depth of greyness is proportional to the X-ray attenuation coefficient of tissue at each part of the scan. Radio-opaque tissues appear white and radiolucent tissue appears black. Attenuation values are given for the small elements which make up the cross-sectional slice and they are expressed as Hounsfield (computed tomography) numbers. The scale is usually from − 1000 for air, 0 for water and + 1000 for dense bone.

Sensitive distinctions can be made between air, fluid, fat, muscle and bone densities and thus bony or soft tissue lesions can be accurately depicted on the reconstructed images. By obtaining successive transverse sections a three-dimensional image can be formed which cannot be obtained by other methods (such as plain films, tomography and arteriography).

Guidelines for the application of CT scanning for the musculoskeletal system have been issued by the Society for Computed Body Tomography (1979) and they are mainly for the evaluation of patients with known or suspected malignant bony or soft tissue tumours.

The value of CT scanning is in determining the intraosseous and soft tissue extent of a tumour and its relationship to the major vessels and nerves. This is of particular importance when en bloc resection of a tumour is being considered (Heelan *et al.*, 1979). CT scanning of the lungs should be a routine staging procedure in those patients who have tumours which metastasize to the lungs. It is also most useful for the identification of a local recurrence.

More recently CT scanning has been used for the evaluation of problems peculiar to the knee joint. The cruciate ligaments have been studied by Pavlov *et al.* (1978; 1979b) and Reiser *et al.* (1981) who have found almost complete correlation between the status of the cruciate ligaments determined by CT scans and clinical or surgical evaluation. The scans were done following double-contrast arthrography and it was found that satisfactory images could be obtained up to 24 hours after the introduction of air into the knee joint and thus the timing of the CT scan was not critical.

CT scanning has also been used very effectively in the study of the patello-femoral joint and the patella, particularly when it is combined with double-contrast arthrography. The advantage of CT scanning is that it can provide multiple transverse images without superimposition of the structures with the knee in a relaxed position. In studying patellar shape, Boven *et al.* (1982a) used Wiberg's (1941) classification in a comparative study of axial radiography and computerized tomography and they found discrepancies in the appearances. In 50% of their cases, the patella shape shown on the CT scan did not correspond to that shown on conventional radiography. They found that a type IV patella was seldom seen on a CT view but it was common for a type III to change into a type IV on a more distal CT slice, and a 'hunter's cap' could be missed on a conventional radiograph. Boven *et al.* (1982b) have also found that CT scanning combined with double-contrast arthrography was a reliable method of detecting chondromalacia patella.

3.10 Nuclear magnetic resonance

Nuclear magnetic resonance is the latest of the imaging modalities. The resonance properties of materials were discovered by two American groups headed by Block and Purcell and for this they received the Nobel Prize for Physics in 1952. In 1973, Lauterbaur demonstrated the possibility of producing cross-sectional images of objects using NMR. He termed the process zeugmatography because of the interaction of two radiation fields, magnetic and electromagnetic, to produce the signal from which images are constructed.

Some of the first images of the human body obtained were those of the forearm (Hinshaw *et al.*, 1979). These authors noted that the highly mobile protons in bone marrow and connective tissue containing fat gave the largest signal, whilst the more solid-like structures such as cortical bone, articular cartilage and tendons have a low density of mobile protons and give a low signal, whilst muscle and fibrous connective tissue produce a moderate signal. Blood within arteries gave a low signal due to its motion which reduces its NMR signal.

A study of normal and abnormal knees with nuclear magnetic resonance has been done in Nottingham by Kean *et al.* (1983). The imaging information was collected such that the high signals from fat and bone marrow appear white, and muscles and fibrous connective tissues appear grey. These structures are well shown on NMR scans (Fig. 3.24). Cortical bone gives a zero signal and thus appears black on the images. Because of this, cortical abnormalities can only be recognized by the detection of alterations in the adjacent bone marrow and soft tissues. Similarly, the cruciate ligaments give a very low signal but can be visualized because they are surrounded by fat which gives a high signal.

Osteosarcomata, secondary neuroblastoma and fractures have all been satisfactorily investigated. The soft-tissue and intramedullary extent of

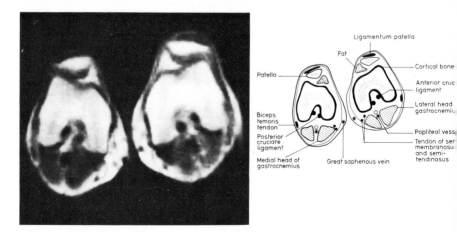

Fig. 3.24 Normal transverse NMR scan through the femoral condyles and the corresponding line diagram. (By courtesy of Professor B.S. Worthington, Dr D. Kean and Mr A. Reyani.)

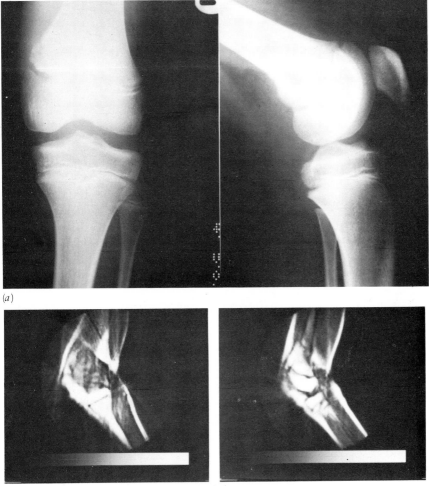

(a)

(b)

Fig. 3.25   Osteosarcoma of lower end of femur. The routine radiographs (*a*) show bone destruction of the medial aspect of the lower femoral metaphysis with soft tissue swelling and some rarefaction of the adjacent epiphysis. (*b*) is a sagittal NMR scan medial to the mid-line and shows destruction of the medial femoral condyle and in the medial part of the lower femoral shaft and a large anterior soft tissue swelling. It can be compared with the scan just lateral to the mid-line showing a normal lateral femoral condyle. (By courtesy of Professor B.S. Worthington and Dr D. Kean.)

tumours is particularly well shown by NMR. Fig. 3.25 shows an osteo-sarcoma of the lower femur where the extensive intramedullary and soft-tissue spread were accurately predicted by the NMR scan. These preliminary studies show NMR, the latest of imaging techniques, to be an ideal modality for evaluating diseases of the knee.

References

Ahlbäck S. Osteoarthrosis of the knee. A radiographic investigation. *Acta Radiol (Diagn) Suppl* 1968;**277**:7–61.

Ahlbäck S, Bauer G C H, Bohne W H. Spontaneous osteonecrosis of the knee. *Arthr Rheum* 1968;**11**:705–73.

Andren L, Wehlin L. Double contrast arthrography of the knee with horizontal Roetgen ray beam. *Acta Orthop Scand* 1960;**29**:307–14.

Blackburne J S, Peel T E. A new method of measuring patellar height *J Bone Joint Surg [Br]* 1977;**59–B**:241–2.

Blumensaat C. Die lageabureichungen und verrenkurigan der kniescheibe. *Ergebr Chir Orthop* 1938;**31**:149–223.

Boven F, Bellemans M A, Geurts J, Potvliege R. A comparative study of the patello-femoral joint on axial roentgenogram, axial arthrogram and computed tomography following arthrography. *Skel Radiol* 1982a;**8**:179–81.

Boven F, Bellemans M A, Geurts J, De Boeck H, Potvliege R. The value of computed tomography scanning in chondromalacia patellae. *Skel Radiol* 1982b;**8**:183–5.

Brower A C, Culver J E, Keats T E. Histologic nature of the cortical irregularity of the medial posterior distal femoral metaphysis in children. *Radiology* 1971;**99**:389–92.

Bufkin W J. The avulsive cortical irregularity. *Am J Roentgenol* 1971;**112**:487–92.

Butt W P, McIntyre J L. Double contrast arthrography of the knee. *Radiology* 1969;**92**:487–99.

Caffey J, Madell S H, Royer C, Morales P. Ossification of the distal femoral epiphysis. *J Bone Joint Surg [Am]* 1958;**40–A**:647–54.

Cooperberg P L, Tsang L, Truelove L, Knickerbocker J. Grey scale ultrasound in the evaluation of rheumatoid arthritis of the knee. *Radiology* 1978;**126**:759–63.

Dalinka M K. (ed.) Knee arthrography. In: *Arthrography*. New York: Springer-Verlag, 1980:71.

Debnam J W, Staples T W. Arthrography of the knee after meniscectomy. *Radiology* 1974; **113**:67–71.

De Haven K E, Collins H R. Diagnosis of internal derangements of the knee. The role of arthrography. *J Bone Joint Surg [Am]* 1975;**57–A**:802–10.

Freiberger R H, Killoran P J, Cardona G. Arthrography of the knee by double contrast method. *Am J Roentgenol* 1966;**97**:736–47.

Genant H K, Wilson J S, Bovill E G, Brunelle F O, Murray W R, Rodrigo J J. Computed tomography of the musculo-skeletal system. *J Bone Joint Surg [Am]* 1980;**62–A**:1088–101.

Genovese G R, Jayson M N, Dixon A S t J. Protective value of synovial cysts in rheumatoid knees. *Ann Rheum Dis* 1972;**31**:179–85.

Ghelman M I, Coleman E Stevens P M, Davey B W. Radiography, radionuclide imaging and arthrography in the evaluation of total hip and knee replacement. *Radiology* 1978;**128**:677–82.

Ghelman M I, Dunn H K. Radiology of knee joint replacement. *Am J Roentgenol* 1976; **127**:447–55.

Gillies H, Seligson D. Precision in the diagnosis of meniscal lesions. A comparison of clinical evaluation, arthrography and arthroscopy. *J Bone Joint Surg [Am]* 1979;**61–A**:343–6.

Goldstein H, McNeil B J, Zufall E, Jaffe N, Treres S. Changing indications for bone scintigraphy in patients with osteosarcoma. *Radiology* 1980;**135**:177–80.

Gristina A G, Wilson P D. Popliteal cysts in adults and children: A review of ninety cases. *Arch Surg* 1964;**88**:357–63.

Hall F M. Epinephrine enhanced knee arthrography. *Radiology* 1974;**111**:215–7.

Hall F M. Radiographic diagnosis and accuracy in knee joint effusions. *Radiology* 1975; **115**:49–54.

Hall F M, Wyshak G. Thickness of articular cartilage in the normal knee. *J Bone Joint Surg [Am]* 1980;**62–A**:408–13.

Harris R D, Hecht H L. Suprapatellar effusions. *Radiology* 1970;**97**:1–4.

Heelan R T, Watson R C, Smith J. Computed tomography of lower extremity tumours. *Am J Roentgenol* 1979;132:933–7.

Hinshaw W S, Andrew E R, Bottomley P A, Holland G N, Moore W S and Worthington B S. An *in vivo* study of the forearm and hand by thin section N M R imaging. *Br J Radiol* 1979;52:36–43.

Hunter J C, Hattner R S, Murray W R, Genant H K. Loosening of the total knee arthroplasty: Detection by radionuclide scanning. *Am J Roentgenol* 1980;135:131–6.

Insall J, Salvati E. Patella position in the normal knee joint. *Radiology* 1971;101:101–4.

Ireland J, Trickey E L, Stoker D J. Arthroscopy and arthrography of the knee. *J Bone Joint Surg [Br]* 1980;62–B:3–6.

Johansen J G, Lilleas F G, Nordshus T. Arthrography of the knee joints with amipaque. *Acta Radiol* 1977;18:523–8.

Jones D C, Cady R B. 'Cold' bone scans in acute osteomyelitis. *J Bone Joint Surg* [Br] 1981;63–B:376–8.

Kean D M, Worthington B S, Preston B J, Roebuck E J, McKim Thomas H, Hakes R C, Moore W S. Nuclear magnetic resonance imaging of the knee: Examples of normal anatomy and pathology. *Br. J Radiol* 1983;56:355–64.

Lancourt J E, Cristini J A. Patella alta and patella infera. *J Bone Joint Surg* [Am] 1975;57–A:1112–5.

Langloh N D, Hunder G G, Riggs B L, Kelly P J. Transient painful osteoporosis of the lower extremities. *J Bone Joint Surg [Am]* 1973; 55–A:1118–96.

Laurin C A, Dussault R, Levesque H P. The tangential X-ray investigation of the patello-femoral joint. *Clin Orthop Rel Res* 1979;144:16–26.

Lauterbur P C. Image formation by induced local interactions: examples employing nuclear magnetic resonance. *Nature* 1973;242:190–1.

Leach R E, Gregg T, Siber F J. Weight bearing radiology in osteoarthritis of the knee. *Radiology* 1970;97:265–8.

Lequesne M, Kerboull M, Bensasson M, Perez C, Dreiser R, Forest A. Partial transient osteoporosis. *Skel Radiol* 1977;2:1–9.

Lisbona R, Rosenthall L. Observations on the sequential use of 99m Tc-Phosphate complex and ⁶⁷Ga imaging in osteomyelitis, cellulitis and septic arthritis. *Radiology* 1977;123:123–9.

Lotke R A, Ecker M L, Alari A. Painful knees in older patients. *J Bone Joint Surg [Am]* 1977;59–A:616–21.

Meir H B, Lindsay D J, Swinson D R, Hamilton E B D. Comparison of ultrasound and positive contrast arthrography in the diagnosis of popliteal and calf swelling. *Ann Rheum Dis* 1974;33:221–4.

Moore T M, Harvey J P. Roentgenographic measurement of tibial plateau depression due to fracture. *J Bone Joint Surg [Am]* 1974;56–A:155–60.

Murray I P C. Bone scanning in the child and young adult. *Skel Radiol* 1980;Part 1,5:1–14.

Nicholas J A, Freiberger R H, Killeran P J. Double contrast arthrography of the knee. *J Bone Joint Surg [Am]* 1970;42–A:203–20.

Pavlov H, Freiberger R H. An easy method to demonstrate the cruciate ligaments by double contrast arthrography. *Radiology* 1978;126:817–8.

Pavlov H, Freiberger R H, Deck M F, Marshall J L, Morrisey J K. Computer assisted tomography of the knee. *Invest Radiol* 1978;13:57–62.

Pavlov H, Freiberger R H, Kaye J J. The cruciate ligaments. In: *Arthrography*. New York: Appleton-Century & Crofts, 1979a.

Pavlov H, Hirschy J C, Torg J S. Computed tomography of the cruciate ligaments. *Radiology* 1979b;132:389–93.

Prentice A I D. Variations on the fibrous cortical defect. *Clin Radiol* 1974;25:531–3.

Reing C M, Richin P F, Kenmore P I. Differential bone scanning: The evaluation of a painful total joint replacement. *J Bone Joint Surg [Am]* 1979;61–A:933–6.

Reiser M, Pupp N, Karpt P M, Feuerbach St, Anacker H. Evaluation of the cruciate ligaments by

CT. *Europ J Radiol* 1981;1:9–15.

Ricklin P, Ruttiman A, Del Buono M S. Meniscus lesions. In: *Practical problems of clinical diagnosis and therapy.* New York and London; Grune and Stratton, 1971.

Roebuck E J. Double contrast knee arthrography. Some new points of technique including the use of Dimer X. *Clin Radiol* 1977;28:247–57.

Rosenthall L, Lisbona R, Hernandez M, Hadjiparlou A. 99m Tc-PP and ⁶⁷Ga imaging following insertion of orthopaedic devices. *Radiology* 1979;133:717–21.

Rovekamp M R, Hardeman M R, Van der Schoot J B, Belfer A J. III Indium-labelled leucocyte scintigraphy in the diagnosis of inflammatory disease – first results. *Br J Surg* 1981;68:150–3.

Scotti D M, Sadhu V K, Heinberg F, O'Hara A E. Osgood–Schlatter's disease: an emphasis on soft tissue changes in Roentgen diagnosis *Skel Radiol* 1979;4:21–5.

Society for Computed Body Tomography. New indications for computed tomography. *Am J Roentgenol* 1979;133:155–9.

Stoker D J. *Knee arthrography.* London: Chapman and Hall, 1980.

Subramanian G, McAfee J G, O'Mara R E, Rosenstreich M, Mehter A. 99m Tc polyphosphate PP46: a new radiopharmaceutical for skeletal imaging. *J Nucl Med* 1971;12:399–400.

Swett H A, Jaffe R B, McIff E B. Popliteal cysts presentation as thrombophlebitis. *Radiology* 1975;115:613–5.

Tait G B W, Bach F, Dixon A S t J. Acute synovial rupture. Further observations. *Am Rheum Dis* 1965;24:273–7.

Tegtmeyer C J, McCue F C, Higgins S M, Ball D W. Arthrography of the knee: a comparative study of the accuracy of single and double contrast techniques. *Radiology* 1979;132:37–41.

Thijn C J P. Accuracy of double contrast arthrography and arthroscopy of the knee joint. *Skel Radiol* 1982;8:187–92.

Thomas R H, Resnick D. Alazraki N P, Daniel D, Greenfield R. Compartmental evaluation of osteoarthritis of the knee. *Radiology* 1975;116:585–94.

Toghill P J, Waugh W. Personal communication, 1982.

Weissberg D L, Resnick D, Taylor A, Becker M, Alazraki N P. Rheumatoid arthritis and its variants: analysis of scintiphotographic, radiographic and clinical examinations. *Am J Roentgenol* 1978;131:665–73.

Weston W J. The extra synovial and capsular fat pads on the posterior aspect of the knee joint. *Skel Radiol* 1977;2:87–93.

CHAPTER 4

Diagnostic Arthroscopy

D. J. Dandy

When arthroscopy was first introduced some surgeons considered the procedure to be possibly dangerous and at best a waste of valuable operating time. With the advent of arthroscopic surgery, the value of arthroscopy became more obvious and the technique gradually came to be accepted. It was then found that arthroscopic surgery was a difficult technique to learn and some surgeons found it physically impossible to progress beyond simple diagnostic arthroscopy. In the fullness of time, it seems likely that all surgeons with a serious interest in the knee will be skilled at both arthroscopy and arthroscopic surgery, but until then there is room for at least two levels of competence. The first, which will be described in this chapter, involves only the basic skills of diagnostic arthroscopy and the second, which will be described in Chapter 11, involves arthroscopic surgery. Many surgeons will be content to restrict their arthroscopic work to diagnosis and perhaps a few of the simpler arthroscopic operations such as synovial biopsy and the removal of meniscal flaps. Some surgeons will progress to arthroscopic surgery, but all must start at the beginning with basic diagnostic arthroscopy.

4.1 Advantages and disadvantages

The advantages of purely diagnostic arthroscopy, apart from its role in relation to arthroscopic surgery, are real but hard to measure. Several studies have shown that clinical diagnosis alone is correct in about two-thirds of patients (Jackson and Abe, 1972; Jackson and Dandy, 1976; Noble and Erat, 1980) and that arthroscopy makes a real difference to the management of the patients in the remaining third, either by disproving the original diagnosis, adding to it, or suggesting different treatment. To advocate arthroscopy on the basis of increased diagnostic accuracy is to suggest that the non-arthroscopist is making diagnostic errors, an assumption that can lead to argument and even resentment. In general, however, it is fair to say that if a clinician is good without an arthroscope, he will be even better with it.

A practical consequence of the improvement in diagnostic accuracy is the reduction in the number of unnecessary arthrotomies performed. To accept that an unnecessary operation has been performed or a normal structure needlessly excised requires considerable intellectual honesty on the part of the surgeon. Most surgeons who have become competent arthroscopists will agree that they have been able to reduce the number of such arthrotomies in their practice.

A less well-defined advantage of arthroscopy is that the 'feedback' of arthroscopy improves the diagnostic skill of the clinician. Without the arthroscope, there is a tendency for patients to be divided into those who have meniscal lesions and need meniscectomy, and those who do not. The information derived from arthroscopy makes it possible to recognize not only those patients who are unlikely to have a meniscal lesion, but also the clinical features of individual patterns of meniscal tear, articular cartilage lesions and synovial disorders.

The disadvantages of diagnostic arthroscopy as a preliminary to arthrotomy are easier to describe and quantify than the advantages. Firstly, the time taken for diagnostic arthroscopy can be measured with some precision and is a source of irritation to the staff of the operating theatre. There is no doubt that learning arthroscopy both adds to the time taken for operation and reduces the number of patients who can be treated. Criticism will quickly be overcome as soon as the surgeon feels confident enough in his arthroscopic findings to send the patient back to the ward without arthrotomy.

A second disadvantage is the need to set aside time to learn the technique and to reorganize one's work accordingly. To introduce arthroscopy to a practice that is already functioning well without it can be disruptive. The number of patients treated on each operating list is reduced; the number of patients admitted is less; waiting lists for admission may become longer and corresponding changes in practice must be made by the nurses and physiotherapists. A third disadvantage is the cost of the arthroscope and the associated equipment.

4.2 Indications

The indications for arthroscopy will vary from surgeon to surgeon but the usual indications are as a preliminary to any arthrotomy for internal derangement or anterior knee pain, in the assessment of the 'problem knee', or following ligament injury or previous surgery. It is also likely to be helpful in the 'doubtful knee' of hysterics, possible malingerers and those involved in medico-legal claims and in assessing the prognosis of patients with degenerative joint disease.

The suggestion that every patient with a bucket-handle tear of the medial meniscus should undergo arthroscopy before arthrotomy is sometimes questioned. Although the diagnosis of a locked bucket-handle tear of the medial meniscus is usually obvious, every surgeon will one day open a knee convinced that there was a tear of the medial meniscus, only to have the diagnosis proved wrong. To learn by the mistakes of others is difficult and most surgeons will need to make their own diagnostic errors before becoming convinced that arthroscopy is indeed an essential preliminary to arthrotomy for any supposed internal derangement. A lady of 24 fell, twisted her knee, experienced pain on the medial side, had an effusion, and a block to both extension and flexion. On the basis of the history and clinical examination, the author was certain that she had a locked bucket-handle tear of the medial meniscus and arthroscopy was omitted. At arthrotomy, she was found to have intense synovitis with normal menisci, but histological examination of the synovial biopsy suggested that she had early rheumatoid arthritis. Three weeks later the opposite knee swelled and this was soon followed by swelling of the small joints of the hands and feet.

In the evaluation of the problem knee, arthroscopy is a useful addition to the range of techniques already available but does not replace any of them. While the clinical history and examination are of paramount importance in the assessment of any knee, examination under anaesthesia and arthroscopy will frequently yield valuable additional information that will complement the findings of other techniques and thus help in planning the incision if arthrotomy is necessary.

In the assessment of joints affected by degenerative disease, arthroscopy is useful in assessing the state of the articular cartilage in each compartment and the relief likely to be obtained by osteotomy. Although examination of the articular surface is useful in the assessment of joints under consideration for osteotomy or total joint replacement, there is as yet no evidence to show that such information improves the long-term results of osteotomy. Such studies will take many years to complete and until the results are available, it will still be necessary to rely on common sense and basic principles which suggest that arthroscopic assessment of the knee is more likely to be helpful than otherwise.

4.3   Who should perform arthroscopy?

The suggestion that every orthopaedic surgeon should perform arthroscopy is debatable. In the present state of knowledge, it would seem as unreasonable to expect every orthopaedic surgeon to perform arthroscopy as it would be to expect every orthopaedic surgeon to be competent in the management of scoliosis and other specialized techniques. On the other hand, it seems unlikely that it will be possible for any surgeon who operates upon the knee regularly to continue doing so unless he is familiar with the basic principles of arthroscopy and can offer a confident opinion on the state of the menisci and the articular surfaces. Although attempts to predict the future are always fraught with uncertainty, there seems little doubt that arthroscopy will eventually come to be regarded as an essential part of the assessment of internal derangements, ligament instability and degenerative joint disease. It is, of course, the task of the individual surgeon to decide whether he will learn arthroscopy or not, but it is a personal view that a surgeon who operates upon the knee without being able to perform an arthroscopy will soon find himself in a similar position to a urologist who is unable to perform a cystoscopy.

4.4   Relationship to arthrography

The relationship between arthroscopy and arthrography is a fruitful source of discussion (Gillies and Seligson, 1979; Thijn, 1979; Ireland *et al.*, 1980). A competent radiologist can achieve the same degree of accuracy in the diagnosis of meniscal lesions as the average arthroscopist, but when a thorough assessment of synovial disorders and ligamentous instability is required, the arthrogram has less to offer. Arthroscopy will show if the fronds of synovial proliferation are thick, thin, filled with cartilaginous deposits, or tipped with fibrin; partial ruptures of the anterior cruciate can be distinguished from complete ruptures and irregularities of articular cartilage which would have escaped detection on arthrographic examination will be identified and assessed with considerable accuracy. While arthrography is probably as effective as arthroscopy in the assessment of meniscal lesions, it is not particularly helpful in the investigation of other knee disorders.

The attractions of arthrography are obvious. The only additional effort needed on the part of the surgeon is to complete a request form, but arthroscopy requires admission of the patient to the hospital and an operation which may take as long as an hour. Against arthrography it can be argued that the skill of radiologists varies just as much as that of surgeons. The interpretation of arthrographic films is by no means as straightforward as it might seem at first sight. To suggest that arthrography is an alternative to arthroscopy is an over-simplification. While arthrography may give as much information about the menisci as a full arthroscopic examination, it cannot yield as much information about the synovium, the ligaments or articular surface.

4.5   Equipment

The basic equipment for diagnostic arthroscopy is simple (Jackson and Dandy, 1976; O'Connor, 1977). A robust 5 mm arthroscope, with appro-

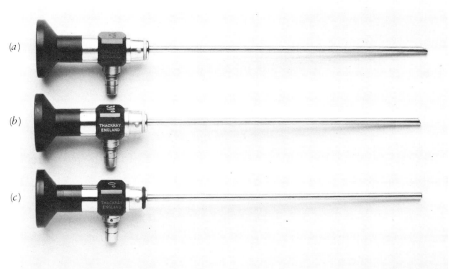

Fig. 4.1 (a) the 70° fore-oblique, (b) 30° fore-oblique, and (c) 0° straight-ahead telescopes for use in diagnostic arthroscopy.

priate sheath, trocar, light cable and light source is all that is required. Most arthroscopes are available as 0° (straight ahead), 30° and 70° fore-oblique patterns (Fig. 4.1). Of these, the 0° is best for beginners but most will quickly gain enough skill and expertise to use the 30° arthroscope with confidence. The 30° arthroscope is the work-horse of arthroscopic surgery, and it should be the aim of all surgeons to use the 30° instrument for routine examination.

In addition to the arthroscope itself, a blunt probing hook and intravenous needle (21 gauge) are invaluable (Fig. 4.2). The hook can be inserted either directly through a short (5 mm) skin incision or through a cannula and can be used to probe areas of soft articular cartilage or suspicious areas of meniscus, as well as to rehearse the manipulations that will be required if the lesion were to be dealt with arthroscopically. The use of a blunt hook is an essential prelude to arthroscopic surgery and any surgeon who considers embarking on this technique should be completely confident of his ability to use the hook before inserting cutting instruments of any type into the knee.

4.6   Technique

Arthroscopy can be conducted under local or general anaesthesia but if there is a chance that arthroscopic surgery is to be performed, general anaesthesia is preferable. Although local anaesthesia is acceptable for diagnostic arthroscopy (McGinty and Matza, 1978), it does have the disadvantage that the

107

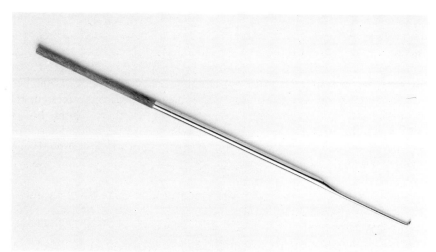

Fig. 4.2   A blunt probing hook for arthroscopic examination of the menisci.

patient is awake throughout the operation. General anaesthesia permits complete relaxation and avoids any possible discomfort or embarrassment if attempts at arthroscopic surgery are prolonged or unsuccessful.

Arthroscopy should always be the last stage in the investigation of a knee disorder and be considered together with the patient's history and the findings of clinical and radiological examination, as part of the general assessment of the knee. If general anaesthesia is used, the arthroscopic examination should be preceded by a thorough examination of the ligamentous stability of the joint, including the pivot–shift test of MacIntosh.

The use of a tourniquet will prevent unnecessary bleeding which might obscure vision, but will not interfere with the assessment of the vascularity of the synovium unless an Esmarch bandage is used to exsanguinate the limb. It is the author's preference to elevate the limb for 2–3 minutes before inflation of the tourniquet unless there is good reason to suppose that the principle pathology lies in the synovium, in which case inflation of the tourniquet is delayed until the initial examination of the knee has been completed.

The limb should always be prepared and draped as if arthrotomy were to be performed. A standard skin preparation consisting of two washes of 70% alcohol containing 0.5% chlorhexidine or similar antiseptic is quite sufficient. The draping technique for a standard arthrotomy of the knee is also perfectly adequate for arthroscopy. To perform arthroscopy without the sterile precautions that are routine for any operation on the knee is to court disaster.

There are many points of insertion of the arthroscope, but the one most commonly used for the routine initial examination is the anterolateral approach. An alternative approach is the central approach described by Gillquist and Hagberg (1976) but most surgeons prefer to avoid routine penetration of the patellar tendon, although this approach may be necessary if technical difficulties are encountered during arthroscopic surgery. The advantages and disadvantages of the different arthroscopic approaches are described elsewhere (Dandy and Jackson, 1975; Whipple and Bassett, 1978). In summary, it can be said that the anterolateral approach offers the best overall view of the knee; the central approach offers easier access to the posteromedial and posterolateral compartments, but there is some loss of mobility of the arthroscope in the suprapatellar pouch. Detailed description of the exact technique for examining the knee from the anterolateral approach is described in other texts but an important point of detail which is often overlooked is the need to insert the arthroscope as close to the patellar tendon as possible and a little above the anterior horn of the lateral meniscus. Incorrect insertion of the arthroscope – even 1 cm off target – makes examination unnecessarily difficult. Other details of technique, including the manipulation of the leg, the balance of the saline inflow and outflow, the height of the operating table and other factors are also of great importance in simplifying the operation. The precise arthroscopic technique will, like other surgical techniques, vary from one surgeon to another, but some of the satisfactory starting points for development of an individual technique are described elsewhere (Jackson and Dandy, 1976; O'Connor, 1977).

Although the technique of arthroscopic examination may vary from one surgeon to another, it is essential to have a routine method if the joint is to be examined thoroughly. Complete assessment of the knee should include a good view of the suprapatellar pouch, the whole of the undersurface of the patella and the region of the medial synovial shelf. In the medial compartment, the free margin of the meniscus can be seen throughout its entire length in every patient with the help of a valgus and external rotational force in 30° of flexion. The intercondylar notch should be carefully assessed, including the anterior cruciate ligament throughout its length, and the femoral attachment of the posterior cruciate ligament.

In the lateral compartment, the meniscus should be visible from one end to the other and the popliteus tendon should also be identified (Fig. 4.3). In most patients, the posteromedial and posterolateral compartments can be entered from the anterolateral approach and the posterior surfaces of both menisci inspected, with a 70° telescope if necessary.

Any arthroscopic examination which does not demonstrate these areas is incomplete. If there are any arthroscopic blind areas in the knee, they are more likely to be the result of defects in the surgeon's technique than the visual field of the arthroscope.

If a meniscal lesion is suspected, a percutaneous needle or a blunt hook can be used to lift, push or tug the meniscus until it is clear whether the meniscus is ruptured or intact (Fig. 4.4). The exact point of insertion of the probing needle and hook is, like the point of insertion of the arthroscope itself, critical and must be decided with as much care as the point of incision for any other

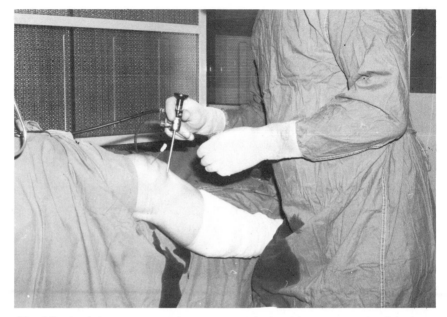

Fig. 4.3 Applying a varus strain to open up the lateral compartment of the knee using the edge of the operating table as a fulcrum.

operation. There is no room for poor technique or wrong incisions in arthroscopy as in any other field of orthopaedic surgery. A full arthroscopic examination of the knee is a dynamic event that involves movement of the joint in different positions and with different stresses. To regard the arthroscopy as a series of still pictures is an error of technique that can only lead to diagnostic mistakes.

4.7 Learning arthroscopy

Learning arthroscopy can be a frustrating experience. There is no complete substitute for the live, bleeding, human knee but alternatives exist. Cadaveric knees are stiff, messy, smelly, difficult to obtain and the leakage of fluid across the cell membrane causes distension of the subcutaneous tissues and obscures vision. Model knees are quite good enough to practise the basic manipulations and to acquire the necessary experience to interpret distance, perspective and size, all of which can be difficult to appreciate at first with monocular vision. Models will not reproduce the technical difficulties of bleeding, or the feel of handling living tissue (Fig. 4.5).

Books provide information on details such as irrigation and manipulation and can eliminate needless difficulties. For example, a method of irrigation can be described so that a reverse flow of fluid, which might cause joint debris and blood to be washed towards the lens of the arthroscope rather than away from it is avoided. However carefully written or dutifully read, books can never give 'hands on' experience, but should ensure that the basic principles of examination are sound. Video tapes help in becoming familiar with the arthroscopic view but, like books, are of little help in acquiring basic techniques and skills.

Learning arthroscopy should begin, as with other surgical techniques, with basic bookwork, followed by practise on models, if possible with the help of video tapes. When the arthroscope is first used on patients, it is helpful to put a strict limit on the time – 15 minutes perhaps – before the joint is opened. If no such limit is set, it is surprisingly easy to spend as long as an hour in

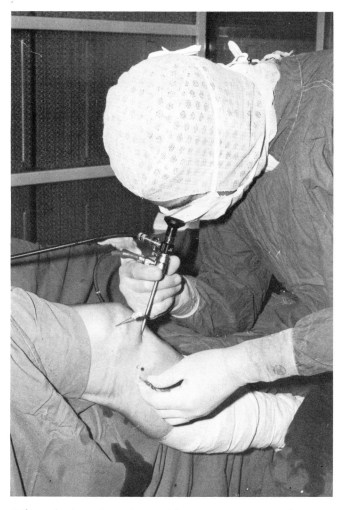

Fig. 4.4 Lifting the lateral meniscus with a percutaneous needle to examine its undersurface.

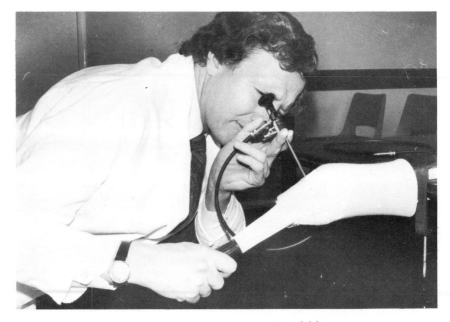

Fig. 4.5 Practising arthroscopic examination on a model knee.

fruitless examination of the knee, a practice that will not only antagonize the operating theatre staff but will have serious implications for the number of patients that can be treated. With experience, more and more of the knee will be seen in the time allowed for examination and the surgeon will have grown accustomed to the discipline of examing the knee without unnecessary delay. If this procedure is not followed, it is all too easy to fall into the bad habit of spending too long on a procedure that should never last more than 20 minutes.

Although the 30° fore-oblique arthroscope is the standard instrument for diagnostic arthroscopy and arthroscopic surgery, the offset in its direction of vision can complicate learning, and orientation may be simpler with a 0° telescope, in which the field of vision is directly in front of the instrument itself. When familiarity with the 0° telescope has been achieved, which should not take more than 20 or 30 examinations at the most, the 30° telescope should be used.

As soon as confidence in the basic diagnostic technique has been gained, it is safe to manipulate structures in the knee with a percutaneous needle or probing hook. The time taken to develop these skills varies so much from one person to another that no firm timetable can be given, but it is unusual to become confident in these techniques until 40–50 arthroscopies have been performed. At this stage, when skill in manipulation of the hook and needle has been acquired, the surgeon may wish to insert cutting instruments and undertake some of the simpler arthroscopic operations such as synovial biopsy and the removal of small meniscal flaps. The borderline between diagnostic arthroscopy and arthroscopic surgery is ill-defined and the extent to which the surgeon involves himself with arthroscopic surgery is a matter of personal choice.

References

Dandy D J, Jackson R W. The impact of arthroscopy on the management of disorders of the knee. *J Bone Joint Surg [Br]* 1975;**57–B**:346–8.

Gillies H, Seligson D. Precision in the diagnosis of meniscal lesions: a comparison of clinical evaluation arthrography and arthroscopy. *J Bone Joint Surg [Am]* 1979;**61–A**:343–6.

Gillquist J, Hagberg G. A new modification of the technique of arthroscopy of the knee joint. *Acta Chir Scand* 1976;**142**(2):123–30.

Ireland J, Trickey E L, Stoker D J. Arthroscopy and arthrography of the knee. A critical review. *J Bone Joint Surg [Br]* 1980;**62–B**:3–6.

Jackson R W, Abe I. The role of arthroscopy in the management of disorders of the knee. *J Bone Joint Surg [Br]* 1972;**54–B**:310–22.

Jackson R W, Dandy D J. *Arthroscopy of the knee.* New York: Grune & Stratton, 1976.

McGinty J B, Matza R A. Arthroscopy of the knee. Evaluation of an out-patient procedure under local anaesthesia. *J Bone Joint Surg [Am]* 1978;**60–A**:787–9.

Noble J, Erat K. In defence of the meniscus, a prospective study of two hundred meniscectomy patients. *J Bone Joint Surg [Br]* 1980;**62–B**:6–11.

O'Connor R L. *Arthroscopy.* Philadelphia and London: J B Lippincott, 1977.

Thijn C J P. *Arthrography of the knee joint.* Berlin and New York: Springer-Verlag, 1979.

Whipple T L, Bassett F H. Arthroscopic examination of the knee. Polypuncture technique with percutaneous intra-articular manipulation. *J Bone Joint Surg [Am]* 1978;**60–A**:444–52.

PART TWO

Injuries and Related Disorders

CHAPTER 5

The Meniscus

J. P. Jackson

The knee is injured more frequently than any other joint in the body because it is part of a weight-bearing limb and, secondly, does not have the stability produced by the joint congruity of the hip and ankle. The menisci are thus especially vulnerable and meniscectomy is one of the more common operations performed by orthopaedic surgeons.

5.1 Function

For many years there has been debate about the exact function of the menisci.

(a) Load bearing (see page 39)

Load bearing is now thought to be the most important function of the menisci and meniscectomy will lead to change in load distribution and in the course of time, osteoarthritis in the affected compartment. Walker and Erkmann (1975) have shown that when the knee is not under load there is only very limited contact between the femoral and tibial articular cartilage, most being through the menisci (Fig. 5.1). Even when the joint is loaded with 150 kg not all the exposed articular cartilage on the tibia is immediately in contact. As the knee flexes the load shifts posteriorly; the major part still falling on the menisci. This loading of the posterior horns may well be a factor in explaining the predominance of posterior horn tears.

(b) Stability

Stability of the normal knee is maintained by a combination of the menisci, collateral and cruciate ligaments and the capsule (Markolf et al., 1976).

When any of these structures is cut, either alone or in combination, there is a progressive increase in joint laxity. Removal of the menisci alone has relatively little effect on laxity, either at full extension or 30° of flexion, whether or not the joint is under load. Cutting both cruciate ligaments, when the knee is under a load equal to body weight and at 30° (a position in which many meniscal tears take place), produces anteroposterior laxity of 6 mm. Removal of the menisci in addition increases this to 14.6 mm (Hwa Hsin and

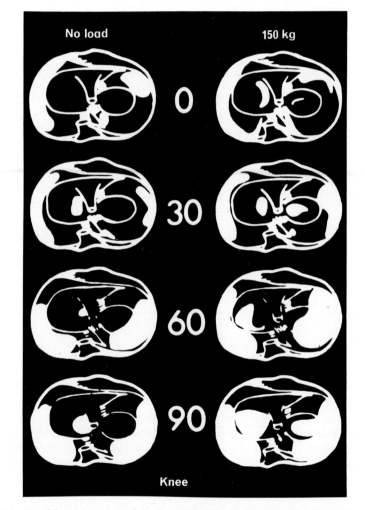

Fig. 5.1 Load bearing areas of the knee (Walker and Erkmann, 1975). The white areas represent contact with the femur. On the left, with no load, no contact with the medial area of articular cartilage takes place. On the right increasing contact is seen as the knee flexion increases to 90°. In both columns the area of contact moves posteriorly as the flexion increases. (From Walker and Erkmann, 1975, with permission.)

Walker, 1976). The effect of meniscectomy on a joint in which there is already some ligamentous laxity may, therefore, cause significant instability.

(c) Nutrition of articular cartilage

For many years it has been thought that the menisci play a role in spreading a film of synovial fluid over the articular surface during movements of the joint (MacConaill, 1932). They may not only play a part in lubrication but may also help in the nutrition of the articular cartilage by spreading the fluid over the surface.

(d) Protection

Bennett *et al.* (1942) drew attention to the fact that in knees showing degenerative changes in the articular cartilage, the damage was most obvious in the tibiofemoral contact area and only later did the area in relation to the meniscus, particularly on the tibial surface, appear to become degenerate.

Removal of the meniscus results in loss of function and should only be undertaken if there is persistent or recurrent disability. The use of arthrography and arthroscopy has meant that there is no excuse for removing a normal meniscus. The importance of the meniscus in the normal knee will be futher emphasized when the association between meniscectomy and osteoarthritis is discussed later in this chapter.

5.1.1 MECHANISM OF TEARING

This remains a matter of speculation. Unfortunately factual information is difficult to obtain.

(a) Longitudinal tears

Longitudinal tears vertical to the tibial plateau occur most commonly in younger patients, often as a result of sporting activity (Fig. 5.2(a) and (b)). This type of tear most frequently follows a single injury. Experiments using cadaveric knees are not particularly helpful in reproducing a tear, since the normal muscular control of the joint is not present. Most patients, who can recall the circumstances of the injury, will state that the knee was semi-flexed and underwent a valgus and rotational stress whilst under compression. Often the incident is related to a change in direction when running, but in other cases the joint may in addition be submitted to external force, such as another player falling on the side of the knee. The anterior and posterior horns of the meniscus are firmly anchored and as the load is suddenly increased a split occurs in the line of the circumferential fibres. The initial split may be small but with further injuries, increases in size so that eventually the

119

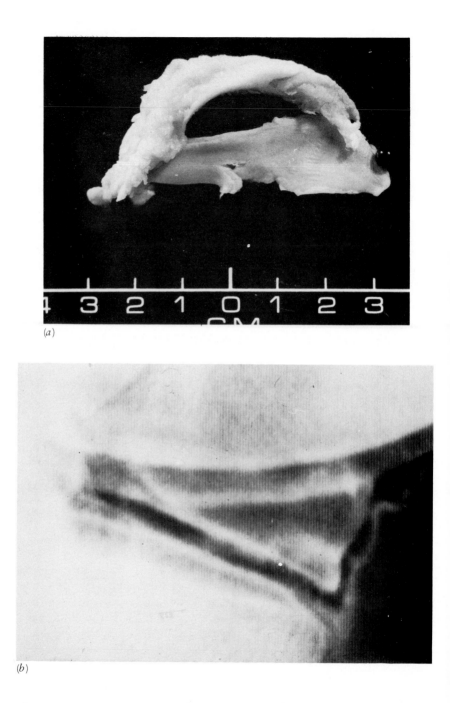

(a)

(b)

Fig. 5.2 (a) Longitudinal tear and (b) arthrogram showing vertical tear.

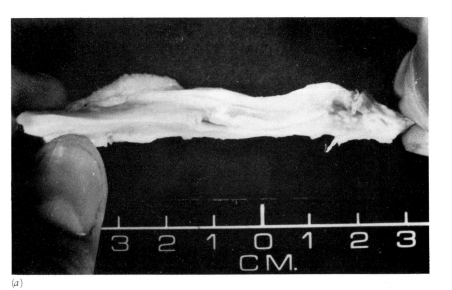

(a)

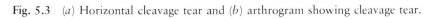

(b)

Fig. 5.3 (a) Horizontal cleavage tear and (b) arthrogram showing cleavage tear.

central portion can be displaced to the inner side of the femoral condyle, locking the joint. The displaced portion is known as a bucket-handle, and may become detached at either end or tear in the middle so that it forms a tag based either anteriorly or more often posteriorly. If a significant amount of peripheral meniscal rim remains, further bucket-handle tears or tags may occur so that a variety of shapes of tears may be encountered. Longitudinal tears are more frequent in the medial than the lateral meniscus. Wynn Parry (1958) gave a ratio of 2.2:1 and Smillie (1978) in his series of a thousand meniscectomies found the ratio was 2.5:1. Both agreed that tears were most common in the posterior horn of the medial meniscus.

(b) Horizontal cleavage tears

These tears occur in older people when there is usually macroscopic evidence of degeneration of the meniscus (Fig. 5.3(a) and (b)). The split, which is parallel to the tibial plateau, occurs as a result of sheering stresses. Noble and Hamblen (1975) examined and reported on a hundred cadaveric knees with an average age of 65 years: 29% of the menisci had cleavage tears and 60% of patients had one or more menisci affected. They suggested that it was unlikely that such a high proportion of patients would have symptoms. The presence of a meniscal cleavage tear, they argued, was not necessarily an indication for meniscectomy. This type of tear is most common in the posterior third of the medial meniscus, which is the thickest part. The outer and peripheral part of the meniscus may get adequate nutrition from an arterial supply but most of the meniscus depends on the diffusion of nutrients from the synovial fluid (Bullough *et al.*, 1970). The deepest part of the posterior horn, which is about 7.5 mm in thickness, is situated at a distance from the surface which puts it at the upper limit for the efficient diffusion of nutrients. As a result, degeneration may ensue, so that this part is particularly vulnerable to injury. Of meniscal tears 8% do not give a history of a traumatic incident (Saugmann-Jensen, 1963) and the symptoms may be gradual in onset.

5.2 Diagnosis

5.2.1 SYMPTOMS

(a) Pain

Pain is commonly present and is usually associated with the original injury. The onset, however, may be more insidious, particularly with cleavage tears. The pain, which is normally well localized, is most often felt on the side of the joint of the meniscus which has been damaged. Tears of the lateral meniscus may be associated with pain on the medial side, though the converse is rarely

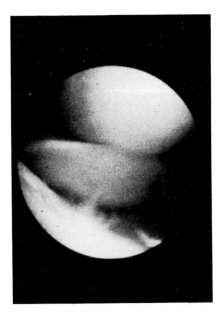

Fig. 5.4 Knee locked by short tear under tension. During arthroscopy the bucket-handle has been displaced forward.

true. Generalized aching of the knee may be related to stretching of the synovium by an effusion or haemarthrosis.

(b) Swelling

Swelling is almost invariably present. The initial injury is followed within hours by an effusion, though it may not always be noticed by the patient until the next day. The quantity of fluid is maximal after the first episode, but becomes less in amount after each succeeding incident. Caution should be exercised in diagnosing a meniscal tear if no effusion is present and if there has been no history of swelling.

(c) Giving way or buckling

Giving way or buckling of the knee may occur if the meniscus is trapped and the sudden pain causes reflex inhibition of the quadriceps muscle. On the other hand, ligamentous laxity may be the cause; the instability being lateral or more frequently rotatory, and the torn meniscus an incidental finding. Episodes of giving way occur more often when the patient is on an uneven surface or coming downstairs when the posterior horn of the meniscus is trapped more easily as the load is increased on this part as the joint flexes (Walker and Erkmann, 1975).

(d) Locking

Locking is caused by the torn part of the meniscus, usually a bucket-handle, being trapped in front of the femoral condyle. Typically, on getting up from a kneeling position the patient finds that the knee will not straighten, although it will flex and there is pain on the side of the trapped meniscus. Alternatively, locking may follow a sporting injury and occasionally the patient finds the knee is locked on waking in the morning. Pain is worse on bearing weight and the patient cannot get the heel to the floor. The angle at which locking occurs varies with the length of the bucket-handle tear. If the split is short so that the bucket-handle is only just long enough to displace to the centre of the joint the knee may be locked at some 50° or 60° (Fig. 5.4). The meniscus is under considerable tension in this position due to the short tear, so that the pain may be severe. Most often the tear is longer so that the knee locks in 10° or 20° of flexion and, although pain is experienced, it is not usually so severe. Unlocking, like locking, is dramatic and confirms that there has been true locking. Patients will often claim that the knee has locked, although the subsequent operative findings make this seem doubtful. Wynn Parry (1958) reported that half the patients in whom a normal meniscus was found complained of locking. For this reason a history of unlocking may be a better indication that a tear is present. As the knee straightens, it does so with a clunk, which may be audible, and at the same time the pain disappears. In most cases a small effusion will develop. Patients often feel that the joint has momentarily dislocated during these episodes.

(e) 'Loose body'

Meniscal tags may be tucked up into the gutter at the side of the femoral condyle. They are small, firm and move slightly with some of the characteristics of a loose body.

5.2.2 PHYSICAL SIGNS

(a) Swelling

Swelling may be due to an effusion, which is confined to the synovial cavity, giving a characteristic appearance. More generalized swelling is due to involvement of the periarticular tissues by oedema or bleeding. If the effusion becomes chronic the synovium may be thickened. Small effusions are most easily recognized by smoothing the fluid away from the medial gutter, which then appears as a hollow. Compression of the suprapatellar pouch and the lateral side of the joint will result in a small visible wave of fluid passing back into the gutter. Larger quantities of fluid are more easily fluctuated across and behind the patella.

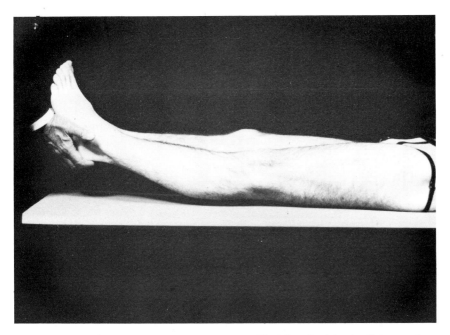

Fig. 5.5 Loss of passive extension. Demonstrated by lifting both heels off the couch.

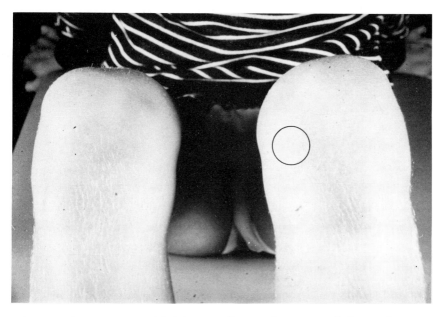

Fig. 5.6 There is an area of ill-defined swelling on the anteromedial aspect best seen with the knee flexed. The area is outlined with a circle.

(b) Muscle wasting

Muscle wasting can appear within a few days of an acute injury which is painful enough to restrict knee movement, especially if the knee cannot be fully extended. This wasting is most easily seen in the oblique fibres of the vastus medialis which are normally prominent. The lateral part of the quadriceps is covered by thick fascia and is not so visible. Some patients, if the interval between episodes is long, may show very little wasting.

(c) Movement

Movements must be compared with the opposite knee since there may be only minor degrees of limitation. Loss of passive extension can be assessed by lifting both heels off the examination couch with the patient relaxed (Fig. 5.5). If there is a flexion deformity of 15° or 20°, then it is probable that the knee is locked. Smaller degrees of fixed flexion may also indicate locking but can be due to reflex muscle spasm associated with such conditions as ligamentous injury or inflammatory disease. Rotation, although difficult to assess, should be compared in both knees. This is most easily done with the joint at a right angle. The thigh is held in one hand to fix it, whilst the other hand rotates the tibia using the foot as a lever. Locked knees will invariably show some loss of rotation and forced external rotation causes pain.

(d) Tenderness

Tenderness is localized over the meniscotibial ligament at or just below the joint line. Comparison with the opposite knee may often show that the normal hollow at the joint line has been obliterated by localized swelling at the point of tenderness (Fig. 5.6). A haemarthrosis may give rise to more generalized tenderness.

(e) Ligament laxity

This should be assessed by carrying out the tests outlined in Chapter 7. If the joint is very painful, anaesthesia may be necessary.

(f) McMurray's test

McMurray's test (1928) is carried out by fully flexing the knee, rotating it internally and extending the joint. The test is then repeated with the tibia in external rotation. The fingers, which are placed over the joint line, may feel a clunk as the femoral condyle passes over the torn meniscus. Saugmann-Jensen (1963) found the test to be positive in 21% of knees in which no tears were found. Wynn Parry (1958) gave an even higher figure of 65%. The test may be of limited value, particularly in equivocal cases.

(g) Apley's test

Apley's test (1959) is carried out with the patient lying on his face with the knee flexed to 90°. The tibia is rotated whilst a compression force is maintained through the length of the bone. If a grinding sensation is felt, this suggests that the meniscus is torn. This test is also open to misinterpretation.

5.3 Investigations

5.3.1 RADIOGRAPHY

Radiography will exclude other disorders but gives little positive help in the diagnosis of a meniscal tear. A decrease in the cartilage space may sometimes be observed in a compartment in which there is a large displaced bucket-handle tear. Conditions such as osteochondritis dissecans and stress fractures will be excluded. Osteoarthritic changes should be noted as their presence may affect the subsequent recovery and prognosis.

Arthrography can be of value, particularly in the area which is more difficult to assess by arthroscopy, i.e. the posteromedial compartment. An experienced radiologist is needed since the technique and interpretation may be difficult (Chapter 3).

5.3.2 ARTHROSCOPY

Arthroscopy is a valuable investigation and its value is related to the skill of the surgeon. Its use is discussed in Chapter 4. Whilst tears may be seen, experience is necessary to decide, particularly with cleavage lesions, as to what contribution they make to the patient's symptoms. As Noble and Hamblen (1975) have observed, the occurrence of tears after 45 or 50 years of age is common and many of them in all probability do not cause symptoms.

5.3.3 DIFFERENTIAL DIAGNOSIS

(a) Pain

Pain over the medial and lateral side of the joint must be distinguished from collateral ligament injuries. Stressing the damaged ligament will reproduce the pain and, although there may be tenderness over the joint line, it is usually not so localized and is more often maximal at the attachment of the ligament to bone.

On the *medial* side of the joint, inflammation of the small bursa between the superficial and deep parts of the ligament and occasionally the semimembranosus bursa can give very similar symptoms. An injection of hydrocortisone into the bursa will often relieve the pain and help to confirm the diagnosis. On the *lateral* side injury to the popliteus tendon or inflammation of its sheath must be distinguished from a meniscal tear. Stressing the muscle by resisted flexion or internal rotation will cause pain.

Anterior knee pain due to a variety of causes may be confused with meniscal injury. The commonest conditions are chondromalacia, malalignment of the patella and degenerative arthritis; all of which tend to give pain more localized to the infrapatellar region. Synovial plicae and lesions of the fat pads should be considered in the differential diganosis.

Stress fractures of the tibial and femoral condyles may confuse but careful examination will show that the pain and tenderness is more localized to the condyle rather than the joint line (Engber, 1977). Confirmation by radiograph is not usually present for several weeks.

(b) Locking

Locking is most frequently due to a torn meniscus, but loose bodies should be excluded by radiographs. Various conditions preventing full extension of the knee either by muscle spasm, capsular contracture or oedema of the anterior soft tissues must be considered. Momentary catching of the joint due to surface irregularity of the condyles can give the patient the impression that the joint has locked. These conditions should not confuse the surgeon, provided a proper history is taken and is followed by careful examination.

5.3.4 ASSOCIATED CONDITIONS

Before proceeding to treatment, it is important to assess the knee joint fully. The meniscal tear may be simple and uncomplicated but is frequently associated with one or more of the following conditions.

(a) Haemarthrosis

A haemarthrosis may arise as a result of damage to any of the structures in the joint. Most commonly the bleeding arises from a tear of the anterior cruciate ligament (Noyes *et al.*, 1980; Gillquist *et al.*, 1977). Bleeding may be suspected if the knee swells within minutes of the initial injury and becomes tense and very painful. In some cases the bleeding is more gradual and diagnosis can only be made by aspiration.

(b) Ligamentous injury

Ligamentous injury may often accompany damage to the meniscus, particularly those cases arising as a result of high speed injuries or occurring in body contact sports. If damage to the ligaments is suspected, the joint should be examined under anaesthesia so that any laxity can be assessed.

(c) Fractures of articular cartilage

These either alone or with the underlying bone should be excluded, since their presence will affect the management of any meniscal tear.

Osteoarthritic changes are of importance in determining the management. Although more common in relation to cleavage tears, the association is not constant (Noble and Hamblen, 1975).

5.4 Treatment

5.4.1 CONSERVATIVE

Some peripheral tears may heal. There is evidence that this will occur in dogs (King, 1936). More recently Heatley (1980) has been able to obtain healing in lesions of the menisci in rabbits. Some were sutured but other menisci healed spontaneously, if the meniscus was in contact with the synovium. Whether healing will occur in the human knee under similar circumstances is not known. There does, however, seem to be a possibility that many knees with localized joint-line tenderness after injury may have suffered a peripheral tear of the meniscus. Following a period of rest, symptoms and signs may disappear (absence of pain, absorption of effusion and return of full movement), which could indicate healing or quiescence. If symptoms are improving, it would seem reasonable to continue with a regime of limited activity unless there is good reason for surgical intervention. Should the symptoms not subside within a few weeks or if they return on the resumption of full activity, then arthroscopy is indicated so that a more definite diagnosis can be made.

(a) Physiotherapy

Surgeons for many years have advised that quadriceps exercises may help in the patient's rehabilitation by building up the muscles and this may encourage absorption of fluid. Patients with an occupation which does not require strenuous activity may find that their symptoms and signs subside with rest and that they can do their work without difficulty. If more vigorous exercise produces further complaints, then the patient may be prepared to give up strenuous sport in order to avoid an operation.

(b) Locking

Locking of the joint may be present when the patient is first seen and in this case manipulation should be carried out at the earliest opportunity. This is likely to be successful in the first 24 hours or even after longer periods. In the first few hours after locking it is usually possible to unlock a joint in the conscious patient but as the joint becomes increasingly painful, then anaesthesia is likely to be necessary. With the passage of time the possibility of unlocking becomes less likely since the meniscus loses elasticity and will not easily spring back to the periphery of the joint. To reduce the displaced meniscus the joint is first fully flexed and rotated both internally and externally as the joint is straightened, initially with a valgus and then, if unsuccessful, with a varus stress. When the joint is unlocked it will extend fully without difficulty and no attempt should be made to force full extension. This may result in an extension of the tear further forward and render unlocking more difficult, or in damage to the anterior cruciate ligament.

5.4.2 OPERATIVE

Meniscectomy should only be done if the diagnosis is confirmed and it is reasonably certain that the tear which is seen is causing the patient's symptoms. If possible, arthroscopy should always precede the operation.
Indications for operation are:

1. Locking
2. Repeated giving way
3. Recurrent effusion
4. Pain

If the patient presents with a locked knee and manipulation has failed to restore full extension easily, then operation should be carried out as soon as possible. Should there be delay for any reason, the patient will need crutches since weight bearing is difficult and painful. If the diagnosis is in doubt, arthroscopy should certainly be advised and the need for meniscectomy based on the results of the investigation and the clinical findings. The following methods of arthrotomy are outlined below.

(a) Medial meniscectomy

The patient is positioned so that both legs are flexed at a right angle over the end of the table. The vessels and nerves behind the knee are protected by soft cushions or sand bags. The surgeon is seated so that the foot of the limb for operation is comfortably held between his knees and the tibia can be rotated. A vertical incision is made about a finger's breadth from the medial side of the patella with two-thirds of the incision above the joint line and one-third below (Fig. 5.7). An advantage of arthroscopy is that this incision can be kept small if it is known as a result of the arthroscopy that only a bucket-handle or some tags are to be removed. The infrapatellar branch of the saphenous nerve should be seen in the lower part of the wound passing laterally and should be preserved. The capsule and the synovial membrane are incised in the same line with minimal dissection. A bucket-handle tear or tag should be separated from the peripheral part of the meniscus by an incision in the line of the circumferential fibres. Care should be taken to ensure that the inner margin of the meniscus is smooth after the removal.

Total meniscectomy should only be carried out if the meniscus is very degenerate with multiple tags or splits so that partial meniscectomy is difficult or impossible. In this event the meniscus should be divided in its outer part after the anterior horn has been detached. The tissue peripheral to the meniscus should not be cut or incised, since this will result in unnecessary bleeding. When the anterior two-thirds has been detached, the meniscus can then be dislocated into the intercondylar notch. Whilst it is kept under tension by means of a Kocher's forcep, the posterior horn can be cut with a tenotome or Smillie's knife. If the meniscus should tear in the middle leaving a large

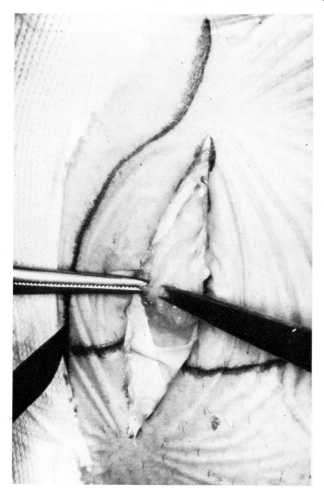

Fig. 5.7   Vertical incision for medial meniscectomy. The position of the joint line and the patellar tendon have been marked. The saphenous nerve is indicated.

posterior tag or if, indeed, other large posterior tags are seen, then it may be necessary to remove any meniscal remnants through a posteromedial incision. A second incision, however, should rarely be required since most large tags can be removed through the anterior approach. If they cannot be easily seen from the front, the tags are probably small and so need not be removed. During the 1939–45 war it was considered unwise to leave any of the posterior horn *in situ* (Campbell, 1956). As a result, attempts were made to remove remnants, which often inflicted unnecessary damage on the joint. Dandy and Jackson (1975) in a review of 174 knees with continuing symptoms after meniscectomy found that retained posterior horn fragments were the cause in only 13% of the cases. A conservative attitude should, therefore, be maintained since further surgery may often do more harm than

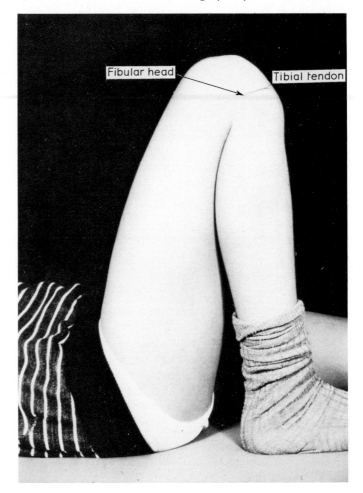

Fig. 5.8 Position of patient for removal of lateral meniscus by Bruser's method.

good. Should it for any reason be necessary, the incision must be made far enough posteriorly so that a retractor can be placed in the pouch of synovium, which appears when the knee is flexed. Placing the incision, which also should be vertical, is most easily made after passing a dissector through the anterior incision to the back of the joint.

(b) Lateral meniscectomy

Lateral meniscectomy can also be carried out through a vertical incision but access is not so good as on the medial side. The transverse incision of Bruser (1960) is preferred, since it not only makes the operation easier but also allows the whole of the meniscus to be seen. The popliteus tendon is visible and perhaps more important the lateral geniculate artery can be protected. This is close to the meniscus and if damaged in this operation will cause considerable bleeding. The incision is made with the foot flat on the table so that the knee is fully flexed and the hip at 90° of flexion (Fig. 5.8). This relaxes the iliotibial tract and allows wide retraction. Anteriorly the incision extends from the patellar ligament and runs backwards towards the tip of the styloid process of the fibula at the level of the joint line. The iliotibial tract can be divided in the line of the skin incision; care being taken not to damage the fibular collateral ligament. This incision is particularly useful if a cyst of the lateral meniscus is being removed. The cyst can first be exposed and then if it is considered necessary, the operation continued to remove the meniscus.

5.4.3 TOTAL OR PARTIAL MENISCECTOMY

For many years there has been debate as to whether it is wiser to remove the whole or just part of the meniscus.

Robert Jones advocated partial removal in 1909. From then onwards there was a gradual swing to total meniscectomy, which was strongly advised by Timbrell Fisher (1933) and Watson Jones (1946). Perhaps the most influential advocate was Smillie (1946). The reasons given to support the need for total meniscectomy were the necessity to avoid leaving posterior tags and, secondly, to allow regrowth of a meniscus by removing the whole of the avascular part. The danger of leaving posterior tags which cause symptoms has been exaggerated (Dandy and Jackson, 1975). Furthermore, the occurrence of degenerative changes which so often follow meniscectomy suggests very strongly that the reformed meniscus has little, if any, functional value.

Cargill and Jackson (1976) have shown that the short- and long-term results of partial meniscectomy are better than those achieved by removal of the whole meniscus. Removal of the bucket-handle fragment only, produced better results compared with total meniscectomy both clinically and in a study of the radiographs (Tables 5.1–5.3). There is also theoretical evidence from bioengineering studies (Hargreaves and Seedhom, 1978) to suggest that

Table 5.1 The frequency of symptoms in the two groups

	Excision of bucket-handle alone (37 knees)	Excision of whole meniscus (50 knees)
Discomfort	13 (35.0)*	26 (52.0)
Episodes of locking	1 (02.7)	1 (02.0)
Sensation of instability	6 (16.2)	10 (20.0)

* Percentages in parentheses

Table 5.2 The frequency of physical signs in the two groups

	Excision of bucket-handle alone (37 knees)	Excision of whole meniscus (50 knees)
Effusion	2 (05.4)*	11 (22.0)
Quadriceps wasting	6 (16.2)	17 (34.0)
Medial collateral instability	4 (10.8)	6 (12.0)
Anteroposterior laxity	27 (72.9)	34 (68.0)
Quadriceps lag	0	0
	(28 knees)	(35 knees)
Restricted range of movement†	9 (32.0)	24 (69.0)

* Percentages in parentheses
† Unilateral operations only. $p < 0.05$

Table 5.3 The frequency of abnormal roentgenographic changes in the two groups

	Excision of bucket-handle alone		Excision of whole meniscus	
	Overall (37 knees)	5-year follow-up (13 knees)	Overall (50 knees)	5-year follow-up (29 knees)
Marginal osteophytes	13 (35.0)*	3 (23.0)	18 (36.0)	11 (37.9)
Tibial spine deformation	15 (40.5)	3 (23.0)	26 (52.0)	15 (51.7)
Condylar flattening	7 (19.9)	3 (23.0)	20 (40.0)	14 (48.2)
Anteroposterior ridge	17 (45.0)	6 (46.1)	25 (50.0)	13 (44.8)
Cartilage space narrowing	2 (05.4)	0	8 (16.0)	5 (17.2)

* Percentages in parentheses

the load on the articular surface was four times as great after total meniscectomy but only twice as much after partial meniscectomy. Removal of the bucket-handle only is much easier and accomplished with less trauma to the joint, so that the convalescence is quicker and less troublesome.

5.4.4 POST-OPERATIVE CARE

Many surgeons advise bed rest for a number of days after operation. The author is of the opinion that patients should be encouraged to walk and bend the knee as soon as possible, since this minimizes muscle wasting and preserves the nutrition of the articular cartilage. To this end partial meniscectomy is carried out so that a limited incision is used. Splinting is unnecessary and only a crepe bandage rather than a pressure dressing is used. Plaster immobilization has been used but does not appear to offer any advantage in recovery either of strength or motion (Bryan et al., 1969). For many years quadriceps exercises have been carried out as a routine in the rehabilitation period. There is now some evidence (Forster and Frost, 1982) that supervision by a physiotherapist is unnecessary and wasteful of time and resources. The recovery is just as rapid and as satisfactory if the patient is simply instructed in how to carry out the exercises on their own and encouraged to gradually increase their activity. If there are no complications, full flexion returns gradually. Patients should be encouraged to regain full extension since only when this had been achieved will the quadriceps power build up again. Oedema of the fat pad or bleeding into it may make this difficult in some patients but careful surgery will minimize this problem.

5.4.5 REPAIR OF THE MENISCUS

The long-term results of the first recorded meniscal repair which was published by Annandale (1889) are unknown, although the patient, a Newcastle miner, was back at work six months later. However, since the long-term ill-effects of removing the meniscus have become recognized, there have been attempts at repair.

Palmer (1938) drew attention to the fact that the medial meniscus might become loosened in combination with ligamentous injuries and advocated fixing it by suture to the posterior part of the collateral ligament. Price and Allen (1978) investigated tears of the meniscus in relation to ligament injury in more detail and advised that any peripheral tear should be sutured unless the meniscus was irreparably damaged. They reported good function after a follow-up period of 2.7 years in knees in which this policy has been carried out.

King (1936) and Heatley (1980) have both shown that healing of meniscal tears in animals occurs if a vascular supply is available. The meniscus has for many years been regarded as a relatively avascular structure, but Arnoczky and Warren (1982) demonstrated that not only is there a good peripheral blood supply but this penetrates the meniscus for 10–30% of its width. In view of the deleterious effects of removal of the meniscus, in the last few years attempts have been made to preserve this structure wherever possible.

Wirth (1981) obtained good results in a small series of ten patients. De Haven (1983) in a larger number of meniscal tears (104 menisci) has advised suture in those cases in which there is a vertical tear at or near the periphery of the meniscus with the body of the meniscus remaining intact. Arthroscopy is necessary in all cases to determine the suitability of the tear for suture, and arthrography has also been found to help in the assessment, particularly in chronic cases. De Haven, as far as possible, plans the approach to this tear to avoid major stabilizing structures. Where there is a rim of meniscus still attached to the capsular structures, this is excised. Sutures are placed 2–3 mm apart and tied inside the joint. Post-operatively the knee is immobilized in 45° of flexion for four weeks and then knee movements are commenced; the patient still remaining on crutches for a further two weeks. No strenuous activity is allowed for a period of six months from the operation.

Repair of the meniscus has been attempted arthroscopically (Ikeuchi, 1975) and it is probable that with improvements in instrumentation and technique this route will be used more frequently.

5.5 Complications

5.5.1 IMMEDIATE

(a) Haemarthrosis

Severe pain after operation may be caused by bleeding into the joint, which can occur in the first 24 hours. The wound should be inspected on the day following operation. If the joint is swollen and tense, then aspiration should be carried out. Removal of blood from the joint will not only relieve the patient's pain but lead to a more rapid convalescence. Aspiration should be repeated if there is thought to be a further collection of blood in the joint. Very occasionally bleeding may be more severe and there should be no hesitation in reopening the joint to wash out any clot and endeavouring to ligate any bleeding points.

(b) Infection

Infection is fortunately rare after meniscectomy. If it is suspected, the joint should be aspirated and the fluid sent for examination and culture. A broad spectrum antibiotic should be given. This may later have to be changed in the light of any bacteriological findings. If the aspirated fluid is turbid, arthrotomy and washing out the joint is indicated. Adequate and early treatment will avoid the long-term problems of chronic joint infection and stiffness. The joint should be immobilized as long as pain and pyrexia persist. When the condition is quiescent movement should begin but stopped if symptoms recur.

(c) Division of the saphenous nerve

The infrapatellar branch is frequently divided and this will result in an area of anaesthesia 5 or 6 cm across, just below the knee. Subjective symptoms are, however, uncommon. In the series of 577 patients investigated by the author, nearly half had patches of anaesthesia. Many of the patients were unaware of the sensory loss until it was pointed out to them. A proportion were miners who were engaged in working on their knees but, despite this, they had no symptoms. Neuromata causing pain and disability have been reported but in the author's experience this is a rare complication.

(d) Persistent effusion

Persistent effusion can delay the patient's recovery. Neither suction drainage at wound closure nor application of a cast affects the incidence of effusion (Bryan et al., 1969). Aspiration may be carried out initially to exclude the presence of blood but if the fluid is clear there is nothing to be gained by repeated aspiration, since the effusion will recur. Wynn Parry (1958) suggested that, providing the knee was stable, patients with an effusion were quite fit for duties in the RAF, though they might need to avoid vigorous physical activity and sport. Nearly 9% of all the patients he reviewed were returned to duty with an effusion without any ill-effects. If the effusion is large and troubles the patient, then it may be necessary to apply a back splint and to immobilize the knee which will encourage absorption of the fluid.

5.5.2 DELAYED

(a) Instability

Instability may occur following removal of a meniscus. When this occurs it seems likely that joint laxity must have been present before the operation, though the patient may not have complained of the knee giving way. The posterior third of the meniscus blocks rotation, particularly if weight is being borne. Repetitive impingement of the femoral condyle on the meniscus in a lax joint may result in a late secondary tear and removal of the meniscus can unmask rotatory instability (Slocum and Larson, 1968). The patient may not complain of the knee giving way until he resumes sporting activities.

(b) Meniscal tears and osteoarthritis

Noble and Hamblen (1975), in their review of elderly cadaveric knee joints, came to the conclusion that osteoarthritis was not necessarily directly associated with degeneration of the meniscus. Out of 39 severely degenerate knees 15 had a normal meniscus. On the other hand 18.4% of normal knees had a cleavage lesion present; of which a third were massive. Noble considered that it was unlikely that all patients with cleavage lesions had symptoms and that, secondly, many of them did not require operation. Lotke *et al.* (1981) found that in the older patient with normal radiographs before operation and a short duration of symptoms, meniscectomy gave a good result. Other patients who had a good prognosis after operation were those in whom there was a history of specific trauma; the pain was sudden in onset and the degenerative changes were not marked. They suggested that it was wise to leave the meniscus if there was only a minimal split and a considerable degree of degenerative change, since the results of removal were not satisfactory. If, on the other hand, the meniscus was badly frayed and the femoral and tibial condyles were smooth, meniscectomy was recommended (Fig. 5.9).

5.5.3   OSTEOARTHRITIS

The most important function of the meniscus is the distribution of load.

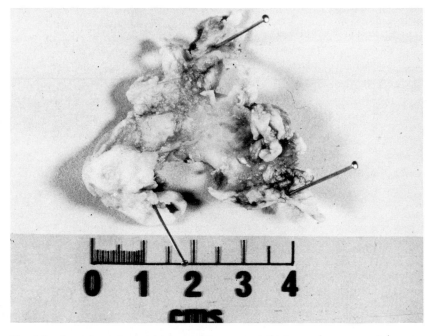

Fig. 5.9   Frayed meniscus which requires removal if joint surfaces are satisfactory.

Fairbank (1948) drew attention to the fact that comparison of radiographs of knees before and after prolonged load bearing showed joint narrowing of up to 2 mm (Fig. 5.10). He pointed out that the meniscus was attached firmly at its two ends, though the peripheral attachments were lax. From these observations he concluded that the circumference of the meniscus must be forced centrifugally when weight is borne and that there must be increasing tension in the stretched and elastic meniscus. At the same time that the meniscus was being stretched the articular cartilage was being deformed. If the meniscus was removed, excessive loads might be placed on the articular cartilage which might not recover fully. Hirsch (1944) had previously found that articular cartilage was perfectly elastic only for small loads applied for a short time and that when greater loads were applied for longer periods, the recovery might not be complete.

Fairbank also described the appearance of the radiographs of knees which had previously had a meniscectomy and found various changes, alone or in combination:

'. . . formation of an antero-posterior ridge on the femoral condyle, generalised flattening of the femoral articular surface, and narrowing of the joint space.'

These radiographic appearances might appear as early as five months after operation and followed the loss of the load-bearing function of the meniscus. He did not believe that these changes were those of osteoarthritis, though they might predispose to degenerative change.

Effect on meniscus of joint compression

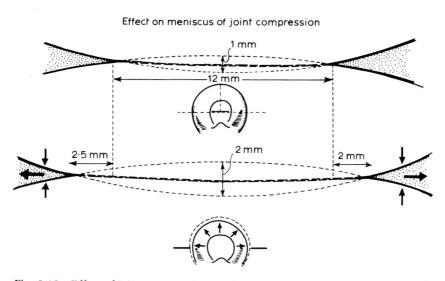

Fig. 5.10   Effect of joint compression on the meniscus. (From J.T. Fairbank, with permission.)

Vandendorp *et al.* (1939) assessed the long-term results of meniscectomy and reported osteoarthritis in some cases. The author reviewed a series of 640 cases at Harlow Wood Orthopaedic Hospital (Jackson, 1967; 1968). The shortest follow-up was five years. In 133 patients (23%) well marked degenerative changes were present (Fig. 5.11). In 382 patients the opposite knee had not been operated on and as far as could be ascertained had not suffered any significant injury. These knees were, therefore, used as a control group. It was found that well-established degenerative changes were present in the radiographs of 23% of knees after meniscectomy and only 5% in the control group. The incidence of degenerative changes increased with time, but there were fewer changes in the control group (Fig. 5.12).

The Harlow Wood Orthopaedic Hospital records showed that 107 normal or near normal menisci had been removed. Examination of the follow-up radiographs showed 23% had degenerative change – no different from those patients with significant tears.

Damage to the articular cartilage is frequently seen in relation to a torn meniscus (Fig. 5.13). The author (Jackson, 1968) noted these changes in 29%

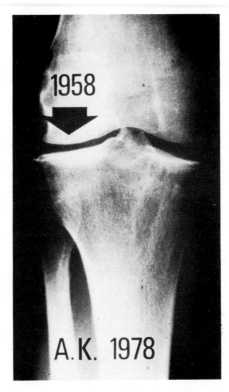

Fig. 5.11 Degenerative changes in the medial compartment ten years after meniscectomy.

140

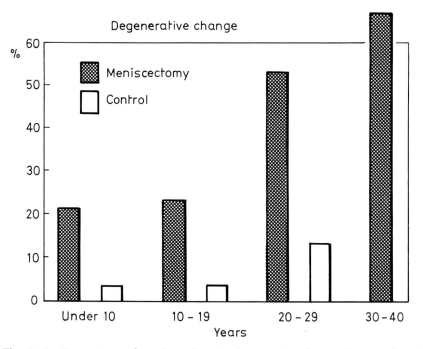

Fig. 5.12 Comparison of numbers showing degenerative changes in control and operated knees five years or more after meniscectomy.

of an unselected group of 100 patients undergoing meniscectomy. If this damage were important in determining the onset of osteoarthritis, comparison of groups with a differing length of history from the time of initial injury to the meniscectomy operation would be more likely to show evidence of osteoarthritis the longer the pre-operative history. The incidence was the same in patients whether or not the injury had occurred within six months of the meniscectomy or at a longer interval. Operative delay is unlikely, therefore, to lead to an increased chance of developing osteoarthritis.

Appel (1970) in a similar review of the long-term joint changes after meniscectomy reported very similar figures to the author. Of the cases he followed up 10% showed evidence of osteoarthritis after meniscectomy, but in the opposite knees, which he used as controls and which had not undergone surgery, only 1% were affected.

Meniscectomy is not an innocuous procedure (Fairbank, 1948) and should not be carried out unless the diagnosis is confirmed before operation by arthroscopy or arthrography. Ireland and his co-workers (1980) achieved an accuracy of 98% using a combination of these methods. Whether the meniscus is removed by arthroscopic surgery or arthrotomy will depend on the skill and experience of the surgeon. Every effort should be made to limit the amount of dissection and to remove the minimum amount of meniscal

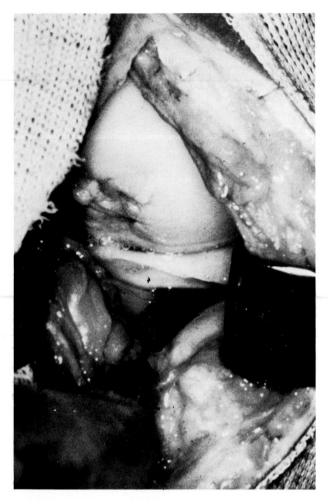

Fig. 5.13 Damage to articular cartilage on the femoral condyle in relation to a meniscal tear.

tissue compatible with obtaining relief of the patient's symptoms. When there is doubt about the diagnosis, operation should be deferred. Noble and Erat (1980) found in a series of 250 patients listed for meniscectomy that 50 had no symptoms by the time they were admitted to hospital and a further 50 had no significant tear at operation. Goodfellow (1980) summed up the situation in his editorial in the *Journal of Bone and Joint Surgery*

> '. . . meniscectomy is only justifiable if a meniscus is causing more trouble than it is worth and that it is probably better to underestimate than to overestimate the significance of minor lesions.'

5.6 Cystic menisci

Ebner (1904) is credited with the first description of meniscal cysts and since then there has been much debate about their aetiology. Ollerenshaw (1921) was of the opinion that they were congenital in origin but at no time has there been any real evidence to support this theory, since the cyst rarely appears before maturity. Bonnin (1952) reported that 30% of patients he examined gave a history of trauma. This was a clinical survey of patients in whom the cysts were large enough to give rise to symptoms.

Barrie (1979) examined 1571 menisci, of which 112 showed evidence of cystic change. All the cysts could be shown to communicate with either a horizontal cleavage tear or a longitudinal tear if there was a horizontal component. Previously Gallo and Bryan (1968) had described two cases in which there was continuity between the cyst and a cleavage lesion of the meniscus and speculated that fluid from the joint might penetrate the meniscus and produce cystic changes. Barrie's evidence was much more convincing and as a result of his examination of cystic menisci he suggested that cysts first appeared in the inner avascular zone and were small. They then migrated to the periphery of the knee as a result of the pumping action of the synovial fluid caused by movements of the joint. An increase in size occurred due to more fluid being pushed into the cyst and because of the looseness of the parameniscal tissues allowing expansion. The mechanism was in all probability a central shearing stress produced by rotation of the knee under load. Of the 112 menisci examined there was a history of injury in 5% of those appearing in the lateral meniscus and 54% of those in the medial. Wroblewski (1973) had reported an incidence of tears in 50% of 299 cases, and there is undoubtedly a close relationship between trauma and the cyst, but there is still some doubt as to whether injury is the cause or just an aggravating factor. In many cysts there may be blood or blood pigments. This may be due to bleeding from neighbouring blood vessels. Barrie (1979) points out that in the outer vascular portion of the meniscus and the parameniscal tissues the blood vessels are susceptible to rupture.

5.6.1 CLINICAL

The cyst is characterized by aching pain which is often described by the patient as like toothache. The pain, which is episodic, is increased by exertion. Night pain is a frequent complaint and is aching in nature.

Cysts in the parameniscal tissues may be large enough to be noticed by the patient, but often they are unaware of the swelling. A blow may cause bleeding and bring the cyst to clinical attention by producing pain and increase in size.

Symptoms associated with a tear of the meniscus, such as giving way and occasionally locking, may occur. Tears are commonly associated with cystic change (Wroblewski, 1973). The mobility of the meniscus may be impaired by the size of the cyst and render it more liable to tearing. Characteristically, the tears are of the parrot-beak type (Figs 5.14 and 5.15).

The cysts are usually detectable at or near the joint line but occasionally may migrate anteriorly into the fat pad. The swelling is more easily seen with the knee in extension but tends to disappear in flexion. Most cysts feel hard because they are tense, so much so that fluctuation may be difficult to elicit. There is often localized tenderness.

5.6.2 DIFFERENTIAL DIAGNOSIS

Marginal exostoses and tags of meniscus overlying the joint line may appear similar. Other cysts around the joint, such as enlarged bursae and ganglia, must be considered. Arthroscopy may be helpful since the meniscus may show evidence of cystic degeneration and be thickened and yellowish in colour. Furthermore, a tear may often be seen and give a view of the substance of the meniscus in which small cysts may be visible.

Coker and Kent (1967) have described two cases which gave rise to irritation of the peroneal nerve, which were relieved by removal of a cystic meniscus and a cyst arising from it in relation to the nerve. Ganglia arising from the tibiofemoral joint and in one case from the knee were reported by Stack *et al.* (1965) as affecting the peroneal nerve and must be considered in the differential diagnosis. Radiographs may occasionally show pressure erosion on the side of the tibial plateau (Enis and Ghandur-Mnaymneh, 1979).

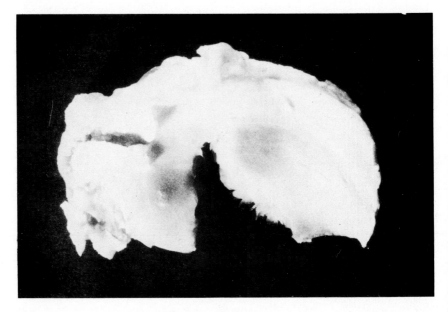

Fig. 5.14 Cystic meniscus with parrot-beak tear.

5.6.3 TREATMENT

Many patients will be prepared to tolerate the continued presence of the cyst since the episodes of pain may be short. All that is required is reassurance that the swelling is harmless. If symptoms are continuous, surgical treatment will be indicated. Removal of the cyst alone has the advantage of a shorter rehabilitation period and a more comfortable convalescence. The meniscus is preserved and the possibility of osteoarthritis avoided. Flynn and Kelly (1976) reported on 22 patients, of whom 12 had only a local excision of the cyst. No recurrence was noted over an average follow-up period of 7.5 years. Some of these cysts may perhaps have been true ganglia and unconnected with the meniscus.

Should the patient be averse to surgery but suffering enough to demand treatment, then aspiration and steroid injection may be tried. Recurrence of the cyst is the most likely outcome.

5.7 Discoid menisci

5.7.1 AETIOLOGY

For some years as a result of investigations by Smillie (1948) the discoid meniscus was thought to be due to lack of absorption of the central part of a disc which separated the tibial and femoral condyles. Since then work by

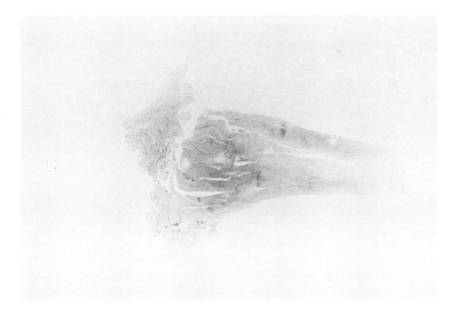

Fig. 5.15 Section of cystic meniscus.

145

Kaplan (1955) has shown that the meniscus at a very early date in the development of the embryo has an adult conformation. As a consequence it is now accepted that the discoid meniscus is a true congenital malformation.

5.7.2 INCIDENCE

Noble and Hamblen (1975) found 5% of 100 cadavers had a discoid meniscus and this probably gives a fairly accurate indication of the incidence. Most other accounts are based on series of meniscectomies and assess the frequency with which it gives rise to symptoms. Jeannopoulos (1950) found an incidence of 0.17% out of 580 meniscectomies, though when lateral menisci only were considered this rose to 15.5%. Smillie reported 4.74% of discoid menisci in 10 000 meniscectomies.

The condition affects the lateral meniscus almost totally, although medial discoid menisci have been described. In Smillie's series there were only seven cases out of 474. Jeannopoulos (1950) reported an unusual case of a young girl, aged ten, from whom both a medial and lateral discoid meniscus were removed from the same knee at different times, both having given rise to symptoms.

5.7.3 TYPES

Smillie (1978) differentiated three types. These were based, as he himself points out, on a false premise (the absorption of the central part). The classification is, despite this, valid since it indicates the type of lesion encountered.

He suggested the following types:

(1) *Massive*: this occupies the entire space between the femoral and tibial condyles so that there is no contact between the articular cartilage (Fig. 5.16). He points out that there is often a very large lateral geniculate artery in relation to this, which may give rise to troublesome bleeding during meniscectomy.

(2) *Intermediate*: this is less complete and the central zone is quite thin.

(3) *Analogous*: this is similar in shape to the normal meniscus but the middle segment is greatly increased in breadth.

5.7.4 LESIONS

The most common is a horizontal cleavage tear which probably arises, as Smillie (1978) points out, by continuous movement of the relatively free superior surface on the relatively fixed inferior surface. Since the discoid meniscus is often very thick, the central part may well degenerate because of the poor nutrition resulting from the distance that the nutrients have to travel from the surface of the meniscus. Once a horizontal split has occurred then

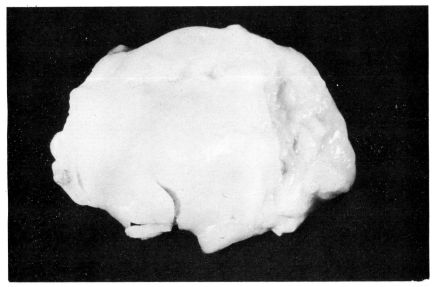

Fig. 5.16 Discoid meniscus.

the inferior portion may disappear as a result of continued wear, and eventually central fenestration follows if the upper layer disappears in addition.

Longitudinal tears will occur but are less frequent. The analogous type is liable to parrot-beak tears (Smillie, 1948).

5.7.5 CLINICAL

The classical sign which is attributed to the discoid meniscus is a loud clunk felt during the last 15° of flexion and extension of the knee joint. This sign is not, however, very frequently present and Jeannopoulos (1950) reports its presence in only three out of 21 cases. Patients who are usually in the second decade complain of a mild intermittent ache, usually of insidious onset. Giving way is a frequent complaint and locking may be reported. In some cases the patient does not have episodes of locking but may be unable to fully extend the knee.

Examination will reveal a localized swelling on the lateral aspect of the knee which moves during flexion. The appearances may resemble that of a cyst.

5.7.6 RADIOGRAPHIC CHANGES

There may be widening of the affected compartment and if the condition is suspected, it is advisable to take comparable views of both knees on the same film. Jeannopoulos (1950) reported two of his cases as showing dysplasia of the lateral femoral condyle.

5.7.7 TREATMENT

This is similar to that for any meniscal lesion. If the symptoms are sufficiently troublesome, then meniscectomy should be advised. It is probable that many patients will have no symptoms. Noble and Hamblen's (1975) cadavers which they dissected were all in an older age group, mostly 60–80 years. Since the discoid menisci were still *in situ* in 5%, it seems unlikely that all the patients were much troubled during life.

References

Annandale T. Excision of the internal semilunar cartilage resulting in perfect restoration of the joint movements. *Br Med J* 1889;i:291–2.

Apley A G. *A system of orthopaedics and fractures.* London: Butterworth, 1959.

Appel H. Late results after meniscectomy in the knee joint. A clinical and roentgenological follow-up investigation. *Acta Orthop Scand Suppl* 1970;133H.

Arnoczky S P, Warren R F. Microvasculature of the human meniscus. *Am J Sports Med* 1982;10:90–5.

Barrie H J. The pathogenesis and significance of meniscal cysts. *J Bone Joint Surg [Br]* 1979;61–B:184–9.

Bennett G A, Waine H, Bauer W. *Changes in the knee joint at various ages with particular reference to the nature and development of degenerative joint disease.* New York: The Commonwealth Fund, 1942.

Bonnin J G. Cysts of the semilunar cartilage of the knee joint. *Br. J Surg* 1952;40:558–65.

Bruser D M. A direct approach to the lateral compartment of the knee joint. *J Bone Joint Surg [Br]* 1960;42–B:348–51.

Bryan R S, Dickson J H, Taylor W F. Recovery of the knee following meniscectomy. *J Bone Joint Surg [Am]* 1969;51–A:973–8.

Bullough P G, Munera L, Weinstein A M. The strength of the menisci of the knee as it relates to their fine structure. *J Bone Joint Surg [Br]* 1970;52–B:564–70.

Campbell W C. *Campbell's operative orthopaedics.* New York: C V Mosby Co. 1956;I:347.

Cargill A O'R, Jackson J P. Bucket-handle tear of the medial meniscus. A case for conservative surgery. *J Bone Joint Surg [Am]* 1976;58–A:248–51.

Coker T P, Kent M. Peroneal nerve irritation associated with cystic lateral meniscus of the knee. *J Bone Joint Surg [Am]* 1967;49–A:362–4.

Dandy D, Jackson R W. The diagnosis of problems after meniscectomy. *J Bone Joint Surg [Br]* 1975;57–B:349–52.

De Haven K E. Peripheral meniscus repair. In: Ward Cassells S. ed. *Diagnostic and surgical arthroscopy.* Philadelphia: Lea & Febiger, 1983.

Ebner H. Ein fall von ganglion amkriegelenksmenisken. *Munchenere Med Wochenschr* 1904; 51:1737–9.

Engber W D. Stress fractures of the medial tibial plateau. *J Bone Joint Surg [Am]* 1977;59–A:767–9.

Enis J E, Ghandur-Mnaymneh L. Cyst of the lateral meniscus causing erosion of the tibial plateau. *J Bone Joint Surg [Am]* 1979;61–A:441–2.

Fairbank T J. Knee joint changes after meniscectomy. *J Bone Joint Surg [Br]* 1948;30–B:664–70.

Forster D P, Frost C E. Cost effectiveness study of out-patient physiotherapy after medial meniscectomy. *Br Med J* 1982;13:485–7.

Flynn M, Kelly J P. Local excision of cyst of lateral meniscus of knee without recurrence. *J Bone Joint Surg [Br]* 1976;58–B:88–9.

Gallo G A, Bryan R S. Cysts of the semilunar cartilages of the knee joint. *Am J Surg* 1968; 116:65–8.

Gillquist J, Hagberg G, Oretorp N. Arthroscopy in acute injuries of the knee joint. *Acta Orthop Scand* 1977;48:190–6.

Goodfellow J. He who hesitates is saved. *J Bone Joint Surg [Br]* Editorial 1980;62–B:1–2.

Hargreaves D J, Seedhom B B. Partial or total meniscectomy? A quantitative study. *Br Orthop Res Soc.*, 1978.

Heatley F W. The meniscus: can it be repaired? *J Bone Joint Surg [Br]* 1980;62–B:397–402.

Hirsch C. A contribution to the pathogenesis of chondromalacia. *Acta Chir Scand* 1944;90 (Suppl 83):1–106.

Hwa-Hsin H, Walker P S. Stabilizing mechanism of the loaded and unloaded knee joint. *J Bone Joint Surg [Am]* 1976;58–A:87–93.

Ikeuchi H. Presented at the *Second Congress of the International Arthroscopy Association*. Copenhagen: Denmark, 1975.

Ireland J, Trickey E L, Stoker D J. Arthroscopy and arthrography of the knee. A critical review. *J Bone Joint Surg [Br]* 1980;62–B:3–6.

Jackson J P. Degenerative changes in the knee after meniscectomy. *J Bone Joint Surg [Br]* 1967;49–B:584.

Jackson J P. Degenerative changes in the knee after meniscectomy. *Br Med J* 1968;2:525–7.

Jeannopoulos E L. Observations on discoid menisci. *J Bone Joint Surg [Am]* 1950;32–A:649–52.

Jones R. Notes on derangement of the knee. *Am Surg* 1909;50:969–1001.

Kaplin E B. The embryology of the menisci of the knee joint. *Bull Hosp Joint Dis NY* 1955; 16:111.

King D. The healing of the semilunar cartilage. *J Bone Joint Surg* 1936;18(2):333–42.

Lotke P, Lefkoe R, Elker M. Late results following medial meniscectomy in an older population. *J Bone Joint Surg [Am]* 1981;63–A:115–9.

MacConaill M A. The function of intra-articular fibro-cartilage with special reference to the knee and inferior radio-ulnar joints. *J Anat* 1932;LXVI:210.

McMurray T P. *The Robert Jones birthday volume*. London: Humphrey Milford, 1928.

Markolf K L, Mensch J S, Amstutz H C. Stiffness and laxity of the knee. The contribution of the supporting structures. *J Bone Joint Surg [Am]* 1976;58–A:583–94.

Noble J, Erat E. In defence of the meniscus. A prospective study of 200 meniscectomy patients. *J Bone Joint Surg [Br]* 1980;62–B:7–11.

Noble J, Hamblen D L. The pathology of the degenerate meniscus lesion. *J Bone Joint Surg [Br]* 1975;57–B:180–6.

Noyes F R, Bassett R W, Grood E S, Butler D L. Arthroscopy in acute traumatic haemarthrosis of the knee. *J Bone Joint Surg [Am]* 1980;62–A:687–95.

Ollerenshaw R. The development of cysts in connection with the external semilunar cartilage of the knee joint. *Br J Surg* 1921;8:409.

Palmer I. On the injuries to the ligaments of the knee joint. A clinical study. *Acta Chir Scand* 1938;Suppl:53.

Price C T, Allen W C. Ligament repair in the knee with preservation of the meniscus. *J Bone Joint Surg [Am]* 1978;60–A:61–5.

Saugmann-Jensen J. Meniscus lesion of the knee joint. In: *Knaets Menisklaesioner*. Copenhagen: Munksgaard, 1963.

Seedhom B B, Dowson D, Wright V. The loadbearing function of the menisci. A preliminary study. In: *The Knee Joint.* Amsterdam: Excerpta Medica, 1974:37–42.

Slocum D B, Larson R L. Rotatory instability of the knee. *J Bone Joint Surg* [*Am*] 1968; 50–A:211–25.

Smillie I S. *Injuries of the knee joint.* 1st ed. Edinburgh: E & S Livingstone 1946.

Smillie I S. The congenital discoid meniscus. *J Bone Joint Surg* [*Br*] 1948;30–B:671–82.

Smillie I S. *Injuries of the knee joint.* 5th ed. Edinburgh, London, New York: Churchill Livingstone, 1978.

Stack R E, Bianco A J, MacCarty C S. Compression of the common peroneal nerve by ganglion cysts. *J Bone Joint Surg* [*Am*] 1965;47–A:773–8.

Timbrell Fisher A G. *Internal derangements of the knee joint.* 2nd ed. London: H K Lewis & Co Ltd, 1933.

Vandendorp, Bastien, Vandecasteele. Résultants eloignées des meniscectomies. *Révue d'ortho-pédie* 1939;26:629.

Walker P S, Erkmann M J. The role of the meniscus in force transmission across the knee. *Clin Orthop Rel Res* 1975;109:184–92.

Watson Jones R. *Fractures and joint injuries.* 3rd ed. Edinburgh: E & S Livingstone, 1946: vol 2.

Wirth C R. Meniscus repairs. *Clin Orthop Rel Res* 1981;157:153–9.

Wroblewski B M. Trauma and the cystic meniscus. Review of 500 cases. *Injury* 1973;4:319–21.

Wynn-Parry C B. Meniscectomy. A review of 1,723 cases. *Ann Phys Med* 1958;IV:201–15.

CHAPTER 6

Acute Ligamentous Injuries

E. L. Trickey

6.1 Introduction

The first serious attempt to understand the problems associated with knee ligament injuries was made by Palmer (1938) in his extensive monograph. He presented the anatomy and physiology of the ligamentous structures and described his experience of operative repair in 58 patients. He rationalized treatment and advised that a high proportion of complete tears could only be satisfactorily dealt with by operation.

Further efforts were made to appreciate the effects of ligamentous injury of the knee in the following two ways.

First, by cadaveric experiments in which individual ligaments, or combinations of ligaments were divided, and then by studying the displacements which resulted after the application of various forces (Abbott *et al.*, 1944; Brantigan and Voshell, 1941; Girgis *et al.*, 1975; Hsieh and Walker, 1976; Markolf *et al.*, 1976; Kennedy *et al.*, 1974; Kennedy and Fowler, 1971). The disadvantage of this method was that it did not reproduce actual joint injuries in which not only may one ligament be torn but where there might also be partial damage to other structures.

Secondly, studies of the consequence of actual injuries have been made which were based on clinical and operative findings (O'Donoghue, 1950; Hughston *et al.*, 1976). The obvious drawback to this approach is the difficulty of assessing the full extent of the injury and relating it to the actual displacements.

Butler *et al.* (1980) attempted to overcome these objections by applying a precise displacement and measuring the restraining force. By cutting a ligament and once more calculating the restraining force it was possible to deduce the contribution made by the ligament since the displacement was controlled. As a result primary and secondary restraints to joint displacement were demonstrated. The clinical relevance is the importance of appreciating that removal of a primary restraint (such as the anterior cruciate ligament) leaves intact the secondary restraining structures which can block clinical tests but do not provide stability as they may stretch under the greater force of activity.

Over the past few decades interest in these studies has been intensified as a result of the increasing number of young people sustaining severe injuries to their knees during sporting activities, particularly in North America (Pritchett, 1982).

Assessment of knee injuries requires not only careful clinical examination but, when complete tears are present which do not easily reveal themselves, surgical exploration may be necessary. Experience and appreciation of the

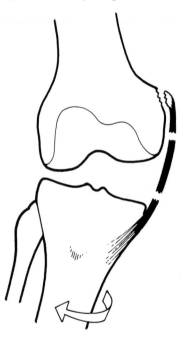

Fig. 6.1 Shows possible sites of tears in the medial collateral ligament and emphasizes the element of external rotation of the tibia which allows the knee to 'open' on the medial side.

Avulsion of a bony fragment or a proximal tear is treated by immobilizing the knee at 40° of flexion in a plaster cast.

Distal tears should be operated on and repaired.

possibilities will help in deciding the need for operation. As O'Donoghue (1950) has pointed out, accurate early diagnosis and appropriate treatment may avoid the need for reconstruction later; the results of such delayed procedures are almost always inferior and often leave the patient with persistent instability.

6.2 Medial ligament

6.2.1 MECHANISM OF INJURY AND ITS CONSEQUENCES

The function of the medial ligament is to control external rotation of the tibia on the femur. It can consequently to be torn by an excess of this rotation, particularly when associated with a valgus strain. Typically, this occurs when a football player rotates away from his foot when it is fixed on the ground and is at the same time struck by another player on the outer side of the knee.

The medial ligament may be torn in any part of its length, most commonly at the femoral or tibial attachments (Fig. 6.1). Tears across the midsubstance occur in the most severe combined injuries and are less common. The superficial part of the ligament extends some 5 cm below the joint line. This distal part on its own provides no stability to the medial side of the joint. If it is found to be avulsed there must be an important tear of the ligament more proximally (usually of the posterior capsular portion).

The abnormal movement which follows a tear of the medial ligament is constant, whatever the level of tear between femoral condyle and the tibial margin, and consists of an excessive degree of external rotation of the tibia on the femur. At the same time the medial tibial condyle will sublux forwards. As the condyle rotates and subluxes in this manner, there is an abnormal opening up of the medial side of the joint (Fig. 6.1). These abnormal movements cannot be produced when the knee is examined in full extension but will be possible with the knee in as little as 10° of flexion. If a valgus strain is then applied in such a manner that external rotation of the tibia is prevented, the joint will hardly open up at all. The joint can open with a valgus strain only because the medial condyle subluxes by rotation.

6.2.2 CLINICAL EXAMINATION

There may be local bruising but this is variable. In the conscious patient the localization of maximal tenderness is a useful indication of the site of damage. This is an important point because it is a guide to the site of operative exposure.

The stability of the medial structures is tested by a valgus force. First this is undertaken in full extension. To determine the position of full extension for one individual the uninjured knee is fully extended. The injured knee is placed in a similar position for this stress examination. With an isolated medial ligament tear there will be no abnormal movement.

The valgus stress is repeated in 10° of flexion and the movement of the medial tibial condyle is carefully observed. When the medial ligament is damaged the medial condyle will rotate forwards and at the same time the medial joint space will open. Any abnormal movement detected must be compared with the results of a similar stress on the uninjured knee.

As with all other soft-tissue injuries of the knee joint, if damage is suspected and examination cannot be carried out because of pain and muscle spasm, adequate sedation is essential and usually this will mean general anaesthesia. Further examination should be made with the joint flexed to the right angle and with the tibia in neutral rotation. An attempt is made to pull the tibia forward. When the medial structures alone are significantly damaged the medial tibial condyle will sublux forward without the lateral condyle. This abnormal rotatory movement can be confirmed by placing both knees in 90° of flexion and exerting maximal external rotation torsion in each tibia. When the medial ligament is torn excessive external rotation is possible.

From this examination it is possible to diagnose a torn medial ligament and to have some idea of the localization of the site and extent of the tear.

Classification of the laxity into degrees by numbers is unscientific. It is better to acknowledge this and state merely that the laxity is mild, moderate or gross. It should be noted that radiographic confirmation and measurement of laxity and abnormal movement is not recommended. The abnormal movement is rotatory and our present radiographic techniques do not measure rotation, unless CT scanning is employed.

6.2.3 TREATMENT

There is some divergence of opinion about the indication for either conservative or surgical management of medial ligament injuries. Nonetheless, it is important to understand that different types of tears need different types of treatment.

When the signs indicate an isolated tear of the ligament at the femoral attachment, it is considered that adequate conservative treatment is as good as surgical repair. This demonstrates the importance of localization of the tear by significant local tenderness.

Surgical repair is indicated in more distal tears which involve the femoromeniscal, tibiomeniscal or posterior capsular portions of the ligament and also when there are signs indicating damage to other ligaments.

It is also important to consider tears at different levels separately, as follows.

(1) *Proximal tears.* The ligament is avulsed from the medial femoral condyle often with a periosteal layer of bone. The normal ligament is tight in

extension and relaxed in flexion. With the knee in the extended position divided ends will separate and approximate in flexion. Therefore, the correct position for immobilization of a torn proximal attachment of the medial ligament is in about 40° of flexion. The avulsed ligament will lie in its bed neatly and join to the bone. It will need protection in a cast for six weeks. Thereafter physiotherapy will be required to obtain return of full knee movements. This may take three to six months, but the knee will be stable.

(2) *Distal tears.* Whether these are of the meniscotibial or capsular portion of the ligament, the tear is not an avulsion from bone but occurs in the ligament close to the bone. It is uncertain that accurate end-to-end positioning and repair will be obtained by flexing the knee. An accurate repair is necessary because these tears can produce a marked instability, particularly when there is a detached meniscus. Surgical repair is recommended with suture to bone if possible.

6.3 Anterior cruciate ligament

The anterior cruciate ligament is large and strong and is commonly injured. Its principle function is to limit the amount of internal rotation of the tibia on the femur when the knee is flexed. The ligament is covered by vascular synovial membrane.

The anterior fibres are tight in forced flexion and the posterior fibres in maximal extension. The whole ligament is tense when the tibia is in forced internal rotation with the knee flexed.

The ligament may be torn in isolation, as discussed below, or in combination with some other ligament, most commonly the medial ligament (see Section 6.4).

6.3.1 MECHANISM OF INJURY

It must be impossible to tear one knee ligament completely without at least some strain to other structures. However, injuries do occur in which the features are of a major injury to the anterior cruciate ligament. This may occur as a result of an excessive force in the direction of movement controlled by the ligament, that is, hyperflexion, hyperextension or forced internal rotation in flexion. A typical example occurs when an athlete falls down from a height, landing on one foot with the tibia internally rotated on the femur while the knee is in slight flexion. The force of landing flexes the knee further and he collapses with the leg under him and actually sits on the foot of the affected leg. The knee joint has thus been hyperflexed in internal rotation. This is a described injury in basketball, netball, trampolining or gymnastics and in soccer to the centre forward in the penalty area.

Hyperextension in sport can occur while on wet ground when the studs get stuck in the ground and the sportsman goes over forwards. A rotational twist can be produced by similar ground conditions. While running and twisting a snap is felt inside the joint. This will stop a man in his tracks but he may not fall immediately. When he attempts to run again he is aware that the knee feels unstable and he then may fall.

The adolescent on a push-bike sustains a similar injury when the bike skids and the child remains on the bike and falls with a flexed knee under the bike. At this age the ligament will avulse its tibial bony attachment.

It is hard to believe that a normal anterior cruciate ligament can be torn by a twist. As with a tendo-Achilles which ruptures, it is reasonable to postulate that there must be a mild degree of degenerative change before the actual rupture.

6.3.2 CLINICAL FEATURES

After rupture the joint will become swollen and painful. The knee may be held in slight flexion and allow very limited movement, but abnormal movement can be detected in the majority of cases. Abnormal anterior gliding of the tibia on the femur can be demonstrated when the knee is examined in about 10° of flexion. Even with a painful swollen knee, the abnormality can be detected because this examination causes so little discomfort. This sign was described by Lachman (Torg *et al.*, 1976) and is the key to the diagnosis. Abnormal anterior gliding when the knee is flexed to the right angle may not be present with the isolated complete tear, and in any case a conscious patient will not allow such an examination to take place. It is not useful for diagnosis. The jerk test of anterolateral instability is not always positive following an acute tear.

Sometimes the joint is emptied of fluid by aspiration to make the knee comfortable. When the anterior cruciate ligament is torn the fluid will look like pure blood because of the tearing of the vascular synovial sheath. The finding of such heavily blood-stained fluid is almost diagnostic of a cruciate ligament tear. When a meniscus is torn the fluid is only tinged with blood. Of course, after evacuation of the fluid the detection of abnormal movement is made easier.

6.3.3 RADIOGRAPHIC SIGNS

A radiograph usually shows no abnormality because the common tear is of the ligament itself. Less commonly in adults, but more commonly in teenagers, the ligament may avulse a fragment of bone from the tibia. The fragment is pulled out from the intercondylar area from under the anterior horns of the menisci and it may be rotated as much as 90°. It is rare to find a bone fragment avulsed from the femoral attachment.

There is one radiographic sign suggestive of an anterior cruciate ligament tear which is not commonly known. A small spicule of bone avulsed from the region of Gerdy's tubercle of the lateral tibial condyle may be visible (Segond, 1879). The fragment is avulsed by fibres of the fascia lata as a result of an internal rotation strain.

6.3.4 TREATMENT

The diagnosis has been made from the history and the detection of a positive Lachman test and the finding of a heavily blood-stained effusion. The other ligaments appear intact.

(a) Avulsion of a bony fragment (Fig. 6.2(a))

The effectiveness of a repair is dependent on the proximity of the lesion to its bony attachment. The best results are in those cases in which bone is avulsed provided that the fragment is replaced correctly. Minor displacements of the tibial bony attachment can be corrected by forced extension of the knee joint under general anaesthesia. The femoral condyle is used to force the tibial fragment back into its bed, but if a radiograph shows that this has not been achieved (and this is quite likely in grossly rotated fractures) operation will be indicated. This can be undertaken using an arthroscope and a hook, or by open arthrotomy through a small incision. In either case, the fragment of bone is slipped back into its bed under the horns of the menisci and usually it will stay in place when the joint is extended. If the fragment is small some

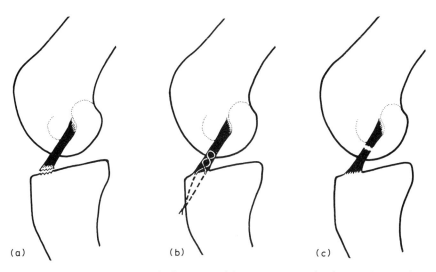

Fig. 6.2 (a) Shows avulsion of a fragment of the anterior spine by the anterior cruciate ligament. (b) Indicates one method of operative repair with a non-absorbable suture tied on the external surface of the tibia. (c) Shows a midsubstance repair in which suture is not successful.

form of internal fixation to bone with a wire or a screw is required. Care must be taken to ensure that the fixation device does not protrude and touch the articular cartilage of the femoral condyle when the knee is extended. After replacement the joint should be immobilized for six weeks.

(b) Tears adjacent to the bony attachment

If bone has not been avulsed a different situation arises. Surgical repair is not possible for midsubstance tears, but partial tears and those immediately adjacent to bone may be reparable. To distinguish the types, an arthroscopic examination with the use of a hook is essential. It may be necessary to probe and look inside the synovial sheath to determine the site and extent of a tear.

If the tear is close to its bony attachment the ligament must be sutured to bone in the normal anatomical position. A figure-of-eight suture of non-absorbable material is taken through the divided ligament and the suture ends are taken through drill holes from the attachment beds in the tibial or femoral condyle and tied on the outer surface of the bone (Fig. 6.2(b)). It must be emphasized that the normal femoral attachment is well posterior on the medial femoral condyle. If a synovial flap is available it should be wrapped round the suture point. After repair the joint should be immobilized in plaster in 20° of flexion for six weeks.

(c) Midsubstance tears (Fig. 6.2(c))

There is considerable debate about the treatment of midsubstance tears. End-to-end suture is not successful. Reconstructive operations are available for late instability and there is a temptation to use these for an irreparable primary lesion. On the other hand, the functional disability of an untreated tear is very variable. Substitution operations involve reconstruction which must be undertaken in ideal circumstances in order to be successful. For these reasons, it is not advisable to undertake a substitution operation as a primary procedure but to reserve it for a later date when it becomes apparent that it is necessary and when it can be undertaken at leisure in the best possible manner.

6.4 Combined injury to medial and anterior cruciate ligaments

6.4.1 MECHANISM OF INJURY

The deforming force is external rotation of the tibia in a flexed knee, with an added valgus strain (Fig. 6.3). First the medial ligament is torn. Because of the circumstances of the injury the deforming force continues and as a result the anterior cruciate ligament becomes angulated over the lateral femoral con-

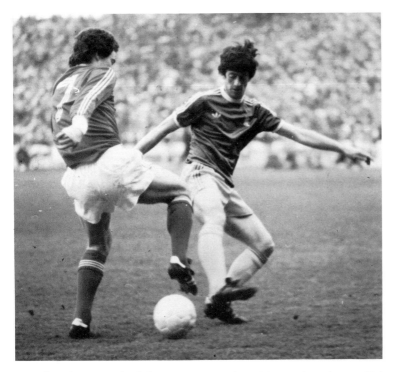

Fig. 6.3 The player on the left is rotating to his right so that there will be a valgus-external rotation force on the flexed knee. This is the mechanism which may produce tears of the anterior cruciate and medial ligaments (as well as the medial meniscus).

The player on the right is likely to fall to his left and since his left foot is fixed, he may damage the lateral structures in his left knee.

dyle and so is stretched to such an extent that it ruptures (Fig. 6.4). The mechanism of tearing is thus quite different from that which causes the isolated tear.

Because of the increase in violence and extent of injury it might be expected that the knee joint would be more distended with fluid, but often the converse is true: due to the increased capsular tearing, knee-joint fluid escapes into the tissues. There may be more bruising, but far less pain because there is less joint tension. The relative comfort can be deceptive in assessing the extent of joint damage.

6.4.2 CLINICAL FEATURES

The physical signs are not difficult to elicit. When the joint is examined in full extension for the stability of the medial structures, it is still stable. But, in a

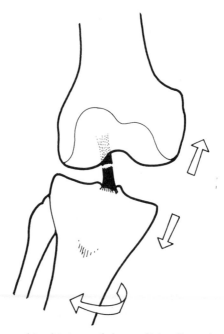

Fig. 6.4 Shows a combined injury of the medial collateral and anterior cruciate ligament. The latter is torn over the edge of the lateral femoral condyle by the external rotation force and valgus strain in a flexed knee.

few degrees of flexion the medial joint space will open more widely than with isolated medial ligament damage. The medial femoral condyle will sublux anteriorly. Lachman test will be strongly positive, and when the joint is flexed to the right angle the tibia can be subluxed forwards without difficulty. This is the classical anterior draw sign.

6.4.3 TREATMENT

Combined lesions should be treated by surgical repair. Arthroscopic examination is not necessary. A long curved anteromedial incision is used through skin and fat and usually because of subcutaneous bruising, it is possible to sweep across the medial side of the joint with a swab until the posteromedial corner of the knee is reached, without the use of a knife. The whole medial side of the knee is easily exposed and the level of capsular and ligamentous damage may be apparent at once, or may be seen when a valgus stress is applied. If the extent of the damage is not clear, the joint should be opened. The exact location and extent of the medial ligament tear is inspected either by reflecting down the capsule attached to the vastus medialis in proximal tears, or for inspection of the lower attachments and posterior capsule by making an incision in the fascia along the upper border of the sartorius tendon and reflecting this fascial layer upwards. It is very important that no incision is made which increases the damage to any intact medial structures. The medial ligament complex is open to full inspection by either of these two methods of exposure.

Before any repair of the medial structures is undertaken, the anterior cruciate ligament is inspected through the arthrotomy incision. The vertical capsular incision can be extended in a proximal direction medial to the patella and rectus femoris tendon so that the patella can be displaced laterally in order to obtain a clearer view of the intercondylar region. As with isolated tears of the anterior cruciate ligament, proximal or distal tears should be repaired, but this is not possible for a midsubstance lesion. A drill director is very useful in order to place correctly the drill holes to take the sutures of the proximal lesion. The sutures in the ligament are passed through the bone but are not tied until after the repair of the medial structures is complete.

The medial meniscus should not be removed if it is possible to preserve it. When the medial tear is distal to the meniscus and through the meniscotibial ligament, retention of the meniscus makes the repair easier and more effective. If the meniscus is detached by injury for a short length, and especially if this is through the vascular periphery, the torn part should be reattached if there is reasonable material to which to attach it. With proximal tears of the medial ligament it should never be necessary to remove the meniscus.

The medial ligament tear is examined now in detail, remembering its exact normal anatomy. A repair must be undertaken starting at the most posterior point and working forwards. Torn structures should be sewn to bone and this may mean drilling holes through the bone for the passage of sutures. It is time consuming, but it is worthwhile.

When the repair is complete the threads of the anterior cruciate ligament repair are tied. Suction drainage is employed. The skin is sutured and the leg immobilized in a padded plaster cast from thigh to ankle for six weeks. The knee should be flexed to about 20°. The plaster should be changed at ten days when the swelling has subsided.

Sometimes it is suggested that repair of the medial structures should be supplemented by a reinforcing procedure, such as a pes anserinus transfer, but this should be reserved for late instability (if such a problem develops).

6.5 Posterior cruciate ligament

This ligament is a structure which is largely hidden from view during many knee operations. The anterior femoral attachment can be identified, but is covered so well by synovial membrane that its presence may not be recognized. When the anterior cruciate ligament has been destroyed by trauma or rheumatoid disease, it is easily identified from the front. The posterior cruciate ligament can be torn in isolation or in a combination with any of the other knee ligaments.

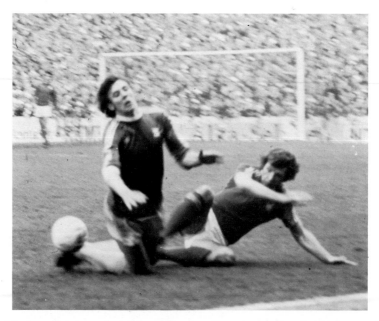

Fig. 6.5 The player on the left has fallen heavily on to his flexed right knee and so could sustain a posterior cruciate injury.

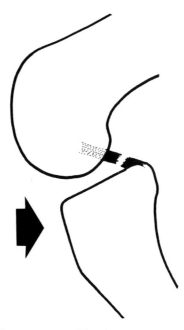

Fig. 6.6 Diagram showing a tear of the posterior cruciate ligament as a result of force applied in a backward direction to the front of the upper part of the tibia.

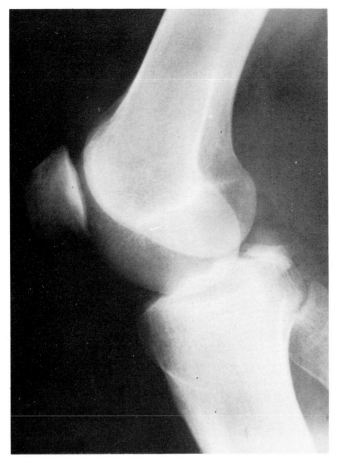

Fig. 6.7 Radiograph showing fragment of bone avulsed by the posterior cruciate ligament.

6.5.1 ISOLATED TEARS – MECHANISM OF INJURY

Accepting the limitations of the word isolated, this is a clinical entity. The tear is caused by a blow or fall on the front of the flexed knee (Fig. 6.5) which results in a posterior displacement of the upper end of the tibia. When this mechanism applies, the injury is to the tibial attachment and the ligament is either pulled off the bone (Fig. 6.6) or a bony fragment is avulsed (Fig. 6.7). It should be remembered that the tibial attachment is just distal to the level of the plateau in the posterior intercondylar area. It is not possible to state the frequency of these two types of injury because the diagnosis is easily missed when a bony fragment is not avulsed. The injury is common in motorcyclists. It can also be produced by the impact of the flexed knee against the dashboard in an automobile accident. The diagnosis should be suspected if the mechanism of injury is known.

Associated injuries may be present because of the force of impact and commonly there is an abrasion or skin laceration on the front of the joint or upper tibia. There may be a fracture of the patella, the tibia, the shaft of the femur or the hip joint may be dislocated posteriorly.

6.5.2 CLINICAL FEATURES

The joint may be tense with a heavily blood-stained effusion because posterior capsular tearing is never gross. However, if there is such a tear the blood escapes into the calf under the deep fascia and then an early symptom is severe calf pain. This may be enough to cause the wrong diagnosis of a calf-vein thrombosis to be made, particularly when no bone fragment has been avulsed.

The physical signs of an isolated tear of the posterior cruciate ligament are straightforward. However, in the presence of a tense effusion in a conscious patient, or when there are associated fractures in the vicinity, it may be difficult to elicit them. Aspiration of the joint effusion and general anaesthesia may be essential.

The knee joint is stable in full extension and remains so until the joint is flexed more than 40°. It is most unstable at 90°. At this point the tibia can be subluxed posteriorly on the femur. The subluxation is directly posterior but sometimes this is associated with a slight rotatory movement due to external rotation of the tibia. It must be emphasized that in an isolated tear of this ligament the rotatory movement is very slight. Each abnormal physical sign is different from that which is seen in tears of the anterior cruciate ligament.

6.5.3 TREATMENT

The posterior cruciate ligament is important and isolated tears should be repaired whenever possible. It is true that the disability from an unrepaired rupture of the ligament is variable but it can be serious and at the time of injury the final prognosis cannot be predicted.

Associated injuries may take precedence and preclude any attempt at an early ligament repair. Skin abrasions on the front of the knee are not a contraindication to repair within six hours as long as they are not too contaminated. However, the necessary treatment for a femoral shaft fracture or a dislocated hip joint can delay the treatment of the less serious knee injury until the optimum time has passed. If a bone fragment has been avulsed this can be repositioned without difficulty up to four weeks after the injury. However, if the ligament has been avulsed from bone, an effective repair is possible only within ten days.

The details of the surgical technique have been described elsewhere

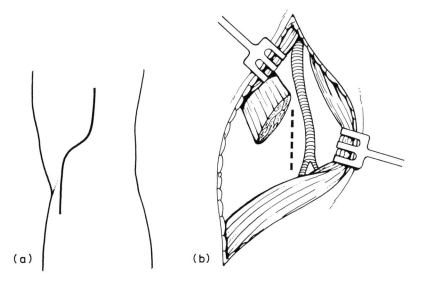

Fig. 6.8 (*a*) Skin incision indicated. (*b*) The medial head of the gastrocnemius has been cut and the lateral head has been retracted. A dotted line indicates the incision through the capsule.

(Trickey, 1968). The approach is shown in Fig. 6.8. A bone fragment is fixed in place with a screw. A detached ligament is reattached to its bed by a suture passing through the tibia to be tied anteriorly. It will be noted during the exposure that there rarely is a significant tear of the posterior capsule. This is not surprising since the injury is sustained with the knee is flexion, at which time the posterior capsule is completely relaxed. The posterior capsule is thus rarely stretched by the force of this type of trauma, but it can be torn by gross hyperextension of the joint.

6.6   Lateral structures of the knee joint

The lateral side of the joint consists of the fascia lata, the lateral ligament, the popliteus and the biceps femoris tendons, and between these structures there are numerous fascial bands. In the posterolateral corner of the knee there is the lateral head of the gastrocnemius and the popliteus muscle. The lateral popliteal nerve lies close to the biceps femoris tendon. Any of these structures may be damaged and an injury to this region can be complex.

6.6.1   MECHANISM OF INJURY

The lateral structures are injured by a varus strain to the joint when the knee is slightly flexed (Fig. 6.9). The pattern of damage to the various structures is dependent on the direction of the strain, so that either the posterolateral or anterolateral corner are predominantly injured. It is usual for the lateral ligament also to be torn when the main injury is to the anterolateral or posterolateral corner. It is only in the most severe injuries that all the structures are involved.

6.6.2 CLINICAL FEATURES

The predominant physical sign of injury to these structures is the opening of the lateral side of the joint when the knee is stressed into varus. The joint will not open with this stress when it is applied in full extension but it will do so when the knee is flexed. The amount of opening will not be gross; understandably, this is a vague term, but the joint will open on the lateral side to a marked degree only if either cruciate ligament is also damaged.

If the injury is mainly to the posterolateral corner (that is to all ligamentous structures except the fascia lata) a varus stress will allow the lateral tibial condyle to drop back slightly and the tibia will externally rotate. This can be observed by picking up the leg by the heel to extend the knee fully; the joint will then hyperextend slightly and the tibia will rotate externally.

The lateral popliteal nerve is vulnerable in injuries in which the lateral structures and either cruciate ligament is damaged, and the extent of injury to the nerve will depend on the degree to which the joint has opened on the lateral side (Fig. 6.10).

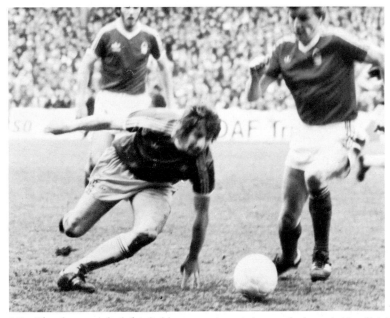

Fig. 6.9 The player on the left is liable to sustain an injury to the lateral side of his left knee.

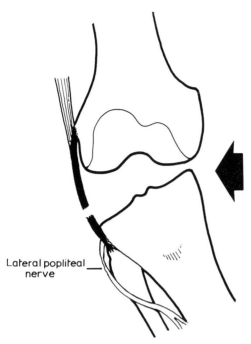

Fig. 6.10 Diagram showing the knee opening on the lateral side as a result of a varus force. The lateral structures are ruptured and the lateral popliteal nerve may be damaged.

6.6.3 TREATMENT

Whenever a serious injury to the lateral structures is suspected, surgical treatment is advised. There are some exceptions to this; for example, when the laxity is mild and particularly when the normal stance for that individual is in slight genu valgum. It seems that such a person can tolerate mild laxity of the lateral structures. If there is any suspicion that the fascia lata or the biceps femoris tendon are avulsed (Fig. 6.11), it is essential to explore, because muscles will cause gross retraction of these structures immediately.

(a) Exposure

The lateral side of the joint is exposed by a long curved anterolateral incision which begins proximal to the patella as a vertical parapatellar incision. Below the joint line it curves posteriorly to reach the fibula 5 cm distal to its proximal end. The subcutaneous plane is swept with a swab through the bruised tissue until the posterolateral corner is reached. In most cases the site of major damage will be clear immediately. In case of severe disruption there is no structure between skin and articular cartilage, because the torn tissues will have retracted.

167

The damage to the posterolateral corner can be a little difficult to sort out because of the normal fascial attachments of one structure to another. Furthermore, one structure may be torn at the femoral level and another from the tibia. A large muscle may present in the wound and this is the popliteus which may have been completely avulsed from the posterior surface of the tibia. If there is a difficulty in identifying the structures, there should be no hesitation in reflecting the fascia lata upwards and this should be done by using an osteotome to remove the tibial insertion with a slither of bone. This structure now can be turned upwards to expose the entire lateral side. The slither of bone is fixed back in position with a staple at the end of the operation.

(b) Repair

All torn structures should be repaired if possible. The joint should be opened by a varus strain so that the lateral meniscus and the cruciate ligaments can be seen. As with operations on the medial side of the joint, the meniscus should be preserved and the cruciate ligaments repaired if possible, and this is undertaken before the lateral repair.

The lateral repair starts posteriorly with a repair of the posterior capsule which should be fixed to bone. A tear of the gastrocnemius is an indication of very severe trauma and an attempt should be made to repair it. When the popliteus muscle has been torn from its tibial origin there is very little that can be done because the muscle will have lost its nerve and blood supply. If the femoral insertion is avulsed, it can be reattached. The biceps femoris muscle may avulse its tendon from the fibula or pull off the styloid process. In either case these structures can be sutured to bone because the tendon is a strong structure and will take sutures easily. Usually, if the styloid process is avulsed, the inferior attachment of the lateral ligament is on the bone. The lateral ligament can be a little difficult to identify in the midst of the torn structures, but time should be taken to do so and to ensure that it is effectively reattached to bone.

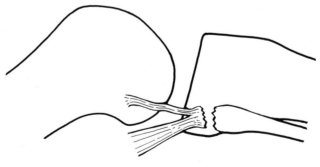

Fig. 6.11 Diagram showing avulsion of a bony fragment from the head of the fibula by the biceps tendon.

(c) The lateral popliteal nerve lesion

Clinical examination will have shown whether or not there is a nerve lesion, but in all cases the lateral popliteal nerve must be inspected. It is remarkable how much macroscopical bruising can be observed in a nerve which is still functioning. A bruised intact nerve should be freed but otherwise left alone. The nerve can be torn apart and commonly this occurs about 12 cm proximal to the joint level. The distal portion will be found lying in a rolled-up ball near the joint. There is no point in attempting repair since there is always extensive intraneural damage. In this case it is recommended that the lateral knee structures are repaired primarily and two weeks later a tendon transplant operation is undertaken because the foot drop will otherwise be permanent. The posterior tibial tendon is detached from its distal insertion, passed anteriorly through the interosseous membrane between tibia and fibula and reinserted to the middle of the dorsum of the foot. The transplant should be protected in plaster cast for six weeks without weight bearing.

6.7   Dislocation of the knee joint

This injury is caused by severe violence and it is not unusual for both knee joints to be injured at the same time. Road accidents are the commonest cause. Because the injury is so violent and because displacement can be gross, there may be serious damage to the skin, injury to the popliteal vessels by avulsion of the artery or intimal damage resulting in thrombosis.

6.7.1   TREATMENT

The primary treatment must be undertaken urgently and the dislocation should be reduced as soon as possible.

(a) The vascular injury

Attention is next given to the circulation of the leg and if this is deficient, as demonstrated by severe pain in the calf and a white pulseless foot, immediate exploration of the popliteal fossa is essential. Assuming that there are no other gross injuries to the leg, arteriography is not necessary and the performance of such an investigation may delay the essential operative treatment. However, if facilities are immediately available and there is no objection to such an examination, it is useful if there is real doubt about the extent of arterial damage. The details of the surgical management of the arterial lesion are a matter for a vascular surgeon, but at the same time the fascial compartments of the leg should be decompressed to prevent the development of a compartmental syndrome.

(b) The ligamentous damage

The management of the damaged ligaments is next considered. It is most usual that some ligamentous structure is undamaged and it is uncommon for all the ligaments to be torn. More often both cruciate ligaments are torn with either medial or lateral structures. The initial radiograph may give a clue to the pattern, otherwise an examination at the time of the reduction will allow an accurate diagnosis to be made.

6.7.2 ARE THE LIGAMENT INJURIES TO BE TREATED CONSERVATIVELY OR BY SURGERY?

The state of the skin or the severity of associated injuries will influence this decision and if operation is contraindicated, the joint should be immobilized in plaster. The final result can be one of reasonable stability.

There are some clear indications for operation:

(1) If the *lateral* structures are injured, repair is advised early because the various structures are usually widely separated by the pull of muscles and a late repair after two weeks can be impossible.

(2) If the *medial* structures have sustained major damage, there are two positive indications for operation: namely, if complete reduction cannot be achieved and there is a depression at the joint line. Both these signs indicate that a flap of the medial capsule with ligament has been turned into the joint.

Finally it should be emphasized that when conditions are ideal as much repair as possible of the damaged ligaments should be undertaken.

References

Abbott L C, Saunders J B D e C M, Bost F C, Anderson C E. Injuries to the ligaments of the knee. *J Bone Joint Surg* 1944;26:503–21.

Brantigan O C, Voshell A F. The mechanics of the ligaments and the menisci of the knee joint. *J Bone Joint Surg* 1941;23:44–66.

Butler D L, Noyes F R, Grood E S. Ligamentous restraints to anterior-posterior drawer in the human knee. *J Bone Joint Surg [Am]* 1980;62–A:259–70.

Girgis F G, Marshall J L, Al-Monagem ARS. The cruciate ligaments of the knee. Anatomical, functional and experimental analysis. *Clin Orthop Rel Res* 1975;106:216–31.

Hsieh H–H, Walker P S. Stabilising mechanism of the loaded and unloaded knee joint. *J Bone Joint Surg [Am]* 1976;58–A:87–93.

Hughston J L, Andrew J R, Cross M J, Moschi A. Classification of knee ligament instabilities. Part I. The medial compartment and cruciate ligaments. Part II. The lateral compartment. *J Bone Joint Surg [Am]* 1976;58–A:159–79.

Kennedy J C, Fowler P J. Medial and anterior instability of the knee. *J Bone Joint Surg [Am]* 1971;53–A:1257–70.

Kennedy J C, Weinberg H, Wilson A. Anatomy and function of the anterior cruciate ligament. *J Bone Joint Surg [Am]* 1974:56–A:223–35.

Markolf K L, Mensch J S, Amstutz H C. Stiffness and laxity of the knee. The contribution of the supporting structures. A quantitative *in vitro* study. *J Bone Joint Surg [Am]* 1976;**58–A**:583–94.

O'Donoghue D H. Surgical treatment of fresh injuries to the major ligaments of the knee. *J Bone Joint Surg [Am]* 1950;**32–A**:721–38.

Palmer I. On injuries to the ligaments of the knee joint. A clinical study. *Acta Chir Scand* 1938;Suppl 53.

Pritchett J W. A statistical study of knee injuries due to football in High School athletes. *J Bone Joint Surg [Am]* 1982;**64–A**:240–2.

Segond P. Recherches clinique et expérimentales sur les epanchements sanguin du genou par entorse. *Prog Méd* 1879;**VII**:297, 319, 340, 379, 400, 419.

Torg J S, Conrad W, Kalen V. Clinical diagnosis of anterior cruciate instability in the athlete. *Am J Sports Med* 1976;**4**:no.2.

Trickey E L. Rupture of the posterior cruciate ligament of the knee. *J Bone Joint Surg [Br]* 1968;**50–B**:334–41.

171

CHAPTER 7

Chronic Ligamentous Injuries

E. L. Trickey

7.1 Introduction

Damage to any of the knee ligaments which results in less than perfect healing will produce some instability and, because ligament damage is never completely isolated, this instability can be complex. It is advisable to dissect and examine specimens of knee joints personally in order to understand the basic problem. The complexities will not be unravelled clearly by clinical experience, operative surgery or reading text books.

Ligaments control passive stability of the joint but active stability is controlled by muscles. In some situations this active control is strong enough to compensate for instability but active stability is controlled by muscles (Noyes *et al.*, 1980). It is essential to appreciate that instability which can be detected on clinical examination does not always produce a disability. Disability is a functional deficit produced by instability. It is dependent on many factors, such as the extent and exact nature of the instability, the presence or absence of a fixed deformity, and the physical demands made on the joint. Obviously a professional sportsman demands more from his knee than a middle-aged sedentary person.

A full history and a knowledgeable clinical examination are essential in order to assess the extent and significance of the disability. Ancillary investigations will follow and this should always include a plain radiograph.

Arthrography and/or arthroscopy may be necessary.

Every aspect of assessment demands the greatest care and accuracy. This point has to be emphasized because the knee is considered by some surgeons to be an easy joint on which to operate. There is no difficulty of access such as in some vertebral injuries or fracture dislocations of the pelvis. It is very easy to assess the knee incorrectly, arrive at the wrong diagnosis and consequently undertake a valueless operation. It should never be forgotten that the commonest cause of an unstable knee in the male is a torn meniscus, and in a young woman a patellofemoral disorder.

The groups of chronic instability to be described are as follows:

(1) Anterolateral instability due to anterior cruciate insufficiency.
(2) Medial laxity due to medial ligament complex damage.
(3) Posterior subluxation due to posterior cruciate ligament damage.
(4) Lateral laxity due to lateral ligament complex damage.
(5) Posterolateral subluxation due to posterolateral corner damage.

It can be stated with complete confidence that the instability from old ligament injury, which causes the largest number of patients to seek advice, is that produced by a damaged anterior cruciate ligament. This may be an isolated injury, but if it is associated with other damage the medial ligament complex is most commonly affected. The medial meniscus may also be torn.

7.2   The natural history of rotatory instability

Much of the credit for drawing attention to rotatory instability belongs to Slocum who described an operation for the control of anteromedial instability (Slocum and Larson, 1968a). Whilst this is common, most surgeons consider that anterolateral laxity causes most disability to the athlete. The starting point of instability is the common injury which occurs with the knee in flexion and abduction and with the tibia externally rotated. This happens when the athlete turns to his left with his weight on the fixed right foot. The long levers of the femur and tibia throw great stress on the medial collateral and anterior cruciate ligaments producing complete or partial tears as a result of the abduction and external rotation of the tibia. O'Donoghue (1955) has drawn attention to the injury and pointed out that the medial meniscus may also be damaged to form an 'unhappy triad'. Should repair of the ligaments, either by conservative or surgical measures be incomplete, there will be a tendency for the joint to be lax on the medial side and for the anterior cruciate ligament to fail in its function of guiding the tibia into external rotation as the joint extends. At this stage anteromedial laxity can be demonstrated by Slocum's (Slocum and Larson, 1968a) test which will allow anterior subluxation of the medial tibial condyle. This is a variant of the anterior drawer sign and assesses the presence or absence of anteromedial instability. The

173

knee is put in 90° of flexion with the hip at 45°. The tibia is maintained in internal rotation by fixing the foot in this position. This has the effect of tightening the posterior cruciate ligament (Fig. 7.1) and compressing the femoral condyle against the tibial plateau. As a result forward movement of the tibia on the femur is prevented. If the tibia is then placed in 15° of external rotation the posterior cruciate ligament is relaxed so that increased forward and outward displacement of the medial tibial condyle occurs, indicating anteromedial instability.

At first the subluxation may be slight, but with recurring stress the abnormal movement becomes more evident. Since the muscles producing internal rotation of the tibia are strong, the athlete may be able to compensate. Slocum's anserine muscle transfer may improve this power and help to overcome this particular instability should the symptoms become troublesome (Slocum and Larson, 1968b).

Many patients will continue in active sport indefinitely with a degree of anterior cruciate instability. Chick and Jackson (1978) followed up a group of competitive athletes who were found to have an absent or non-functional anterior cruciate during a meniscectomy operation. Of these 80% were able to return to full time athletics and were still participating when interviewed an average of 2.6 years later. Six out of their group of 30 patients had developed positive pivot shift, although four of these were still taking part in unrestricted athletic activity. On the other hand, Fetto and Marshall (1980) have shown that almost all patients who suffered anterior cruciate insufficiency tended to deteriorate. Of their patients 92% were significantly worse than they were before their knee was injured. Furthermore, when examined five years after injury 85% of the patients were classified as having only a poor functional result.

There seems every reason to suppose that with continued athletic activity a knee with a damaged anterior cruciate ligament will gradually worsen. Once anteromedial laxity has become established, and the athlete attempts to compensate by internal rotation of the femur on the fixed tibia, there is progressive damage to the menisci, particularly the posterior horn of the medial meniscus. If, therefore, this structure has not been previously removed, because of damage in the initial injury, there is every possibility that sooner or later meniscectomy will be undertaken. Although this operation may relieve the immediate symptoms, it has the effect of increasing the instability of the knee. As a result the screw-home movement becomes progressively deficient and the mechanism of full extension is no longer normal. In turn this puts increasing stress on the structures on the outer side of the joint. As the iliotibial band and lateral capsule become progressively stretched anterolateral laxity becomes established. The end result is that pivot–shift appears so that the patient is increasingly disabled by the knee giving way and some form of operation may become indicated. At first the giving way may only occur under stress, such as in active sport, so that it may

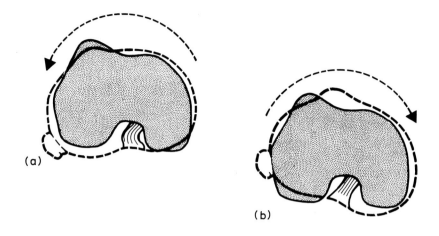

Fig. 7.1 The sectional diagram shows the lower end of the femur (stippled) superimposed on the upper tibia (broken line). In (*a*) the tibia is externally rotated and the posterior cruciate ligament is slack. When the tibia is internally rotated (*b*) the posterior cruciate ligament is made tense so that the tibia can no longer be pulled forward.

therefore be sufficient simply to restrict activity. In some patients the giving way of the joint occurs more frequently and interferes with their employment and daily living so that the need for operation becomes overriding. If the joint is not stabilized then osteoarthritis will supervene (Fetto and Marshall, 1980; Jacobsen, 1977) and since reconstructive procedures are at best inefficient, osteoarthritic changes in the joint will continue, even after reconstruction, though perhaps more slowly and less severely. This reinforces the view that early and adequate repair of the original injury is the best treatment (O'Donoghue, 1955). Attempts to supplement early repair by extra-articular procedures are unwise.

7.3 Anterolateral subluxation of the tibia

When the anterior cruciate ligament is deficient the lateral tibial condyle can be made to rotate anteriorly which implies a rotatory subluxation. The combination of anterior cruciate and medial ligament deficiency will cause an increase in the ease of rotation of the lateral tibial condyle together with the physical signs attributable to the medial ligament damage.

There will be a history of an injury as outlined in the chapter dealing with acute injuries (Chapter 6). The acute injury may have been recognized and treated, but in some instances the diagnosis is not made initially and some torn anterior cruciate ligaments never heal. The cause of the recurring instability may have been wrongly diagnosed for years.

7.3.1 SYMPTOMS

The patient complains that the knee gives way. This may occur only with sporting activities, though in more gross cases it may arise from a minor twist during normal walking. The symptom is produced by movement and the classical description is that the foot is fixed and the body is rotated outwards over it. If considered from the point of view of the tibia, this is an internal rotation of the tibia on the femur.

This rotation occurs with the knee in a few degrees of flexion and results in a forward rotation and subluxation of the lateral tibial condyle. If now the knee flexes a little further the lateral tibial condyle is made to snap back and relocate. The reason for this is the relative shapes of the surfaces of the lateral tibial and femoral condyles. The snap is the essence of the jerk test. It is painful and sudden and so may make a man fall. If such a person is asked to describe what happens he may say 'it is as though the knee comes out of joint and snaps back in', or he may demonstrate the feeling with his hands by rubbing his knuckles one hand over the other. This suggests that the jerk test will be positive and that the anterior cruciate ligament is torn. Commonly the knee swells after such an incident.

The jerk test (Hughston *et al.*, 1976), or its variant the lateral pivot–shift test, is based on the sudden subluxation of the lateral tibial condyle in a knee with anterolateral rotatory instability. The test is most easily carried out by using the technique described by Losee *et al.* (1978). The patient is supine and must be relaxed. The hip and knee are flexed to 45° and the knee slowly extended whilst a valgus stress is applied. To examine the left knee, the examiner supports the foot and ankle with his left hand and holds the leg externally rotated and braced against his abdomen. The right hand is placed with the palm and fingers over the patella and the thumb placed behind the head of the fibula (Fig. 7.2). As the joint is extended the foot and leg drift into internal rotation; at about 20–30° of flexion the lateral tibial condyle subluxes anteriorly and the patient will recognize the sudden movement as the cause of his instability (Fig. 7.3).

The Lachman test is elicited by grasping the leg with one hand above and the other below the knee; and, with the knee in 20° or 30° of flexion, an attempt is made to move the tibia forwards and backwards on the femur. The value of this test is that it is possible to detect partial damage to the anterior cruciate ligament. Since the anteromedial fibres are under maximal tension at 0–30° and again at 90° (Abbot *et al.*, 1944; Girgis *et al.*, 1975), this part of the ligament will prevent anterior movement of the tibia on the femur at both 30° and 90°. Should anteromedial fibres be torn, the posterolateral fibres are under least tension at 40–50° (Kennedy *et al.*, 1974) and do not prevent

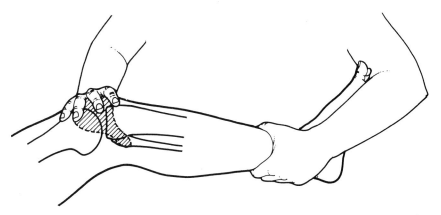

Fig. 7.2 Diagram showing Losee's method of eliciting the pivot–shift test. The surgeon's right palm is placed over the patella with the thumb (cross-hatched) behind the head of the fibula. The left hand exerts a valgus stress on the knee. As the joint is extended the leg drifts into internal rotation; at about 20–30° of flexion the lateral tibial condyle subluxes anteriorly.

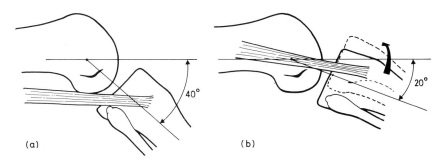

Fig. 7.3 The pivot–shift test. (*a*) Shows the knee at more than 30° of flexion and at this point the iliotibial band stabilizes the lateral tibial condyle. (*b*) As the knee is extended, the iliotibial band passes forward and anterior to the 'centre of rotation' in the femoral condyle so that the lateral tibial condyle can sublux forward with internal rotation.

anteroposterior movement. There is, therefore, significant movement in 30° of flexion, but very little at 90°, so that the anterior drawer sign appears to be negative or at best equivocal (Torg *et al.*, 1976). This has been borne out by cadaveric experiments (Furman *et al.*, 1974).

The symptoms of giving way and locking must be distinguished clearly. Chronic anterior cruciate ligament insufficiency does not cause a knee to lock. Giving way will only occur when weight is borne on the affected leg. A clear history of locking and unlocking, or if the knee gives way while the leg is in the air, or while swimming, indicates that a meniscal lesion is present. Of course, there may be a combination of these disorders.

7.3.2 SIGNS

There is only likely to be an effusion in the knee shortly after the episode. The joint may be scarred from previous operations which may or may not have been helpful. The range of flexion and extension is usually normal.

The clinical diagnosis of anterior cruciate ligament insufficiency causing anterolateral rotatory instability is entirely dependent on two signs: the Lachman sign and the jerk test. If these signs are not present a deficient anterior cruciate ligament cannot be diagnosed as the cause of instability. However, it must be emphasized that in some instances the signs are present and the ligament is deficient, but the disability is due to other causes. The history is all important. When the only complaint is of locking, the disability may be due entirely to a torn meniscus.

Usually it is possible to test for Lachman's sign, however strong the thigh muscles, or apprehensive the patient, but the jerk test examination can be more difficult. This is because it causes discomfort or severe pain. During an examination the Lachman sign can be elicited repeatedly but the jerk test only once because the patient is able to prevent the subluxation occurring by voluntary muscle action.

The stability of the collateral ligaments is next tested and the joint is examined flexed at a right angle. This is not as useful at the previous examinations. An attempt is made to sublux the tibia anteriorly and during this manoeuvre a watch is kept on the knee: is one condyle coming forward or are both being displaced together? The medial condyle is controlled by the medial structures, the lateral by the anterior cruciate ligament.

7.3.3 TREATMENT

There has been a dramatic change in the management of chronic instability from damaged medial and anterior cruciate ligaments. In the 1960s the emphasis was on the importance of the medial structures. MacIntosh (1974) drew attention to the importance of the anterior cruciate ligament insufficiency. As a result, far more operations are undertaken and the success of repair for chronic instability has been advanced considerably. We have come to realize that damaged medial structures produce a gliding instability controlled by good thigh muscles, but the commonest disability is a knee with pivot–shift and this cannot be controlled by strong muscles.

The present approach is to deal with the anterior cruciate insufficiency first and only to consider repair of the medial structures later if it is found to be necessary. It is very rare for the abnormal movement to be so gross that both aspects require attention at the same time.

This approach has a fortunate side to it because it is far easier to achieve a satisfactory repair for anterior cruciate ligament deficiency than it is for medial laxity.

(a) Selection of patients

Operations of this type are major procedures and involve a period in plaster, following by a long period of rehabilitation. The drawbacks of this programme must be weighed against the extent of the disability, the age and physical requirements of the patient, and the financial consequences of the time needed to be taken from work. If the disability occurs only in contact sport in a man of 35 years of age and who is prepared to try other games, operation may not be needed. On the other hand, if the knee frequently gives way when the patient is crossing the road, then a reconstructive procedure will be indicated.

(b) Associated meniscal tears

It is very important to ascertain the state of the menisci prior to any consideration of ligament repair. This may appear to be clear from the history and examination, but either arthrography or arthroscopy are needed. A recurrent abnormal anterior rotatory movement of either the medial or lateral femoral condyle during weight bearing will result eventually in wear of the posterior horn of the respective meniscus and the finding of a posterior horn tear is a measure of the instability. Removal of such a meniscal abnormality alone will not help. However, if the tear is of the displaced bucket-handle type and the complaint is of locking, removal of the torn part without ligament repair can be effective, if the subsequent physical demands are not excessive.

Although meniscectomy may be necessary because of symptoms caused by a tear, removal may accentuate instability since the presence of a normal meniscus makes a positive contribution towards the stability of the joint (Wang and Walker, 1974). As a result the need for a further procedure may become evident.

(c) MacIntosh reconstruction

MacIntosh (MacIntosh and Darby, 1976) drew attention to the symptoms and signs of anterior cruciate insufficiency and devised an operation to correct it. This consists of a tenodesis on the lateral side of the joint which is designed to prevent anterior subluxation of the lateral tibial condyle. A strip of fascia lata is detached proximally (Fig. 7.4) and is threaded under the lateral ligament from a distal position (Fig. 7.5). The strip is then firmly fixed to the lateral femoral condyle and lateral intermuscular septum with the tibia held in external rotation. The knee is immobilized in plaster for six weeks in external rotation. Recovery of movement is quite rapid.

The disadvantage of this operation is that it is not designed to replace the cruciate ligament and that, while it will abolish the jerk test, in most cases it does not abolish the Lachman test. In some patients the tenodesis has un-

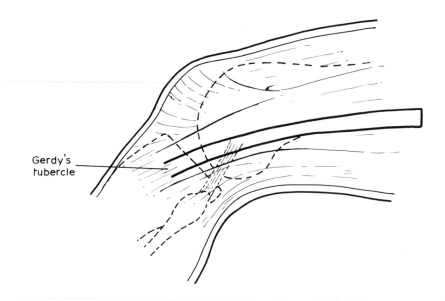

Fig. 7.4 Shows the first step of the MacIntosh reconstruction. A strip of fascia lata outlined and attached distally to Gerdy's tubercle.

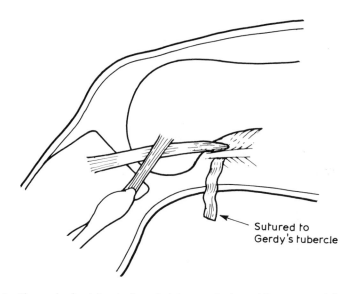

Fig. 7.5 Shows the fascial strip threaded deep to the lateral ligament and through the lateral intermuscular septum. It is seen then sewn back on itself and is firmly attached to the lateral femoral condyle before being finally sutured to the soft tissues in the region of Gerdy's tubercle.

doubtedly stretched in time or ruptured, and it is reasonable to say that this limited operation should only be used for older patients with a relatively slight disability, and when the physical strains are unlikely to be severe.

(d) The modified Jones operation (Fig. 7.6)

It is more logical to consider a direct replacement of the cruciate ligament. A number of procedures have been tried but a modification of the Jones operation (Jones, 1963) is the most satisfactory. In this, part of the patellar tendon is used to replace the deficient ligament. The free proximal part is then taken into the intercondylar area and made to lie in the direction of the normal ligament and is fixed to the intercondylar portion of the lateral femoral condyle. A serious objection to the original procedure is that the normal anterior cruciate ligament is attached far back on the femoral condyle and that despite ingenious methods to prevent it the surgical attachment is often made too far anteriorly. This results in a permanent loss of flexion if the new ligament is under the correct tension. The method to be described overcomes this difficulty.

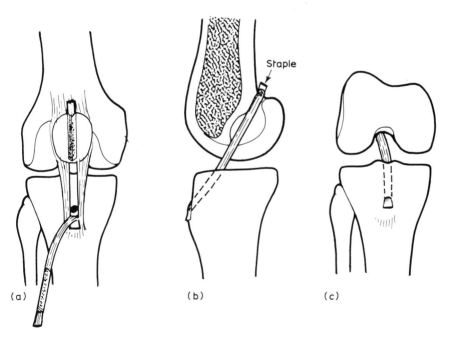

(a)   (b)   (c)

Fig. 7.6 Illustrates the modified Jones procedure. In (a) the strip of patellar ligament, patella and rectus femoris has been separated. In (b) and (c) the strip is shown after it has been passed through a drill hole in the tibia and 'over the top' of the lateral femoral condyle.

(1) A vertical incision is made over the anterior aspect of the knee over the medial third of the patella. It extends from 2.5 cm proximal to the patella to 2.5 cm distal to the tibial tuberosity. The incision is deepened down onto the patella and the patellar tendon sheath which is split longitudinally.

(2) The medial one-third of the patellar tendon is separated and, in line with this, the anterior surface of the patella is detached with an osteotome. The width of the patellar strip is the same as the one-third of the patellar tendon.

(3) A strip of the rectus femoris 1.75 cm long is detached with the patellar tendon strip. At the distal end a wedge-shaped portion of the tibial tubercle is detached with the ligament strip. This provides a free graft of tibial tuberosity, patellar tendon, patellar surface and rectus femoris which measures 13–15 cm in length. There is no biological advantage in leaving the graft attached distally. Length is gained by detaching it.

(4) The graft is laid aside and the inside of the joint is inspected. Removal of the graft has displayed the infrapatellar fat pad which is large and vascular. A generous portion of it is excised, with coagulation of its vessels, to display the intercondylar space. A torn meniscus is partly or wholly removed at this stage. The anterior cruciate remnant is looked for, but it may be absent; in a proportion of cases the distal half is present but adherent to the posterior cruciate ligament. It is not necessary to remove these remnants as they are usually small.

(5) A drill hole is made in the upper tibia, midway between the site of detachment of the tuberosity and the joint line. This advances the distal attachment of the graft. The hole is made large enough for the graft to pass through but not larger than the wedge-shaped distal bone fragment. The fragment is hammered into the hole. It requires no additional fixation because it is wider than the hole.

(6) A second skin incision is made on the lateral side of the lateral femoral condyle from Gerdy's tubercle proximally for about 10 cm. The fascia lata is divided. The lateral head of gastrocnemius is identified and the space posterior to its widened by blunt dissection.

(7) The anterior wound is now used again. A strong pair of forceps with a curved tip, such as Moynihan's cholecystectomy forceps, is passed through the intercondylar space posteriorly and around the posterior aspect of the lateral femoral condyle. The tip of the instrument is felt in the lateral wound and the lateral head of gastrocnemius split to identify the tip of the forceps. The proximal end of the graft is now passed through this hole. The bone of the patellar part of the graft fits over the lateral femoral condyle. The graft is measured for tension by extending the knee fully and is fixed in this portion to the lateral femoral condyle with a staple posteriorly.

(8) The wounds are closed and the leg is immobilized in a long plaster cast with the joint in 20° of flexion. Suction drainage is used for 48 hours and the plaster is retained for six weeks.

(9) After removal of the plaster, physiotherapy is needed to regain movement, redevelop the muscles and to correct any tendency for a flexion contracture of the knee to develop. Contact sport is not allowed for at least six months.

This operation abolishes the instability; the Lachman sign and jerk test can no longer be elicited.

7.4 Chronic medial laxity

The medial ligament is probably the most commonly injured ligament in the knee. In most cases healing takes place and there is very little disability because the abnormal rotatory gliding movement which results is not associated with sudden pain and can be controlled by strong thigh muscles. In late cases the disability may be due to associated cruciate ligament damage (which increases the strain on the medial structures) or because the laxity is associated with a normal standing and walking posture of genu valgum. Body weight accentuates the strain on the medial side so that with every step on the affected foot the joint opens a little on the inner side. Some individuals may consciously walk with the leg in external rotation in order to minimize this strain.

Despite all that has been written, chronic medial joint instability is very difficult to abolish, but a very careful operation may diminish the laxity.

The medial structures are physically wide and the injury may have been to the proximal, middle, distal part of the ligament or to the posteromedial capsule.

7.4.1 TREATMENT

It appears that the only type of direct repair which may help is one in which it is possible to suture the ligament structures tightly onto bone. A direct ligament-to-ligament repair is useless. Reconstruction operations will be considered, therefore, only in general terms. If accurate details of the original injury or of original operation are available, the site of damage is known. Otherwise clinical examination may not contribute very much, except perhaps to detect laxity of the posteromedial capsule. An arthrogram with stress views is helpful. This will demonstrate the site of the laxity in relation to the medial meniscus. The exact details of the proximal and distal repairs have been described elsewhere.

(1) For *proximal* tears, the Nicholas (1973) five-in-one procedure can be used. The basic principle is a proximal and posterior advancement of the femoral attachment of the medial ligament complex, detaching a fragment of bone which can be fixed to bone at the new site. The posterior capsule must also be tightened.

183

(2) For *distal* tears, O'Donoghue's operation (1973) is applicable. The whole tibial attachment of the medial ligament complex is detached with a slither of bone back to the insertion of the semimembranosus tendon. This is advanced distally and anteriorly en bloc and fixed to a new site with a staple. The posterior capsule must again be tightened.

An objection to these operations is that in the descriptions the medial meniscus must be totally removed. This may be necessary because of the meniscal damage. However, it is possible to conserve the meniscus by detaching it peripherally through the vascular margin; then the meniscus can be resutured in place.

At the end of a careful repair, the medial structures should feel tense. The knee is immobilized in a plaster cylinder; it is not necessary to include the foot. If the plaster is removed at six weeks, the tight medial structures are already slightly lax. In order to develop the structure of the medial ligament and prevent it stretching during immobilization, it is a recommended practice now to apply a cast brace at two weeks when the wound is healed, and allow flexion and extension but prevent rotation. This is maintained for six weeks and thereafter a removable knee brace may be used for a further six weeks.

These operations will fail if there is a significant degree of genu valgum. In such a situation, the repair must be combined with a tibial osteotomy to restore normal coronal tibiofemoral alignment.

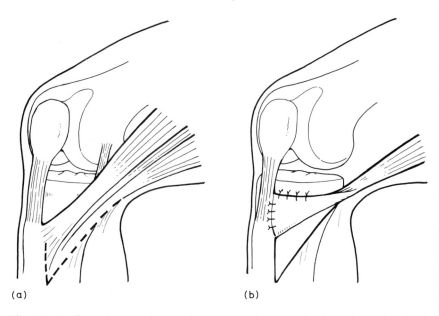

(a) (b)

Fig. 7.7 In Slocum's operation the lower part of the anserine insertion is detached (broken line) in (*a*). It is then freed, turned upwards and sutured to the patellar tendon and the capsule (*b*).

In an attempt to provide active control of the rotatory movement caused by damage to the medial ligament, the operation of pes anserinus transfer was devised (Slocum and Larson, 1968b). This procedure depends on repositioning the insertion of the semitendinosus, gracilis and sartorius, so that their power to internally rotate the tibia is enhanced, but at the same time their power to flex the knee is diminished (Fig. 7.7). Their insertion is transferred to a higher position on the tibia so that their tendons will be directed further from the centre of the tibial plateau. This lengthens the moment arm of the tendons for rotation (Fig. 7.8). It has, however, to be accepted that the operation does not affect the physical signs, but it may improve function and stability. Intensive physiotherapy is given afterwards and this may be more useful than the operation itself.

7.5   Chronic posterior laxity

It is not possible to know how many patients with unrepaired posterior cruciate ligament tears have a subsequent disability. The primary injury is missed very commonly and many cases are sent for consultation late.

7.5.1   SYMPTOMS

There are two main symptoms. First, the abnormal to-and-fro movement is easily noticed when sitting with the knee flexed to the right angle and it is often the first complaint. The second is a feeling of instability occurring characteristically on stairs, steps and ladders. This is easily explained: when the foot is fixed on a step with the knee flexed the tibia is subluxed posteriorly; as weight is taken on this foot, and the knee is gradually

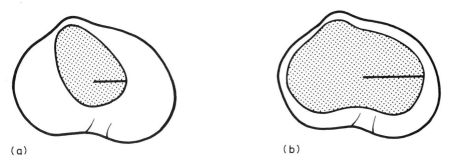

(a)   (b)

Fig. 7.8   Both diagrams show the outline of the upper end of the tibia. In (a) the stippled area represents the outline of the shaft at the level of the normal attachment of the anserine insertion. The short momentum arm of the semitendinosus tendon is indicated. In (b) the stippled area represents the tibial shaft at the level of the new attachment of the semitendinosus and the consequent increase in length of the momentum arm.

straightened, the action of the extensor mechanism is to pull the tibia forward and so the joint feels unstable. Rarely is there a complaint of giving way.

7.5.2 SIGNS

The diagnosis is easy. The posterior subluxation of the tibia is easily seen in the affected knee and it can be corrected to the neutral by pulling the tibia forwards.

7.5.3 TREATMENT

Effective treatment is difficult. Fortunately, the degree of disability in the majority of cases is mild and reassurance is all that is needed. However, there are some cases with a significant disability. Many and various attempts have been made to solve this problem but there is no completely satisfactory operation. One procedure only will be described and it is to reconstruct a new posterior cruciate ligament using two tendons.

(1) A long curved anteromedial incision is used to expose the front of the joint, the tendons of the pes anserinus and the posteromedial aspect of the joint.

(2) The tendons of gracilis and semitendinosus are identified and are divided about 25 cm proximal to their insertion.

(3) Through an incision in the posteromedial capsule behind the medial ligament the normal tibial attachment of the posterior cruciate ligament is identified and a drill hole is made from the front of the tibia to the posterior point and the two tendons are passed through this tunnel.

(4) The tendons are then brought anteriorly in the intercondylar region and passed through a second drill hole in the medial femoral condyle from the site of the normal proximal attachment point of the posterior cruciate ligament. The tendons are then fixed by suture to bone.

(5) If the passive joint instability is gross, it is wise to immobilize the joint by passing a Steinman pin across the joint (for up to four weeks) as well as using a plaster cast for six weeks.

This operation never will produce complete stability but should improve it significantly.

It is known that untreated instability from anterior cruciate ligament insufficiency leads to degenerative joint changes. Such changes are far less common with untreated chronic posterior subluxation. Probably this is because chronic posterior subluxation does not result in damage to the menisci.

7.6 Chronic lateral laxity

Lax lateral structures allow opening of the lateral side of the knee with a varus stress. Apart from the one type of posterolateral laxity, there is no significant rotatory movement.

7.6.1 TREATMENT

This is a difficult problem: when there has been gross disruption in the primary injury the tensor fascia lata and biceps femoris muscles will have retracted the lateral structures widely and these cannot be brought together at a later stage. More usually there is a lesser degree of damage which has been untreated, but this is not much easier to treat.

As with late instability on the medial side all repairs will fail if there is an uncorrected varus posture. This is even more significant on the lateral side because athletes more often have a normal posture of varus than valgus.

Advancement of the proximal or distal attachment of the lateral ligament does not seem to be effective. Sometimes the lateral structures can be reinforced by part of the biceps femoris tendon or a strip from the fascia lata. The most useful treatment is to correct any varus deformity and then the disability is diminished to an acceptable degree.

7.7 Posterolateral subluxation of the tibia

This separate entity must be distinguished from posterior subluxation and from laxity of the lateral structures. It is caused by damage to the posterolateral corner of the knee joint with slight laxity of the posterior cruciate ligament. Such damage as has occurred to the lateral ligament is slight. The major injury is caused by an external rotatory twist to the tibia combined with a posteriorly directed force.

7.7.1 SIGNS

This is suggested by the mechanism of injury. The tibia of a flexed knee can be subluxed posteriorly combined with external rotation of the tibia. The tibia will not sublux posteriorly without this rotation and the main bulk of the lateral structures is not obviously lax. The finer points of this examination can be easily missed by an inexperienced observer.

(a) The posterolateral drawer test (Fig. 7.9)

This is carried out with the knee flexed to 80° and the foot fixed by the examiner as in Slocum's test. Care is taken to obtain muscular relaxation

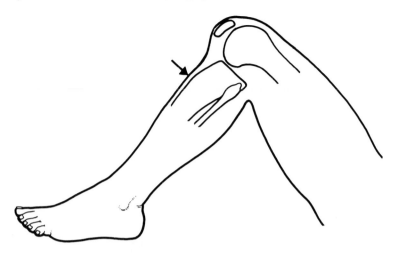

Fig. 7.9 Illustrates the subluxed position of the tibia on the femur in the posterolateral drawer test.

before attempting the test. The tibia is pushed posteriorly in internal, neutral and external rotation. If the test is positive, there will be no movement in internal rotation, since the tibia is fixed by the right posterior cruciate ligament; there is some posterior movement in neutral rotation and this is accentuated by external rotation.

(b) External rotational recurvatum test

Both feet of the patient are lifted from the couch, care being taken to see that the muscles are relaxed. By careful comparison with the normal side, it can be seen that the affected knee goes into hyperextension and the tibia will externally rotate. The rotation can best be observed by noticing the movement of the tibial tuberosity (Hughston and Norwood, 1980).

7.7.2 TREATMENT

The importance of this type of subluxation is that it can be treated by the operation described by Trillat (personal communication). His operative technique is as follows:

(1) A curved anterolateral incision is made which will allow inspection of all the lateral structures.

(2) The tensor fascia lata is detached with a slither of bone from the lateral tibial condyle and turned upwards to expose the lateral structures.

(3) The femoral attachment of the lateral ligament and popliteus tendon is defined and the combined insertion is detached with a block of bone.

(4) The posterolateral capsule is repaired by suture to a roughened area on the back of the tibial condyle.

(5) The detached lateral ligament and popliteus tendon are advanced proximally and anteriorly until tight and fixed in a new bed by a screw, the fascia lata being left in position with a staple.

(6) The leg is immobilized in a plaster cylinder which is changed to a cast brace at two weeks and maintained for six weeks.

It must be emphasized that if there is a complete rupture of the posterior cruciate ligament, this operation alone will not produce much improvement. The diagnosis must, therefore, be accurate.

7.8 Prosthetic repair of ligaments

It is not surprising that surgeons have sought to avoid the complicated reconstruction operations which have been described and believed that it would be simpler to replace a destroyed ligament direct with a synthetic substitute. Such a prosthetic replacement cannot, of course, provide the proprioceptive function of living tissue so that the normal dynamic control of the joint can never be achieved.

Carbon fibre, which was first used to repair old ruptures of the tendo-Achilles (Jenkins *et al.*, 1977), has been reported to give satisfactory results as a substitute material for longstanding damage to the collateral ligaments of the knee (Jenkins, 1978; 1980). The material disintegrates in the body so that it is replaced by fibrous tissue and reorientation of the fibres takes place under stress to reproduce the normal structure of the ligament. The technique of achieving attachment to bone at the correct tension has been improved. Nonetheless it is difficult to see that this material could function effectively for the substitution of a ligament which is in part intra-articular. Although an attempt can be made to cover the implanted fibre with vascular tissue, it is hard to believe that a ligament should be reproduced which would have the subtle spiral arrangement of fibres which is normally present in the anterior cruciate ligament. This means that the new ligament (even if it is strong) can only be a 'second best' since it can never provide the degree of control of the path of movement of the knee which is determined by the anterior cruciate mechanism. It probably has to be accepted that this may also be true of the living substitution used in the modified Jones operation.

Next the problem of the poor biomechanical characteristics must be considered. When a prosthetic material or ligament is lengthened, there is a point beyond which further lengthening will cause plastic deformation, so that the material will not return to its prestressed length. This 'yield point' occurs when the anterior cruciate ligament has exceeded 25% of its original length (Tremblay *et al.*, 1980). During normal flexion–extension this ligament elongates by 14%, so that it will not deform. One of the ligaments (proposed in current medical literature) tested by Tremblay *et al.* had a yield point at 1.5% so that deformation and insufficiency will occur almost immediately. Carbon fibre has a yield point of less than 0.5% and, although the intention is for the fibre to act to produce a normal ligament, this fact may explain some disappointing results when it is used for cruciate replacement.

To overcome this problem of deformation Tremblay *et al.* (1980) have proposed a synthetic ligament made of two materials: a teflon impregnated suture wound around a hollow cylindrical core of silastic 382 medical grade Elastomer, which appears to have the mechanical characteristics of a normal cruciate ligament. There remains the problem of attachment to bone. As yet no results are available.

At the present time the various reconstructive operations which have been described offer better prospects of success than prosthetic replacement of ligaments. However, much research is being done and attitudes may change in the future.

Finally, it is important to repeat that adequate treatment of acute ligamentous tears will achieve better results in most cases than can be obtained by complicated reconstructive procedures at a later date.

References

Abbott L C, Saunders J B d e C M, Bost F C, Anderson C E. Injuries to the ligaments of the knee joint. *J Bone Joint Surg* 1944;26:503–21.

Chick R R, Jackson D W. Tears of the anterior cruciate ligament in young athletes. *J Bone Joint Surg [Am]* 1978;60–A:970–3.

Fetto J F, Marshall J L. The natural history and diagnosis of anterior cruciate insufficiency. *Clin Orthop Rel Res* 1980;147:29–38.

Furman W, Marshall J L, Girgis F G. The anterior cruciate ligament. *J Bone Joint Surg [Am]* 1976;58–A:179–85.

Girgis F G, Marshall J L, Monajem A. The cruciate ligaments of the knee joint: Anatomic, functional and experimental analysis. *Clin Orthop Rel Res* 1975;106:216–31.

Hughston J L, Andrews J R, Cross M J, Moschi A. Classification of knee ligament instabilities Part I. The medial compartment and cruciate ligaments Part II. The lateral compartment. *J Bone Joint Surg [Am]* 1976;58–A:159–79.

Hughston J L, Norwood L A. The posterolateral drawer test and external rotational recurvatum test for posterolateral rotatory instability of the knee. *Clin Orthop Rel Res* 1980;147:82–7.

Jacobsen K. Osteoarthrosis following insufficiency of the cruciate ligaments in man. *Acta Orthop Scand* 1977;48:520.

Jenkins D H R. The repair of cruciate ligaments with flexible carbon fibre. *J Bone Joint Sutg [Br]* 1978;60–B:520–2.

Jenkins D H R. The role of flexible carbon fibre implants as tendon and ligament substitutes in clinical practice. *J Bone Joint Surg [Br]* 1980;62–B:497–9.

Jenkins D H R, Forster I W, McKibbin B, Ralis Z A. Induction of tendon and ligament formation by carbon implants. *J Bone Joint Surg [Br]* 1977;59–B:53–7.

Jones K G. Reconstruction of the anterior cruciate ligament: A technique using the central one third of the patellar ligament. *J Bone Joint Surg [Am]* 1963;45–A:925.

Kennedy J C, Weinberg H W, Wilson A S. The anatomy and function of the anterior cruciate ligament. *J Bone Joint Surg [Am]* 1974;56–A:223–5.

Losee R E, Ennis T R J, Southwick W O. Anterior subluxation of the lateral tibial plateau. *J Bone Joint Surg [Am]* 1978;60–A:1015–30.

MacIntosh D L. *Acute tears of the anterior cruciate ligament over the top repair.* Presented AAOS, Annual meeting, Dallas, Texas, 1974a.

MacIntosh D L, Darby T A. Lateral substitution reconstruction. *J Bone Joint Surg [Br]* 1976;58–B:142.

Nicholas J A. The five-one reconstruction for anteromedial instability of the knee. *J Bone Joint Surg [Am]* 1973;55–A:899–922.

Noyes F R, Grood E S, Butler D L, Malek M. Cruciate laxity tests and functional stability of the knee. Biomechanical concepts. *Clin Orthop Rel Res* 1980;146:84–9.

O'Donoghue D. An analysis of end results of surgical treatment of major injuries to the ligaments of the knee. *J Bone Joint Surg [Am]* 1955;37–A:1–12.

O'Donoghue D. Reconstruction for medial instability of the knee. *J Bone Joint Surg [Am]* 1973;55–A:941–55.

Slocum D B, Larson R L. Rotatory instability of the knee. *J Bone Joint Surg [Am]* 1968a;50–A:211–25.

Slocum D B, Larson R L. Pes anserinus transplantation. *J Bone Joint Surg [Am]* 1968b;50–A:226–42.

Torg J S, Conrad W, Kalen W. Clinical diagnosis of anterior cruciate ligament instability in the athlete. *Am J Sports Med* 1976;4(2):84–93.

Tremblay G R, Laurin C A, Drovin G. The challenge of prosthetic ligament replacement. *Clin Orthop Rel Res* 1980;147:88–92.

Wang C J, Walker P S. Rotatory laxity of the human knee joint. *J Bone Joint Surg [Am]* 1974;56–A:161–70.

Dislocation of the Patella

P. M. Aichroth

Dislocation of the patella occurs in varying circumstances:

(1) It may result from a single *injury*.

(2) The dislocation may be *recurrent* and may follow a relatively slight injury. In these knees there is normally an associated anatomical abnormality which leads to the recurrence. The patella dislocates as the knee flexes and the episodes are likely to occur at increasingly shorter intervals.

(3) Recurrent *subluxation* of the patella occurs when there is partial rather than complete displacement, but is closely related to recurrent dislocation.

(4) *Habitual* dislocation (or subluxation) is present when the displacement occurs at every knee movement.

(5) *Persistent* dislocation implies that the patella is permanently displaced to the lateral side of the knee.

(6) Congenital dislocation is rare but is present at birth.

(7) Subluxation in *extension* is also uncommon, but is an interesting condition which will be considered separately.

8.1 Historical review

Galen (129–200 AD) described dislocation of the patella and indicated a method of bandaging to prevent redislocation. From the Middle Ages to the middle of the last century there were many descriptions of traumatic dislocation but the first series was published by Malgaigne (1836).

Following this, numerous papers were published about the condition and at the beginning of the 20th century many operative methods designed to correct the deformity had been described. Recently the causes of recurrent and habitual dislocation of the patella have been assessed and new methods of treatment continue to be developed.

8.2   Anatomical features

8.2.1   FACTORS AFFECTING THE STABILITY OF THE PATELLA

The displacement is nearly always lateral and this is due to the biomechanical features of the knee joint. The extensor mechanism takes the shortest course between its origin and its insertion and this results in the patella being pulled laterally. The Q-angle is the normal valgus angle which occurs in the extended knee joint between the line of the extensor apparatus in the thigh and the line of the patellar tendon. Many authors have shown that patients with dislocation of the patella often have an increased Q-angle and this may be due to increased genu valgum or where the patellar tendon is attached more laterally than usual.

Medial dislocation is exceedingly uncommon and the author has only seen it in one patient when it occurred as a result of overcorrection of a lateral dislocation.

There are anatomical features which are responsible for active and passive stabilization of the patella. The sulcus between the two femoral condyles contributes to patellar stability (Brattstrom, 1964). The vastus medialis and medial retinaculum balance the tendency of rectus femoris and vastus lateralis to displace the patella laterally.

The patella may dislocate laterally in flexion or in extension and the patient frequently is able to demonstrate the position of the knee in which the dislocation occurs. Dislocation in flexion is most usual because the extensor mechanism takes the shortest course between its origin and insertion and this distance is decreased as the knee flexes. An increased Q-angle is also a factor. The tibia normally rotates internally as soon as the knee is flexed and in the first few degrees of flexion the patella has not completely passed into the sulcus between the two femoral condyles. This is especially so if patella alta is present.

8.2.2   ASSOCIATED ABNORMALITIES IN PATELLAR MALALIGNMENT

Recurrent dislocation and subluxation is usually the result of a minor injury superimposed upon some anatomical abnormality of the knee joint. The initial dislocation may be followed by a deficiency in the medial capsule but it is usually the associated abnormality which allows the recurrence and then possibly habitual dislocation.

In a review of *children's* knees in which a lateral patellar dislocation occurred recurrently or habitually the following associated abnormalities were noted in 35 patients (six with bilateral dislocations – 41 knees assessed):

Congenital lax ligaments	11 patients
Valgus knees	4 patients
Congenital dislocation of the hip	3 patients
Spastic hemiparesis	2 patients
Marfan's syndrome	1 patient
Ehlers–Danlos syndrome	1 patient
Turner's syndrome	1 patient
Peroneal muscular atrophy	1 patient

(a) Soft-tissue abnormalities

Ligamentous laxity
De Palma (1954), Carter and Sweetnam (1958) and Heywood (1961) have described this association. Children with Ehlers–Danlos syndrome with gross ligament laxity frequently have patellar dislocations.

Abnormal attachment to the iliotibial band
Ober (1939), Jeffreys (1963) and Smillie (1974) have observed that the iliotibial band may be abnormally attached to the lateral side of the patella and the lateral patellar expansion pulls the bone towards the lateral side.

Soft-tissue damage following injury
Major damage to the medial patellar retinaculum and the medial side of the patellar tendon may occur in severe traumatic dislocation of the patella. The patellar tendon may be avulsed from the tibial tuberosity and there may also be a fracture through the medial side of the tuberosity. This is likely to be followed by recurrent dislocation if operative repair is not undertaken.

(b) Bony abnormalities

Genu valgum
An increase in the valgus angle will increase the Q-angle (Insall, 1982). Bizou (1966) reported five recurrent dislocations treated by supracondylar osteotomy for correction of genu valgum but this is a rare cause of recurrent dislocation.

Lateral location of the tibial tuberosity
This has been thought an important aetiological factor by Trillat *et al.* (1964). It is difficult to measure and may be associated with external tibial torsion. Brattstrom (1964) could find no statistical significance between the degree of external tibial torsion in his patients with recurrent dislocation of

the patellae and in a control group. Heywood (1961) reported only two examples in his series of 54 cases.

Femoral anteversion
Femoral anteversion occurring in congenital dislocation of the hip does seem to be associated in some children with recurrent dislocation of the patella.

Abnormalities in shape of the intercondylar groove
The lateral femoral condyle is normally more prominent than the medial. When the patella dislocates recurrently the lateral condyle has been said to be underdeveloped and is lower than usual. Brattstrom (1964) used a precise radiological technique for assessing this trochlear abnormality in 131 patients with recurrent dislocation of the patella and compared them with 200 normal controls. He felt that the most important factor in patients with recurrent dislocation of the patella was an abnormality of the trochlea and suggested that the change in the trochlear angle (Fig. 8.1) was due to a decrease in the depth of the sulcus rather than a decrease in the prominence of the lateral femoral condyle.

8.2.3 VARIATIONS IN THE SHAPE OF THE PATELLA

Wiberg (1941) recognized three types of patellar shape:

Type I. Both facets are the same size with both medial and lateral articular facets being concave (10%).

Type II. The medial facet is smaller with the lateral facet concave and the medial slightly convex (65%).

Type III. The medial facet is small and convex (25%). This type may have a greater tendency to recurrent dislocation.

Ficat (1970) stressed the importance of skyline views of the patella in 30°, 60° and 90° flexion and he introduced another classification of patellar shape which was based on the angle which the two patellar facets made with each other (the normal angle being 120–140°).

The groups described were:

(1) A pebble-shaped patella in which the angle was greater than 140°.
(2) Wiberg type III patella in which this angle measures 90–100°.
(3) A hemipatella with one articular facet (alpine-hunter's cap deformity) in which the angle is 90°.
(4) A patella in the form of a half moon with a very acute angle. Ficat considered that this type was most commonly present in persistent dislocation of the patella.

Although absence of the patella has been reported without related musculoskeletal abnormalities, it is most commonly found in the nail–patella syndrome.

195

8.2.4 PATELLA ALTA

There is little doubt that a high patella is an important factor in recurrent patellar dislocation or subluxation. The incidence of patella alta differs from series to series but more than half the patients with a malalignment syndrome have a high patella. There are several ways of assessing patellar height which have their own advantages and disadvantages:

(1) Blumensaat's lines indicate the correct position of the patella when flexed to 30°.

(2) Insall's method of assessment is commonly used but may be inaccurate in the presence of Osgood–Schlatter's or Sinding–Larsen's disease.

(3) Blackburne's method is probably the most reliable and can be easily made on a lateral view of the knee with the joint flexed 30°.

These methods are illustrated in Chapter 3.

8.3 Traumatic dislocation

Most patients describe an injury as the cause of the first dislocation. This may be a direct blow over the patella but more frequently the foot is fixed and the knee rotates in some flexion. Abduction will increase the tendency of the patella to move laterally. Baum and Bensahel (1973) state that 38% of such injuries occur during athletics. The patient experiences a sudden pain, the knee gives way and the patient falls. The effect of patellar dislocation is to produce:

(1) A rupture of the medial capsule and synovium.

(2) A medial tangential osteochondral fracture from the patellar articular facet often occurs.

(3) A lateral femoral condyle osteochondral fracture is less common.

All these features are associated with a haemarthrosis.

8.3.1 TREATMENT

The patient usually presents with a painful swollen joint and a few days rest in a padded bandage is usually required to help decrease the pain and effusion. Quadriceps exercises are then recommended and mobilization may be encouraged by the physiotherapist. The patient rarely presents in the Accident and Emergency Department with the patella dislocated, for spontaneous relocation is usual. If the patient, however, does come in with the patella dislocated, manipulation is necessary. Simple extension of the knee, which is locked in 30–40° flexion, is usually all that is required. Manual reposition of the patella is rarely necessary. If there is a large haemarthrosis it should be aspirated and a plaster cast applied.

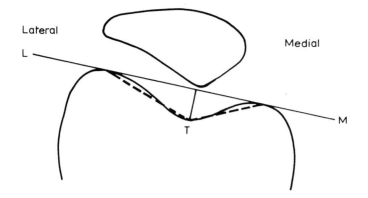

Fig. 8.1 The trochlear angle LTM is normally 141–143°. An angle greater than 143° indicates dysplasia of the trochlear sulcus.

An assessment of the amount of soft-tissue damage must be made. If there is an associated osteochondral fracture or if there is a disturbance of the tibial tuberosity with partial avulsion then the soft-tissue injury is severe. Operative repair of the capsular tear and excision or reposition of an osteochondral fragment may be necessary.

8.4 Recurrent dislocation

Recurrent dislocation of the patella is more common in girls (with a ratio of 2:1; MacNab, 1952) perhaps because of greater ligamentous laxity. A clear family history may be obtained (Bowker and Thompson 1964; Sweetnam *et al.*, 1964) and approximately one-third of cases are bilateral. If the dislocation remains unilateral then the incidence is equal between right and left knees. The most common age of onset of the condition occurs between 15 and 17 years in girls and a year or two later in boys.

Whether the patella dislocates or subluxes recurrently is a question of degree. The subluxing patella rides on the lateral femoral condyle and almost dislocates. The subluxation may be considered minor to major depending upon the degree of lateral movement without full dislocation. All the aetiological factors described above apply.

8.4.1 CLINICAL FEATURES

A few patients may never dislocate or sublux their patella again after a traumatic dislocation but the number is small and Heywood (1961) has indicated a figure of 15%. Most patients, however, have a further dislocation of the patella with much less violence and eventually only minor twists or strains produce the displacement and cause a feeling of insecurity which manifests as 'the knee giving way'. The patient may describe a 'peculiar' feeling or is unable to 'trust his knee' when the patella subluxes. There is a tendency towards a decreased incidence after the age of 26 years (Crosby and Insall, 1976) but some patients have continued patellar dislocations in later life. The decreased incidence with increasing age may be due to decreasing athletic activities.

8.4.2 PHYSICAL SIGNS

In the acute stage the knee is flexed and the femoral condyles appear prominent; the patella may be felt laterally. There may be more tenderness medially and this may lead to an incorrect diagnosis of a torn meniscus. The most important sign is that described by Fairbank (1937) and Apley (1947) and is appropriately called the 'apprehension sign'. An attempt is made to displace the patella laterally, but this is clearly painful and is resisted by the patient whose apprehension is obvious. An abnormality of movement of the patella may also be noted: the knees are flexed while the patient is sitting and as they are then extended *slowly*, the patella jumps medially as full extension is achieved. If an osteochondral fracture has occurred as the result of patellar dislocation a loose body may be palpated in the joint cavity.

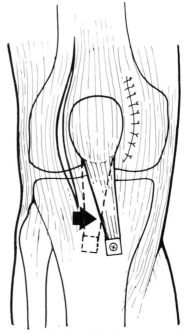

Fig. 8.2 Tuberosity transplant. The bone block incorporating the patellar tendon insertion is transplanted medially and inferiorly in Hauser's (1938) original description.

8.4.3 RADIOLOGICAL FEATURES

Patella alta may be seen as described above. Axial views should be taken in 30°, 60° and 90° of flexion to show the relation of the patella to the femoral sulcus. The shape of the patella and the sulcus can be assessed. A lateral tilt of the patella is seen frequently in patellar subluxation and dislocation.

Osteochondral fractures of the lateral femoral condyle and also tangential osteochondral fractures of the patella may be revealed when the appropriate views are taken.

Although clinical diagnosis of patella subluxation may be easily made, its confirmation requires careful technique by the radiographer. The method requires that the quadriceps is completely relaxed. As the knee is extended from the flexed position it is probable that subluxation does not occur (Laurin et al., 1978). If on the other hand the knee is relaxed in full extension, the patella can drift laterally, and subluxation is evident during the first 20–30° of flexion. Active contraction of the quadriceps or passive stretching which occurs at 40° and beyond will return the patella to the intercondylar groove.

Measurement of the degree of subluxation can be made either by assessment of the congruence angle (Merchant et al., 1974) or more simply by assessing the tilt of the patella as described by Laurin et al. (1979).

8.4.4 TREATMENT

An attempt must be made to realign the patella and also to stabilize the whole extensor apparatus. The stabilization depends upon many factors as described above and if there is substantial dysplasia of the femoral sulcus then centralization of the patella may be difficult.

There have been many procedures described for realignment and stabilization which suggest that there is no *one* adequate for all. Houkom (1942) stated that 'the treatment of recurrent dislocation of the patella has been a fertile field for the growth and development of the surgical ingenuity'. This summarizes the present position after 150 years of surgical effort.

(a) Bony operations

(1) Transfer of the tibial tuberosity. This was described by Hauser (1938) (Fig. 8.2) and modified by Smillie (1946). These procedures will be considered in more detail on p. 201.

(2) Raising of the lateral femoral condyle after osteotomy and insertion of a graft as described by Albee (1919).

(3) Maquet's operation in which the tibial tuberosity is elevated forwards (Maquet, 1976).

(4) A femoral osteotomy. If a valgus deformity is associated with recurrent

dislocation of patella the possibility of realignment by supracondylar osteotomy must be considered.

(5) Patellectomy. The extensor apparatus may still subluxate or dislocate after patellectomy. West and Soto-Hall (1958) added advancement of the vastus medialis to the patella to control this possibility (Fig. 8.3).

(b) Soft-tissue operations

(1) Simple lateral capsular release by open operation. The lateral release must be sufficient in length from the tibial tuberosity to the suprapatellar region. It is best undertaken for simple recurrent patellar subluxation. It is possible to undertake the capsular release using arthroscopic inspection and control but this may make a relatively simple operation more difficult.

(2) Fascioplasty. Campbell's (1921) procedure is the most commonly undertaken (Fig. 8.4). An attempt has been made over the years to graft skin, nylon and other materials to reinforce the medial structures. These procedures however have had dubious success.

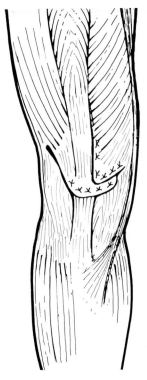

Fig. 8.3 West and Soto-Hall's tendon transposition after patellectomy. The vastus medialis is freed and transferred laterally and distally to partially cover the defect left by excising the patella.

200

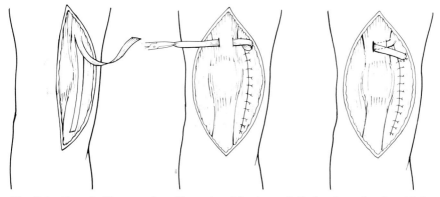

Fig. 8.4 Campbell's operation. The strip of fascia medially has been freed and left attached proximally. It is then pulled laterally through the quadriceps tendon and back on itself to act as a sling which is attached medially.

(3) Patellar ligament procedures. Goldthwaite (1904) and Roux (1888) both described splitting of the patellar tendon with detachment of the lateral half from the tibial tuberosity. This part of the tendon is then rerouted beneath the intact medial part and sutured to the medial capsule.

(4) Tendon and muscle transfers. Gracilis, semitendinosus and sartorius have all been used independently or together to act as a medial tendon transfer to stabilize the patella. Tendon transfers were first described by Galleazzi in 1921. Semitendinosus tendon transfer has gained popularity after Baker *et al.* (1972) described excellent results in 81% of their series of 53 patients. There have been multiple methods of attachment of the medial tendons to the patella: Max Langer (1951) (Fig. 8.5(a)); McCarroll and Schwartzmann (1945) (Fig. 8.5(b) and Lexer (1931) (Fig. 8.5(c)). Baksi (1981) described the transfer of the lower pes anserinus with good results. Medial capsulorraphy with advancement of vastus medialis is an important part of many techniques (Crosby and Insall, 1976).

(c) Transfer of the tibial tuberosity

Although Roux in 1888 first described successful medial transfer of the tuberosity to the medial side in one case, it was not until 1938 that Hauser reported a small series and so popularized the procedure. The tibial tuberosity with the patellar tendon was detached, transferred medially and fixed in position with a screw. Smillie (1974) modified the technique and used an ingenious method of fixation of the tibial fragment in which the bony fragment was locked beneath cortical bone of the tibia (Fig. 8.6). The short-term results have been good but longer follow-up has shown that patellofemoral osteoarthritis frequently follows this procedure (McNab, 1952; Loff and Friedebold, 1969; Crosby and Insall, 1976). There is no doubt that

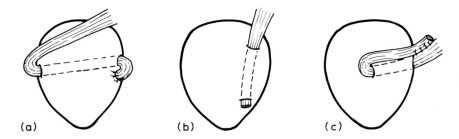

Fig. 8.5 (*a*) The semitendinosus tendon is brought through a transverse patellar tunnel from lateral to medial side (Lang, 1951). (*b*) The semitendinosus tendon is attached by passage through a vertical medial tunnel (McCarroll and Schwartzmann, 1945). (*c*) Lexer's method of attachment of semimembranosus tendon.

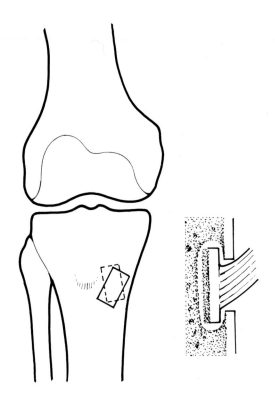

Fig. 8.6 Smillie's modification of Hauser's tibial tuberosity transplant. The rectangle of bone with attached patellar tendon is locked beneath the cortex by rotation.

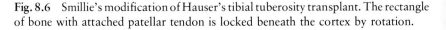

downwards transposition of the tibial tuberosity produces tightness of the patellar tendon and increased patellofemoral pressure causes secondary osteoarthritis. Smillie's modification of Hauser produces a similar effect. The Trillat *et al.* (1964) technique (Fig. 8.7) uses a cancellous screw to fix the tibial tuberosity which is tilted and swung over to the medial side: medialization of the extensor apparatus may, however, sometimes be inadequate with this method.

(d) Tibial tuberosity transfer in the skeletally immature patient

Fielding *et al.* (1960) described a series of 24 skeletally immature patients in whom this operation was performed. Only one case presented with genu recurvatum later due to disturbance of the anterior part of the upper tibial epiphysis. However, this is a well-recognized complication and this type of operation should be avoided in children. The transplanted tibial tuberosity may also migrate downwards and a valgus deformity can occur (Heywood, 1961).

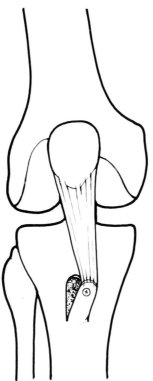

Fig. 8.7 The tibial tuberosity transfer of Trillat leaves an osteoperiosteal flap distally, and the medially displaced tuberosity is fixed with a screw.

(e) Combined lateral release and partial patellar tendon transfer

Any single procedure will not be appropriate for all types of recurrent patellar dislocation and combinations of different methods are frequently necessary. Careful assessment of the cause and type of malalignment will indicate the best operation for any particular patient.

Examination under anaesthesia will allow assessment of the degree of capsular laxity. Arthroscopy is important to exclude associated meniscal tears and it is also helpful to evaluate the state of the patellar and femoral articular surfaces. Osteoarthritis may affect both sides of the joint (particularly the patella). Osteochondral fractures or defect of the patella and/or the lateral femoral condyles may result from recurrent dislocations.

A soft-tissue operation which may be used in recurrent patellar dislocation in the child, adolescent and adult with success is a combination of lateral patellar release together with a Goldthwaite–Roux type of partial patellar tendon transfer. It has also been used in recurrent habitual and persistent dislocations with good effect.

(1) A lazy 'S' incision (with the lateral arm superiorly) is made.
(2) The lateral release must be adequate and should extend from the tibial

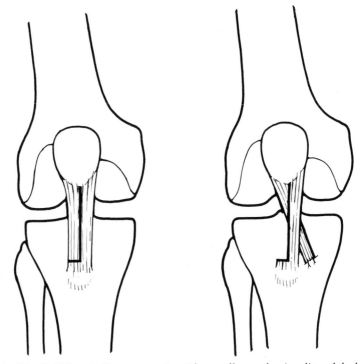

Fig. 8.8 The Goldthwaite Roux operation. The patellar tendon is split and the lateral half is passed under the medial half and sutured under an osteoperiosteal flap.

tuberosity below to the point above the patella where the vastus lateralis muscle merges with the lateral capsule aponeurosis.

(3) Synovial incision and joint exploration; the synovial membrane on the outer side of the joint is often thick and fibrotic (particularly in persistent dislocations and it may need to be divided to allow reposition of the patella). The joint may then be explored if arthroscopy has not been undertaken.

(4) Partial patellar tendon transfer is effected by longitudinal division of the tendon from patella to tibial tuberosity. A little more than one-half of the lateral part of the tendon is detached inferiorly and brought medially beneath, or sometimes over the top of, the intact medial part of the tendon. The site of reattachment of the inferior end of the half patellar tendon is determined by placing it at various points on the tibia medial to the tuberosity and deciding where it produces the best alignment. This should be tested with the knee extended and flexed. The inferior pole of the patella is rotated medially by this manoeuvre and this may be of importance because when the Q-angle is increased, the laterally malaligned patella tends to allow the inferior pole to tilt laterally. The partial patellar tendon transfer therefore may successfully counteract this abnormal tilt. When the correct position has been found, the lateral half of the patellar tendon is inserted under an osteoperiosteal flap. (Fig. 8.8). By adjusting the final tension of the sutures the patellar position may be again confirmed during flexion and extension of the knee joint.

8.5 Habitual dislocation

This occurs with the knee in either flexion or extension. The patella dislocates at every flexion and extension movement of the knee joint. The author has seen an increasing number of patients with habitual dislocation particularly in extension and it seems the more one looks for this condition, the more it is found. McKeever (1954) stated that dislocation in extension did not occur. However, Mayer (1897) and Daunegger (1880) described it as the most usual form. The habitual dislocation in extension has therefore been observed for a very long time. Factors which allow this habitual dislocation to occur are:

(1) Rotation of the knee at full extension produces external rotation of the tibia in a final screw-home mechanism.

(2) Genu recurvatum unloads the patellofemoral joint and allows more patellar laxity.

(3) Patella alta is common in this condition so that the patella lies above the femoral condylar sulcus.

(4) Dysplasias of the femoral condyles and the patella may be present.

The symptoms and radiological features are the same as those described above for recurrent dislocation of the patella.

8.6 Persistent dislocation

The patella remains dislocated through the whole range of knee movement in both flexion and extension.

(1) *Congenital*. This is a rare condition described by Green and Waugh (1968). They pointed out that the diagnosis is usually made rather late. A flexion contracture of the knee is often present at birth and this persists. The patella is not seen radiologically until the age of four to five and the position of the patella is frequently difficult to assess in the earlier years.

(2) *Acquired* (see also Chapter 12). Hněvkovský (1961) described a condition of progressive quadriceps fibrosis in a small series. His cases showed progressive contracture of the quadriceps leading to persistent dislocation of the patella.

Neonatal injections of antibiotics into the lateral thigh region and vastus lateralis muscle in particular may produce contractures of the lateral quadriceps. The injections are usually given for respiratory infections in the neonatal period and progressive contracture of the vastus lateralis ensues (Lloyd Roberts and Thomas, 1964).

Twelve children were reviewed by the author with persistent patellar dislocations and the following causes were suggested:

Nail–patellar syndrome	3 patients
Neonatal injections into the thigh which produced a vastus lateralis contracture	3 patients
Gross congenital ligament laxity	2 patients
Significant trauma	1 patient
Congenital dislocation of patella	1 patient

It was interesting to note that even in the persistently dislocated patella the obvious abnormality of knee shape was regularly recognized very late by the patient's parents and general practitioner. The average age at diagnosis was five years.

8.6.1 TREATMENT

The length of the extensor apparatus may be very short when the patella has been persistently dislocated. The femoral condylar sulcus may also be flat, or even convex, which may make successful repositioning of the patella impossible. Nevertheless, disability from persistent dislocation may be such that if, after full clinical and radiological assessment, repositioning appears possible then realignment should be attempted.

The lateral release must be extensive and all abnormal bands anchoring the patella laterally are divided. It is usually necessary to cut across the fibrotic lower end of vastus lateralis as far as the border of the vastus intermedius. This type of extensive release will usually allow the patella to be centralized. If the knee will still not flex due to shortening of the remaining quadriceps muscle and tendon, then adhesions between the vastus lateralis and vastus intermedius and rectus femoris must be looked for and divided. If full flexion does not occur with the patella centrally placed a Z-lengthening of rectus femoris will be needed. If this is done, the lengthening must be sufficient to allow 90° flexion at the knee. After operation the knee is best immobilized in a cast in 45° flexion. If it is too flexed then an extensor lag will persist. The Goldthwaite–Roux type half patellar tendon transfer is again recommended once the patella is centralized.

A similar operative technique is used in congenital dislocation and the procedure carried out as early as possible.

8.7 Persistent lateral subluxation

Ficat (1970) has suggested that this may be the consequence of the lateral pressure syndrome and the abnormal forces on the patellofemoral joint produce osteoarthritis. He has described three stages of this condition:

Stage 1 – subluxation alone
Stage 2 – subluxation with patellofemoral osteoarthritis
Stage 3 – subluxation with both patellofemoral and tibiofemoral osteo-arthritis.

In stage 1 the symptoms are slight but axial views show a significant sub-luxation. In stage 2 there is an aching pain which is worse on climbing stairs. In stage 3 the osteoarthritis changes have spread to all compartments of the knee.

8.8 Intercondylar dislocation

This occurs when the patella slips on to its side. The condition is rare and the author has only seen it in one child with excessively lax joints and bilateral dislocation of the hips. At the time of dislocation the patella was on its side in the intercondylar notch of the femur in full extension and a radiograph of the knee joint in anteroposterior projection showed the patella in lateral view.

References

Albee F H. *Orthopedic and reconstruction surgery*. Philadelphia: 1919.
Apley A G. The diagnosis of meniscus injuries. *J Bone Joint Surg* 1947;29:78–84.
Baker R H, Carroll N, Dewar P, Hall J E. Semitendinosus tenodesis for recurrent dislocation of the patella. *J Bone Joint Surg* [Br] 1972;54–B:103–9.
Baksi D P. Restoration of dynamic stability of the patella by pes anserinus transposition. *J Bone Joint Surg* [Br] 1981;63–B:399–403.
Baum C, Bensahel H. Luxation recidivante de la rotule chez l'enfant. *Rev Chir Orthop* 1973; 59:583–92.

Bizou H. Contribution a l'etude des desequilibres de l'appareil extenseur du genou dans le plan frontal. Thesis (Toulouse) 1966.

Blackburne J S, Peel T E. A new method of measuring patellar height. *J Bone Joint Surg [Br]* 1977;59–B:241–2.

Bowker J H, Thompson E B. Surgical treatment of recurrent dislocation of the patella. *J Bone Joint Surg [Am]* 1964;46–A:1451–61.

Brattstrom H. Shape of the intercondylar groove normally and in recurrent dislocation of the patella. *Acta Orthop Scand Suppl* 1964;68:134–48.

Campbell W C. Arthroplasty of the knee. Report of cases. *Am J Orthop Surg* 1921;14:430.

Carter C, Sweetnam R. Familial joint laxity and recurrent dislocation of the patella. *J Bone Joint Surg [Br]* 1958;40–B:664–7.

Crosby E B, Insall J. Recurrent dislocation of the patella. *J Bone Joint Surg [Am]* 1976;58–A:9–13.

Daunegger C. *Versuche und Stucken uber die Luxation des patellae.* Zurich; Diss, 1880.

De Palma A F. *Diseases of the knee.* Philadelphia; J B Lippincott, 1954.

Fairbank H A T. Internal derangement of the knee in children. *Proc R Soc Med* 1937;3:11.

Ficat P. Pathologie fémoro-patellaire. Paris: Masson et Cie, 1970.

Fielding J W, Liebler W A, Tambakis A. The effect of a tibial tubercle transplant in children on the growth of the upper tibial epiphysis. *J Bone Joint Surg [Am]* 1960;42–A:1426–34.

Galleazzi R. Nuove applicazion del trapianto muscolare e tendineo. (XII Congress Societa Italiana di Ortopedia). *Arch Ortop* 1922;38.

Goldthwaite J E. Slipping or recurrent dislocation of the patella with the report of eleven cases. *Boston Med Surg J* 1904;150:169–74.

Green J P, Waugh W. Congenital lateral dislocation of the patella. *J Bone Joint Surg [Br]* 1968;50–B:285–9.

Hauser E D W. Total tendon transplant for slipping patella. *Surg Gynaecol Obstet* 1938; 66:199–213.

Heywood A W B. Recurrent dislocation of the patella. *J Bone Joint Surg [Br]* 1961;43–B: 508–17.

Hněvkovský O. Progressive fibrosis of the vastus intermedius in children. *J Bone Joint Surg [Br]* 1961;43–B:318–25.

Houkom S S. Recurrent dislocation of the patella. *Arch Surg (Chicago)* 1942;44:1026.

Insall J. Patellar pain, current concepts review. *J Bone Joint Surg [Am]* 1982;64–A:147–51.

Jeffreys T E. Recurrent dislocation of the patella due to abnormal attachment of the ilio-tibial tract. *J Bone Joint Surg [Br]* 1963;45–B:740–3.

Lange M. Orthopadisch chirurgische. *Operations lehve Munchen* J B Bergmann, 1951.

Laurin C A, Dussault R, Levesque H P. The tangential investigation of the patellofemoral joint. *Clin Orth* 1979;144:16–26.

Laurin C A, Levesque H P, Dussault R, Labelle H, Peides P. The abnormal lateral patellofemoral angle. *J Bone Joint Surg [Am]* 1978;60–A:55–60.

Lexer E. *Weiderherstellung schirurgie*, 2 Aufl Bd II S 822 Leipzig: Ambrosias Barth, 1931.

Lloyd Roberts G C, Thomas T G. The etiology of quadriceps contracture in children. *J Bone Joint Surg [Br]* 1964;46–B:498–502.

Loff P, Friedebold G. Die habituelle patellar luxation als pararthrotische deformit. *Ergeb Chir* 1969;52:60.

McCarroll U R, Schwartzmann J R. Lateral dislocation of the patella. *J Bone Joint Surg* 1945;27:446.

MacNab I. Recurrent dislocation of the patella. *J Bone Joint Surg [Am]* 1952;34–A:957–67.

Malgaigne J F.Memoire sur les determinations des diverses especes de lux de la rotule, leurs signes et leur traitment. *Garz Med* 1836;433–8,465–71,565–9,673–8.

Maquet P G T. Biomechanics and osteoarthritis of the knee. *SICOT XI'e Congres.* Mexico 317, 1969.

Maquet P G T. Advancement of the tibial tuberosity. *Clin Orth* 1976;115:225.

Mayer H N. Congenital absence or delayed development of the patella. *Lancet* 1897;ii:1384–5.

McKeever D C. Recurrent dislocation of the patella. *Clin Orthop Rel Res* 1954;3:55–60.

Merchant A C, Mercer R L, Jacobsen R H, Cool C R. Roentgenographic analysis of patello-femoral congruence. *J Bone Joint Surg [Am]* 1974;56:1391–6.

Ober F R. Recurrent dislocation of the patella. *Am J Surg* 1939;43:497.

Roux. Luxation habituelle de la rotule. Traitement operatoire. *Rev Chir Paris* 1888;8:682–9.

Smillie I S. *Injuries of the knee joint.* Edinburgh: E & S Livingstone, 1946.

Smillie I S. *Diseases of the knee joint.* Edinburgh and London: Churchill Livingstone, 1974.

Trillat A, Dejour M, Coutette A. Diagnostic et traitement des subluxations recidivantes de lad rotule. *Rev Chir Orthop* 1964;50:13–24.

West F E, Soto-Hall R. Recurrent dislocation of the patella in the adult. *J Bone Joint Surg [Am]* 1958;40–A:386–94.

Wiberg G. Roentgenographic and anatomic studies on the femoro-patellar joint. *Acta Orthop Scand* 1941;12:319–410.

CHAPTER 9

Chondromalacia Patellae

John Goodfellow

9.1 Introduction

Because the name of a pathological process has been placed upon a syndrome we are in an impossible position. We do not know to which it applies, the pathology or the syndrome, and so unthinkingly and inevitably we are convinced, *without a shred of evidence*, that the one causes the other.

Richard Asher in *Making Sense*
Pitman Medical, London, 1972

The difficulty in writing a chapter about 'chondromalacia patellae' is to disentangle the several meanings which that title includes. Literally it means softening of the cartilage on the back of the knee cap, but by right of common usage it may be employed to describe fibrillation, ulceration and almost any other defect found on the patella's articular surface. In the outpatient clinic the phrase has become synonymous with the clinical syndrome of pain in the front of the knee in young people, a usage which must hinder not help in the search for a solution to that enigma.

In the following pages an attempt will be made to discuss chondromalacia patellae in both its meanings. Firstly, by assembling and interpreting what is known of the pathology of the patella's articular cartilage and, secondly, by reviewing the clinical syndrome of 'anterior knee pain', the theories of its causation and the attempts which have been made to cure it.

Inevitably the evidence will be given the author's bias, which is towards the belief that the articular cartilage of the patella, though very frequently the site of pathological changes, is seldom the cause of anterior knee pain in adolescence.

9.2 Pathology of articular cartilage

9.2.1 SURFACE DEGENERATIVE CHANGES

The diagrams in Fig. 9.1 demonstrate, in simplified form, the stages of deterioration of articular cartilage exemplified by the microscopical sections in Fig. 9.2(a) and (b). They represent progressive destruction of the cartilage from its surface, through its deeper layers, until the subchondral bone is eventually exposed. Such changes are frequently found in all the joints of the adult human body and they become more frequent, and involve increasingly large areas of cartilage, as the subject's age increases. Harrison *et al.* (1953) described the prevalence of fibrillation around the margins of the cartilage of the femoral head, the central areas being spared. Bennett *et al.* (1942) reported the pattern of cartilage degeneration in the knee joint, and several other joints have been shown to exhibit a distinctive geographical distribution of lesions over the surfaces of their facets.

It is, therefore, no surprise to learn that the patella commonly displays degenerative changes; that they become more common and more extensive with increasing age, and that such changes occur in a distinctive pattern. Figure 9.3 shows the 'normal' distribution of early surface degenerative changes. There is peeling and flaking of the tangential layers all round the periphery and over most of the surface of the medial longitudinal or 'odd' facet.

The prevalence and extent of these changes has been established, at least for the population of Liverpool, by the post-mortem studies of Meachim and Emery (1974). Minor changes, like those in Fig. 9.3, were found in most young adult joints and they became more severe with age. However, there were limits to their progression, both in extent and in severity. Frank ulceration, with exposure of the subchondral bone, was rarely seen in lesions at the periphery. Furthermore, the lesions did not encroach, even in older subjects, on to the more central areas. These observations concur with those made upon the peripheral cartilage lesions of the human hip which are also 'benign' in their prognosis, not necessarily presaging the onset of serious degeneration of that joint (Bullough *et al.*, 1973).

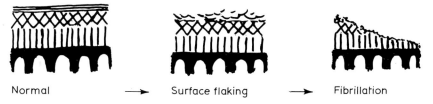

Normal   ⟶   Surface flaking   ⟶   Fibrillation

Fig. 9.1 Diagrammatic representation of the stages of surface degeneration of articular cartilage.

Meachim *et al.* (1954) also recorded the occasional presence of other lesions which lay not at the periphery nor upon the odd facet but centrally upon the medial and lateral facets. These lesions frequently exposed the subchondral bone and were present mainly in old subjects.

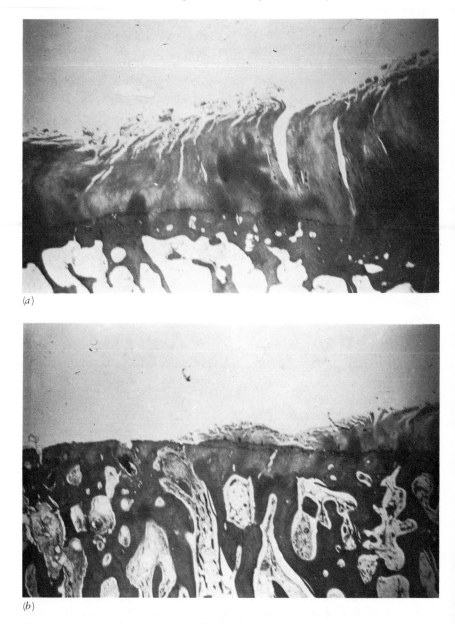

(a)

(b)

Fig. 9.2   (a) and (b) Examples of fibrillation and ulceration.

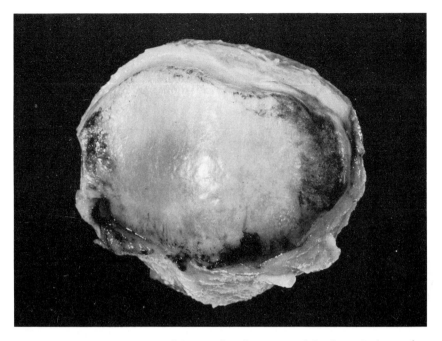

Fig. 9.3 Necropsy specimen of the patella of a young adult, the articular surface painted with indian ink to reveal areas of fibrillation. The cartilage on the 'odd facet' is extensively involved.

Some further evidence of the 'normal' state of the patella's cartilage comes from observations made in the operating theatre. Outerbridge (1961) observed the state of the patella at meniscectomy in 101 patients and recorded 'surface fissuring and fibrillation', predominantly upon the medial facet, in 4 of 12 subjects aged 12–19 years, in 11 of 17 subjects aged 20–29 years and, with increasing frequency at each decade, in 12 of 15 subjects aged 50–69 years.

9.2.2 AETIOLOGY OF SURFACE DEGENERATION

Harrison *et al.* (1953) suggested that fibrillation of the cartilage at the periphery of the human hip joint was caused not by abrasive wear, but by chronic disuse. A similar mechanical explanation has been offered for the patella's peripheral lesions and those upon its odd facet. By contrast, those lesions which occur in central parts of its facets, in areas which are presumably subject to constant and heavy use, may result from excess pressure.

The site and size of the patella's contact area, in various positions of the joint, are therefore of importance if we are to understand the significance of its cartilage lesions.

213

Figures 9.4–9.7 show the changing pattern of contact which the patella makes as the knee bends from 10° of flexion to 135° of flexion. The contact areas are demonstrated by dye exclusion methods on a cadaver joint, mounted in a rig which reproduced the static mechanics of the weight-bearing limb (Goodfellow *et al.*, 1976).

The pictures show how the band of contact moves, from the distal pole of the patella to its proximal pole, as flexion increases from 0° to 90°. At the same time, the band of contact on the trochlear facets of the femur moves distally. During this flexion movement the area of patellofemoral contact progressively enlarges, a feature of the joint's design which tends to maintain

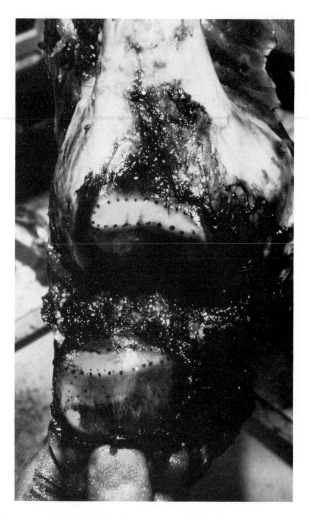

Fig. 9.4 Contact areas at 20° flexion.

the average pressure constant, despite the increase in load which it sustains in flexed postures.

In the range from 0° to 90° of flexion, every part of the medial and lateral facets of the patella and every part of the trochlear facets of the femur is, at some time, employed. The odd facet at no time makes contact with the femur in this range.

The pattern of contact beyond 90° of flexion is quite different. As the patella slides off the trochlear facet, and on to the femoral condyles, its medial facet loses contact with the femur and comes to lie against the retropatellar fat pad in the intercondylar notch. The odd facet, alone, now supports the

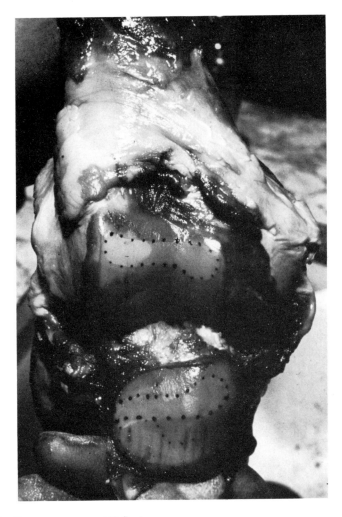

Fig. 9.5   Contact areas at 45° flexion.

215

medial margin of the patella articulating with a small area on the lateral margin of the medial femoral condyle (Figs 9.7 and 9.8).

The photographs in Figs 9.6 and 9.7 show that, beyond 90° of flexion, an extensive contact area develops between the back of the quadriceps tendon and the trochlear facets of the femur, which have been vacated by the patella's translation off them and on to the femoral condyles. Load can now be transmitted across this tendofemoral joint, as well as across the rather diminished contact areas of the patellofemoral joint proper.

The contact studies seem, then, to lend support to the theory that lesions around the periphery and upon the odd facet of the patella may be due to

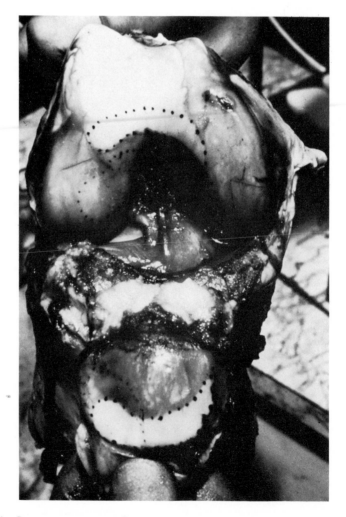

Fig. 9.6 Contact areas at 90° flexion.

habitual disuse. The odd facet must be employed rather little in the knee joints of the urban man who rarely squats or kneels. If such changes arise mainly from disuse it is not difficult to understand why they seldom progress to severe destruction of the cartilage, for their situation protects them from the effects of wear and high-pressure loading.

The gradual increase in the size of the patellofemoral contact areas, as flexion increases from 0° to 90°, matches the gradual increase in the patello-femoral force and tends to maintain the pressure at the joint constant (pressure = force/contact area). Figures 9.9 and 9.10 demonstrate this correlation graphically. Beyond 90° of flexion the diminution in the area of

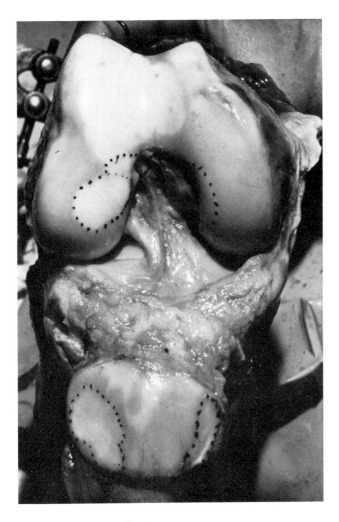

Fig. 9.7   Contact areas at 135° flexion.

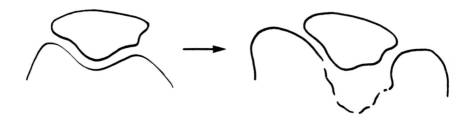

Fig. 9.8 Diagrammatic skyline views of the patella. From full extension to 90° flexion the patella facets of the femur articulate with the medial and lateral facets of the patella. Beyond 90° the patella rotates and the medial femoral condyle articulates with the odd facet.

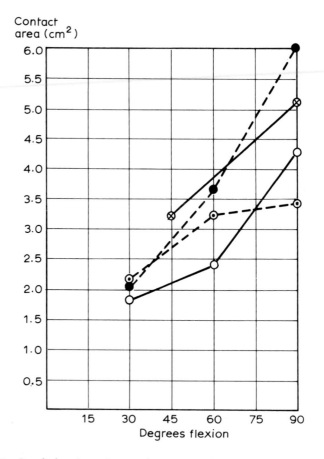

Fig. 9.9 Graph showing unit area of contact in relation to increasing knee flexion for four individual specimens, (with permission from Ficat and Hungerford, 1977).

patellofemoral contact is more than matched by the large tendofemoral contact area.

Unfortunately, these observations only allow the calculation of average pressures. If the pressure is not uniform throughout the contact area some units of cartilage may experience loads much greater than others. Little is known of the range of pressures experienced within the contact areas in this or any other human joint and it is for this reason that we must be cautious in attributing cartilage lesions to overuse or to 'increased pressure'. Figure 9.11 shows that, because of the natural inclination of the patellar tendon, laterally from the line of action of the quadriceps muscle, there is always a force which tends to displace the patella laterally (see Chapter 8, p. 192). However, this

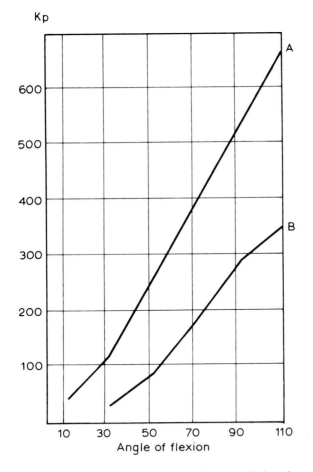

Fig. 9.10 Graph to show the total compressive load applied to the patellofemoral joint with changing knee flexion. A, using the entire length of the femur in the calculation. B, taking into account associated hip flexion.

219

need not imply that the cartilage of the lateral facet of the patella experiences a higher pressure than does the cartilage of its medial facet. The contact studies show that the area of cartilage available for the transmission of the load is greater laterally than medially and the pressures may therefore be similar on both facets.

9.2.3 BASAL DEGENERATION

Surface degeneration, of the kind referred to in previous paragraphs, is not the only disorder encountered on the patella. A number of other changes, confusing in their variety and situation, have been observed. Figure 9.12 shows the most extraordinary of many bizarre kneecaps which the author has encountered!

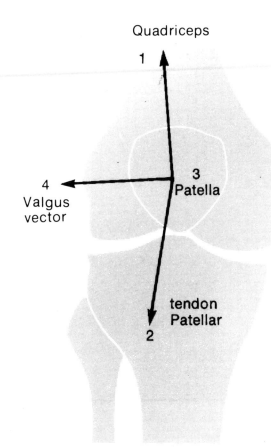

Fig. 9.11 The 'Q' angle imposes a valgus force on the patella near full extension, (with permission from Ficat and Hungerford, 1977).

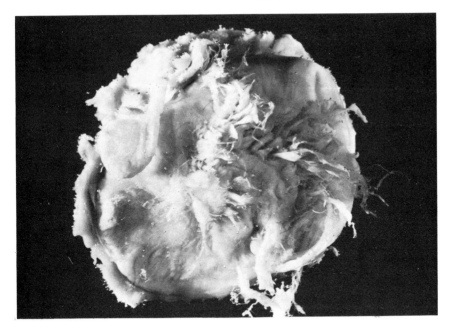

Fig. 9.12 Bizarre cartilage lesion on patella.

An attempt has been made, in Fig. 9.13, to identify a sequence of changes, quite distinct from those of surface degeneration, which would explain some of these appearances. Certainly, lesions having these characteristics have been demonstrated but whether they progress from one to another in the manner suggested by these diagrams, is conjectural.

The articular cartilage of the normal patella is so thick, particularly on its median ridge, that pressure upon it with a blunt seeker will usually produce a dent, analogous to the pitting of other oedematous soft tissues. In some adolescent patellae areas of articular cartilage exhibit this sign to an exaggerated degree, having an appreciably 'spongy' consistency. If an area of cartilage so affected is separated from its surroundings by a circumferential incision the isolated disc of material can be prized off the underlying bone with a rougine. Figure 9.14 shows a disc of cartilage taken in this way. The articular surface of the specimen was shiny and smooth, but the vertical fissuring, seen on the deep surface, suggests lack of cohesion between the coarse bundles, or fasciculi, of the collagen of the deeper layers.

Figure 9.15 exemplifies a similar disorder of the cartilage, yet more advanced. The deep layers beneath the 'blister' have lost all the features of normal cartilage and consist of disorganized fibrous tissues, held together by a thin surface layer of intact collagen.

In such advanced lesions the surface layer of the cartilage may rupture, allowing the degenerate material of the deeper layers to sprout into the joint.

The location of these lesions on the patella is less variable than their morphology. They lie, for the most part, astride either the median ridge or the ridge between the medial and the odd facets.

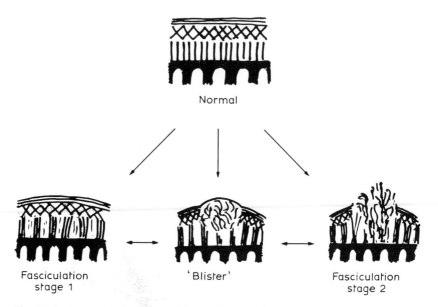

Fig. 9.13 Stages in the lesion of basal degeneration.

All the lesions demonstrated in the foregoing figures were found in the knee joints of adolescents or young adults who were operated upon because they complained of persistent patellofemoral pain. A similar predilection for the medial facet was reported by Wiles *et al.* (1956) and by Outerbridge (1961). However, in contradiction of these authors, Insall *et al.* (1976) reported that the majority of the cartilage lesions, in patients complaining of patellofemoral pain, lay in the central part of the lateral facet.

9.2.4 CHONDRAL FRACTURES

Direct injury to the cartilage may occur when the patella is struck from in front, for instance against the dashboard of a motor car. The full thickness of cartilage may be dislodged, as occurred in the case shown in Fig. 9.16.

Cartilage damage can complicate traumatic dislocation and is common after recurrent patellofemoral dislocation.

9.2.5 OSTEOARTHRITIS

There is, as yet, no distinctive morphological, histological or biochemical feature which can distinguish those cartilage lesions which will proceed, eventually, to osteoarthritis from those, referred to earlier in this chapter, which have a benign prognosis. The generally accepted criteria for the radiological diagnosis of osteoarthritis, joint-line narrowing, osteophyte formation and subchondral sclerosis, all indicate that the joint surface

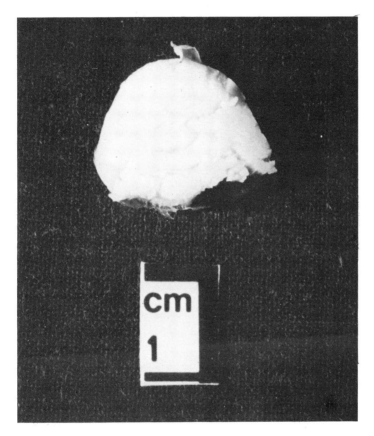

Fig. 9.14 Deep surface of fasciculated cartilage.

involved *has failed* to maintain itself in equilibrium. A critical point of failure has, by then, already been passed, often a long time ago. The prediction, whether a particular joint surface *will fail* depends not so much upon the quality of a cartilage lesion as upon its site and extent. Several authors have suggested that centrally placed cartilage lesions, in which the bone may be exposed, are the first steps towards true osteoarthritis (Byers *et al.*, 1970).

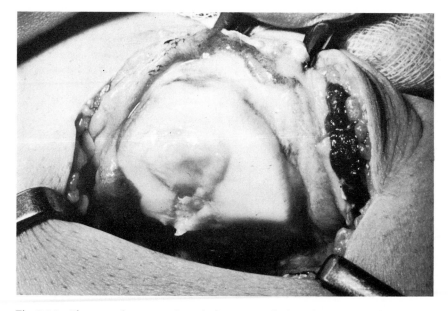

Fig. 9.15 Photograph at operation of a lesion astride the ridge between the odd and medial facets. It is confluent with a second area astride the median ridge. Histologically the lesion consisted of poorly organized fibrous tissue.

In its established form the lesions of osteoarthritis dominate on the patella's lateral facet and are matched by similar lesions on the lateral trochlear facet of the femur. Failure of the lateral facet allows the patella to displace laterally, because of the alignment of the quadriceps mechanism which has already been mentioned.

9.2.6 CONCLUSIONS

The articular surfaces of the patella are commonly the site of cartilage lesions which are, for the most part, similar to those observed in other joints. *Nonprogressive* surface lesions (fibrillation) occur at particular sites, around its periphery and on the odd facet. These lesions are often present in youth and they are the rule in old age. They are probably due to habitual disuse and their frequency may vary between populations with different habits.

At the other end of the spectrum there are *progressive lesions* which are found in the central, heavily used areas. These lesions are found predominately in elderly patients and, when they are associated with reactive changes in the rest of the joint, they justify description as incipient osteoarthritis.

Fasciculation, though it probably does affect the cartilage of other joints, occurs particularly frequently at specific sites on the patella and might justify

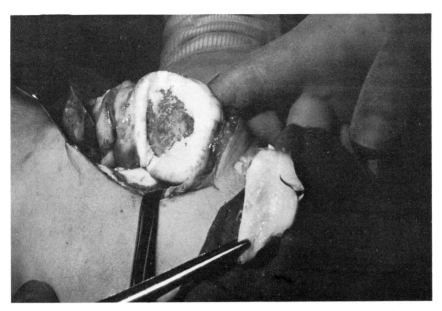

Fig. 9.16 Chondral fracture, resulting from direct injury to the patella during a football match.

the use of the term 'chondromalacia patellae' to describe it if that term could be shorn of its other meanings.

9.3 Anterior knee pain

9.3.1 CAUSES

In its other usage the term 'chondromalacia patellae' has come to signify a well recognized clinical syndrome, the main feature of which is pain in the front of the knee. It would be much better to use another term, which does not presuppose the cause, such as patellofemoral pain syndrome or arthralgia. Best of all we can accept common usage and say 'anterior knee pain', in the same way as we speak of 'lower abdominal pain', or 'headache'.

Anterior knee pain can, of course, arise from a great many causes, some of them situated at a distance from the knee. There comes to mind that 'pons asinorum' of orthopaedics, the young patient whose knee pain is investigated by measurement of the Q-angle, skyline radiographs of the patella and eventually arthroscopy, while all the time the capital epiphysis is slipping slowly off the femoral neck! Lesions of the lumbar spine, the posterior abdominal wall, the proximal end of the femur and the hip joint can all result in anterior knee pain, and they all need to be positively considered if they are not to be overlooked.

225

Pain in the front of the knee may also derive from a number of local causes:

Osteoarthritis of the patellofemoral joint
Osteochondritis dissecans
Meniscal tears
Osgood–Schlatter's disease
Bipartite patella, etc.

All these disorders can occasion similar symptoms but in all of them there is some physical or radiological sign which allows their separation one from another.

There remain, however, a number of patients who complain of anterior knee pain and in whom physical and radiological examination of the limb reveals no abnormality. In civilian practice these are usually adolescent and female but several reports from military sources suggest that the disorder is common in young men in the armed services. Abernethy *et al.* (1978) examined 123 medical students and found asymptomatic patellofemoral crepitus in 62%. Of these 29% admitted to previous transient discomfort and 3% had chronic knee pain.

The classical description of the symptoms strongly incriminates the patellofemoral joint. Pain is localized, fairly accurately, to the region of the knee cap; it is brought on by prolonged sitting with the knee joint flexed and is usually relieved in full extension. Pain is related to activity, particularly climbing and descending stairs; it is accompanied by crunching and grating sensations in the front of the knee.

The most remarkable feature of the physical signs is the lack of them. There is no synovial thickening or effusion, no limitation of movements and, most remarkably of all, there may be no wasting of the quadriceps muscles, even after two or three years of persistent symptoms. The patients are often fearful of any manipulation of the kneecap which is tender to firm palpation of its under surface, particularly medially. The apprehension sign is not usually present.

It is generally believed that the condition has a strong tendency to recover spontaneously; certainly it is unusual in civilian practice to encounter the disorder after the age of 25 years and most cases, in the author's experience, begin between the ages of 13 and 15.

Here, then, is a syndrome in search of a pathology. The hunt for a cause has produced many explanations, a multiplicity of subtle physical and radiological signs and measurements and altogether too many surgical operations.

9.3.2 THE CARTILAGE OPERATIONS

Does anterior knee pain syndrome arise from a lesion of the patellar articular cartilage? Certainly not always, for many patients with all the clinical features described above are found, at arthrotomy or arthroscopy, to have an entirely normal articulation. Nor does it follow, because a patient is found to have a cartilage lesion, that the lesion has caused the symptoms. The postmortem studies referred to above, show that cartilage lesions become more frequent and more severe with advancing age; but the clinical syndrome is a disorder of adolescence and young adulthood.

There is a logical problem, too, in attributing pain to a lesion in articular cartilage, when that tissue is known to be devoid of nerve endings. It is difficult to see how any surface lesion which does not go deep enough to expose underlying bone could give rise to pain; or why such lesions, which are common in many other joints, should cause such symptoms only in the patellofemoral joint. Nevertheless, 'chondrectomy', performed by a variety of means, has been widely employed ever since shaving off the articular cartilage was first described by Wiles et al. (1956).

Whatever the immediate effect upon symptoms may be, paring off the surface of the articular cartilage of any synovial joint is probably a recipe for disaster in the long term. Cartilage has very little capacity to repair after such an injury and the onset of degenerative arthritis would seem to be an inevitable sequel. Repair, by fibrocartilaginous ingrowth, can occur if the whole thickness of cartilage, with its calcified layer, is excised in a circumscribed manner. This procedure, localized full thickness chondrectomy, has been proposed in preference to 'shaving' (Goodfellow et al., 1976). Drilling of the exposed subchondral bone plate may further enhance the repair by facilitating the ingress of fibroelastic tissue from the bone (Childers and Ellwood, 1979). However, the justification for performing any of these procedures in patients with the anterior knee pain syndrome is very doubtful. Surface degenerative lesions, as has been explained in earlier paragraphs, are most unlikely to cause pain, and, even if they were, they could hardly be improved by further damaging the cartilage surface by shaving it. Such lesions are seldom localized and, therefore, cannot be treated by isolated excision.

The lesion called 'fasciculation' may be sufficiently localized to allow removal of an island of cartilage, down to the bone, but its morphology suggests that, at least until the tangential layers rupture, it is a disorder capable of spontaneous recovery. The evidence for attributing pain in the knee to such lesions is slender, but a disorder in the depths of the cartilage might result in altered load transmission to the bone beneath and cause pain by stimulation of the subchondral nerve endings (Goodfellow et al., 1976).

It is the author's view that articular cartilage is a precious commodity, the quantity of which the surgeon is powerless to increase. He should excise cartilage only if he is sure that (1) it is functionally useless and (2) that it is causing symptoms. Figure 9.15 shows one of the very few occasions when a lesion fulfils these criteria. The structure of the cartilage was completely disorganized in a circumscribed area; innumerable fragments were being shed into the joint cavity and the young man, in whose joint it was situated, was experiencing recurrent synovial effusions.

9.3.3 REALIGNMENT PROCEDURES

Dissatisfied with chondrectomy, surgical interest in the relief of anterior knee pain turned to measures aimed at repositioning the patella in its groove. Malalignment has, on the one hand, been blamed for causing cartilage lesions of the patella and, on the other hand, has been thought to be a reason for anterior knee pain in patients whose articular cartilage is normal.

There is, of course, no doubt that some developmental and acquired disorders of tracking occur at the joint and that they can cause instability and occasional dislocation of the patella (Chapter 8). Perhaps less severe abnormalities, insufficient to cause such well recognized symptoms, might nevertheless give rise to altered stresses at the knee and thereby occasion chronic anterior knee pain?

It is from this reasoning that several operations, designed to cure recurrent dislocation of the patella, have been performed upon patients whose knee-caps have never shown any tendency to dislocate. Transfer of the tibial tubercle laterally, or distally, or in both directions has been tried (Devas and Golski, 1973). More popular, at the time of writing, is the less radical procedure of division of the lateral retinaculum. It has no better basis in theory than that incision of the lateral capsular structures is the one common feature of several operations, all of which are more or less successful in curing recurrent dislocation of the patella. The operation has been practised subcutaneously (Harwin and Stern, 1981), as an open procedure (Ceder and Larson, 1979) or via the arthroscope (Metcalf, 1982). It has relieved anterior knee pain in about 7 out of 10 patients followed for one year but the results have not been so good when reviewed at a longer time interval (Osborne and Fulford, 1982).

Several attempts have been made to define and to record the subtle 'subclinical' aberrations of patellar tracking which these and similar procedures purport to correct. The morphology of the patella and its soft-tissue investment has proved to be very variable – there are hardly two alike – but variations from the normal, though numerous, have seldom been proved to have any significance.

One constant feature of the knee's anatomy is the lateral inclination of the patellar tendon from the line of action of the quadriceps muscle (the Q-angle); a feature which varies with the degree of external rotation of the tibia and with the angle of genu valgum. The Q-angle has been found to be greater in those suffering from anterior knee pain than in others. Variations in the length of the patellar tendon, as a proportion of the length of the patella, are described as patella baja and patella alta and the latter is associated with anterior knee pain.

Skyline radiographs allow the categorization of the innumerable forms of the patella into the three common types of Wiberg (1941) and the rare type described by Baumgartl (1964), but there is no evidence to incriminate one form of patella more than another as a cause for knee pain. Axial radiographs of the joint taken in various degrees of flexion have also been used, with and without the injection of contrast medium, to detect minor subluxation. It is evident, from the contact prints shown in Figs 9.4–9.7 that alignment of the X-ray beam at an appropriate angle, tangent to the femur, is essential (Ficat, et al., 1979).

Using meticulous techniques, and careful measurement of radiological joint spaces, it has been shown that some variations in the joint anatomy are often associated with anterior knee pain. The so-called patellofemoral index (the ratio of the width of the medial and lateral radiological joint spaces) was found to be 1, or less, in the normal population and more than 1 in 96% of a group of patients said to have 'chondromalacia patellae' (Laurin et al., 1979). The measurements in this study were made on radiographs taken with the knee flexed no more than 20° and it was stated that, at higher angles of flexion, subluxation often could not be detected. Now, in the fully extended knee the patella is known to lie above the level of the trochlear facets and often lateral to them (Delgado-Martins, 1979); it is only during the first 10–20° of flexion that the patella begins to engage in its groove. Perhaps variations in its position at or near full extension are of little consequence, since the force to be resisted at the patellofemoral joint in that posture is only a small proportion of the quadriceps force.

The case for realigning an apparently normal quadriceps mechanism is, necessarily, rather weak but it can be claimed, at least, that the procedure does little harm. So long as the relationship of the patella with the femur is not altered this may be true, but there is evidence that an increase or decrease of the Q-angle, by as little as 10°, can completely change the pattern of contact, and always for the worse (Fujikawa, 1981). The beautifully matched contours of the natural joint fit one another only in their correct disposition; in any other relative position the contact areas diminish, and the force per unit area of articular cartilage must increase.

The case for attributing anterior knee pain to any of these minor and coincidental anatomical variations remains unproven and the basis for performing realignment procedures is no more than speculative.

9.3.4 THE SYNOVIAL PLICAE

The patellofemoral joint, as the contact studies show, is one of the least congruous articulations in the human body. In any position of the knee only a small proportion of the articular cartilage of the patella is in contact with the femur. Since the normal knee contains only a very small quantity of synovial fluid it follows that the remainder of the cartilage surfaces must be covered, in

229

life, by folds of synovial membrane. As the joint moves, and as the contact areas change, so these synovial folds must rearrange themselves, always squeezed away from the contact area by the opposed cartilage and sucked in to cover the noncontact areas by the joint vacuum. We never see these folds in their natural state because at arthrotomy air fills the joint and during arthroscopy it is dilated with fluid.

Occasionally, a thickened synovial pleat (or plica) causes recurrent clicking and discomfort, during flexion and extension, as it slips back and forth, usually over the medial articular margin of the femur. In the author's experience it is the sensation of clicking, not the pain, which is mainly complained of and is most readily appreciated by the examiner. This uncommon disorder is cured by dividing or excising the thickened synovium. The symptoms are, however, so unlike those of the common anterior pain syndrome as to suggest that the two have little in common. It hardly provides a precedent for the division of any natural synovial folds that may be spied through the arthroscope (Vaughan-Lane and Dandy, 1982).

Nevertheless the author is inclined to think that the common source of the symptoms in adolescent anterior knee pain will probably be found in the peripatellar soft tissues rather than in any other structure of the joint. The creaking and crunching sounds which are so often heard during flexion of the normal, as well as the painful knee, may emanate from the movements of these synovial folds. We have observed that these noises can no longer be produced once the synovial cavity is opened and that they also disappear if the joint is distended, either by a natural effusion or by injection of fluid for arthrography or arthroscopy. The common effect of introducing air or fluid into the joint cavity is to allow the synovial infoldings to retreat from the non-contact areas of the articular cartilage.

It has often been remarked that the symptoms of anterior knee pain are relieved by diagnostic arthroscopy, albeit transiently. Following this clue we have observed relief of pain, for a few days, following the injection of normal saline into the joint.

All these 'cures', and perhaps others achieved by more complex assaults on the joint, have in common that they release the joint vacuum and allow the synovial folds around the kneecap to retreat from between the articular surfaces.

9.3.5 REDUCING PATELLOFEMORAL PRESSURE

Whereas realignment of the quadriceps mechanism, mediolaterally, has been proposed to alter the *distribution* of the pressure on the patella's surface, altering the position of the patellar tendon insertion anteriorly has been suggested as a method of diminishing the *magnitude* of the patellofemoral force which results from quadriceps action. Maquet (1976) has convincingly demonstrated that anterior displacement of the tibial tuberosity by about

2 cm can diminish the patellofemoral force, by as much as 50%, during normal use of the knee. His operation was devised for treating patellofemoral osteoarthritis, and patients seriously disabled may be willing to accept the considerable and irreversible deformity which it induces for relief from pain and a cease to further deterioration. However, the risks involved in altering any feature of the design of the knee should not be minimized. There is theoretical evidence, and some experimental proof, that anteroposterior movements of the femur on the tibia are controlled, not only by tension in the cruciate ligaments but also by that component of patellar tendon force which acts on the tibia in the plane of its plateau (O'Connor et al., 1981). The magnitude of the component of force must be changed by any change in the point of insertion of the quadriceps mechanism. Whether the new pattern of forces then experienced at the tibiofemoral articulation could be damaging to its long-term function no one knows, but the close interdependence which exists between all the loadbearing structures of the knee suggests that the arbitrary movement of a tibial tuberosity, either forwards or from side-to-side, is at least as likely to have a bad as to have a good effect on the mechanics of the joint as a whole.

9.3.6 PATELLECTOMY

If, as seems probable, the patella is not usually the source of the painful sensations of anterior knee pain then its removal would be unlikely to relieve them and, in fact, the results of patellectomy have been usually unhappy. When it is performed as the last (illogical?) act in a series of failed operations it seldom confers any benefit on the patient, though the finality of removing the offending bone may allow the surgeon to wash his hands of the matter! It is better not to initiate such a series of fruitless procedures.

9.3.7 CONSERVATIVE MANAGEMENT

What then is to be done for the young patient who complains of chronic pain in the front of the knee? She (or he) has been carefully examined and no local or distant cause has been found. Radiographs of the knee are normal. The symptoms of the syndrome, though their cause is enigmatic, are so constant that we can confidently advise against the need for any further investigation. In particular, there is seldom any need for arthrography or arthroscopy. If, as is usual, the symptoms have been present for many months, or even years, without producing an effusion or any limitation of movement then such minor abnormalities of the articular cartilage as these investigations may reveal are, anyway, irrelevant.

It is then explained to the patient (and her mother) that the cause of this type of knee pain in adolescence remains a mystery and that medicine can do little if anything to relieve it. Fortunately, it is a symptom which gets better spontaneously in the long run and seldom troubles people much in adult life. It does not presage future arthritis (the parents are relieved to hear) nor will the knee be damaged if the patient continues to play sports and games. Aspirin can be taken if the pain is bad and if it becomes intolerable it can be relieved, temporarily, by a week or two in a plaster back slab or other removable splint. Splintage has no long-term effect on the disorder but it gives the sufferer a period of relief. The wearing of a tight bandage around the knee, or one of the several designs of elastic kneecap, may be of use particularly during athletic activities.

Reassessment at six-monthly intervals is necessary to reassure all concerned that no pathological process is detectable in the knee and to reinforce the assurance that no treatment is necessary.

9.3.8 CONCLUSIONS

1. The syndrome of anterior knee pain, so common in adolescents and young adults, should not be called chondromalacia patellae. Cartilage lesions are not always present on the kneecaps of those complaining of it and, even when they are, those lesions can seldom be held responsible for the pain.

2. Chondrectomy and chondroplasty can, therefore, have little to recommend them. If a localized disorder, with complete degeneration of the full thickness of the cartilage, is encountered its circumscribed excision can occasionally be justified.

3. True malalignment of the quadriceps mechanism may cause dislocation of the patella and require realignment on that score. There is, however, little evidence that the minor variations of anatomy, so commonly found in the knees of sufferers from anterior knee pain, play a causative role. The case for performing the operation of lateral release is not proven in theory nor established in practice. The risks of damaging the joint by altering the position of the patellar tendon insertion may be greater than the chances of improving it.

4. Probably, the painful stimuli of anterior knee pain come from the peripatellar soft tissues. However, no pathological lesion has been regularly demonstrated and the division of normal synovial folds, so tempting to do through the arthroscope, is based more on optimism than logic.

5. Anterior knee pain, like headache, is a common discomfort for which no explanation can usually be found. Since relief of the symptom has been claimed for such a wide variety of operations a non-specific effect of them all must be suspected. The risk of damaging the joint makes surgery an inappropriate placebo.

References

Abernethy P J, Townsend P R, Rose R M, Radin E L. Is Chondromalacia Patellae a separate clinical entity? *J Bone Joint Surg [Br]* 1978;**60–B**:205–10.

Baumgartl F. *Das Kniegelenk*. Berlin: Springer-Verlag, 1964.

Bennett G A, Waine H, Bauer W. *Change in the knee joint at various ages with particular reference to the development of degenerative joint disease*. New York: The Commonwealth Fund, 1942.

Bullough, P G, Goodfellow J, O'Connor J J. The relationship between degenerative changes and load-bearing in the human hip. *J Bone Joint Surg [Br]* 1973;**55–B**:746–58.

Byers P D. Contepomi C A, Farkas T A. A post mortem study of the hip joint. *Ann Rheum Dis* 1970;**29**:15–31.

Ceder L C, Larson R L. Z-Plasty lateral retinacular release for the treatment of patellar compression syndrome. *Clin Orthop Rel Res* 1979;**144**:110–13.

Childers J C, Ellwood B C. Partial chondrectomy and subchondral bone drilling for chondro-malacia. *Clin Orthop Rel Res* 1979;**144**:114–20.

Delgado-Martins H. A study of the position of the patella using computerised tomography. *J Bone Joint Surg [Br]* 1979;**61–B**:443–4.

Devas M, Golski A. Treatment of chondromalacia patellae by transposition of the tibial tubercle. *Br Med* 1973;**1**:589–91.

Ficat R P, Hungerford D S. *Disorders of the patello-femoral joint*. Baltimore: Williams and Wilkins, 1977.

Ficat R P, Philippe J, Hungerford D S. Chondromalacia patellae: A system of classification. *Clin Orthop Rel Res* (1979) **144**:55–61.

Fujikawa K. Biomechanics of patello-femoral articulation with special reference to the influence of femoro-tibial angular deformity. MSc Thesis (University of Leeds) 1981.

Goodfellow J, Hungerford D S, Zindel M. Patello-femoral joint mechanics and pathology: Functional anatomy of the patello-femoral joint. *J Bone Joint Surg [Br]* 1976;**58–B**:291–9.

Harrison M H M, Schajowicz F, Trueta J. Osteoarthritis of the hip: A study of the nature and evolution of the disease. *J Bone Joint Surg [Br]* 1953;**35–B**:598.

Harwin S F, Stern R E. Subcutaneous lateral retinacular release for chondromalacia patellae *Clin Orthop Rel Res* 1981;**156**:207–10.

Insall J, Falvo K, Wise D W. Chondromalacia patellae. *J Bone Joint Surg [Am]* 1976;**58–A**:1–8.

Laurin C A, Dussault R, Levesque H P. The tangential X-ray investigation of the patello-femoral joint. *Clin Orthop Rel Res* 1979;**144**:16–26.

Maquet P. *Biomechanics of the knee, with application to the pathogenesis and the surgical treatment of osteoarthritis*. New York: Springer-Verlag, 1976;134–43.

Meachim G, Emery I H. Quantitative aspects of patello-femoral cartilage fibrillation in Liverpool necropsies. *Ann Rheum Dis* 1974;**33**:39–47.

Metcalf R W. An arthroscopic method for lateral release of the subluxating and dislocating patella. *Clin Orthop Rel Res* 1982;**167**:11–18.

O'Connor J, Goodfellow J, Biden E. Designing the human knee. In: *Mechanical factors and the skeleton*. London: John Libbey, 1981.

Osborne A H, Fulford P C. Lateral release for chondromalacia patellae. *J Bone Joint Surg [Br]* 1982;**64–B**:202–6.

Outerbridge R E. The aetiology of chondromalacia patellae. *J Bone Joint Surg [Br]* 1961;**43–B**:752–7.

Vaughan-Lane T, Dandy D J. The synovial shelf syndrome. *J Bone Joint Surg [Br]* 1982;**64–B**:475–6.

Wiberg G. Roentgenographic and anatomic studies of the femoro-patellar joint. *Acta Orthop Scand* 1941;**12**:319–410.

Wiles P, Andrews P S, Devas M B. Chondromalacia of the patella *J Bone Joint Surg [Br]* 1956;**38–B**:95–113.

CHAPTER 10

Osteochondritis Dissecans

P. M. Aichroth

10.1 Introduction

Osteochondritis dissecans is a condition in which a segment of articular cartilage together with subchondral bone separates completely or partly from a joint surface. It is most common in the knee where the femoral condyles are usually affected and although often unilateral, symmetrical and bilateral lesions are sometimes seen.

Ambroise Paré recognized the disease in the 16th century and is given credit for the first reported case of the surgical removal of a loose body from the knee joint. In 1870 Paget produced a classic account of the condition and described a girl who had the habit of breaking thick pieces of wood across her thigh and knee; he felt that the loose fragment was produced by local trauma. König (1887) called the disease 'osteochondritis dissecans' and although a bad name because osteochondritis suggests an inflammatory condition, he believed that the cause of this 'dissection' was traumatic. Sir Thomas Fairbank (1933) earlier this century noted the association with sporting activity and suggested that the lesion was frequently sustained during sports in the 'heat of the game'.

Since then there have been many theories seeking to explain the aetiology of osteochondritis dissecans: some have put forward trauma as the cause and others an embolic origin producing a localized area of avascular necrosis with later separation. In 1952 Watson-Jones suggested that osteochondritis dissecans in multiple sites in the adolescent was due to bone infarcts caused by the clumping of red cells. Indeed, such conditions as the haemoglobinopathies, renal transplant arthropathies, alcoholism and steroid therapy do produce avascular areas of the femoral condyle due to embolism. The avascularity of the femoral condyle results in osteonecrosis which must be differentiated from osteochondritis dissecans. Smillie (1960), in a major treatise on osteochondritis dissecans, felt that there were four types and that they were all interrelated aetiologically:

(1) The lesion seen at the age of ten or younger was an anomaly of ossification.
(2) The lesion seen at fifteen was described as a juvenile type.
(3) The lesion appearing in the adult was termed adult osteochondritis dissecans.
(4) Certain other lesions were tangential osteochondral fractures.

Experimental and clinical features seem to suggest that the fourth category is the most important.

10.2 Aetiology

The clinical characteristics of this condition are taken from a survey of 200 patients with osteochondritis dissecans of the knee (Aichroth, 1971; 1977). The femoral condyles were most commonly affected; the patella infrequently was the site of osteochondritis dissecans and rarely the upper tibial plateau was involved. The medial femoral condyle was the most common site and the positions of the fragments seen in this survey are shown in Fig. 10.1. Unilateral lesions were present in 74% and bilateral lesions in 26%. Males were affected twice as frequently as females and in 46% of patients a loose body

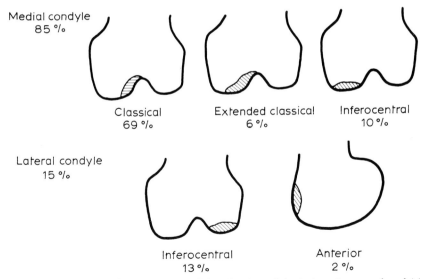

Fig. 10.1 Diagram showing sites and distribution of the lesions in osteochondritis dissecans in the medial and lateral femoral condyles. (Reproduced from Aichroth (1971) with permission.)

235

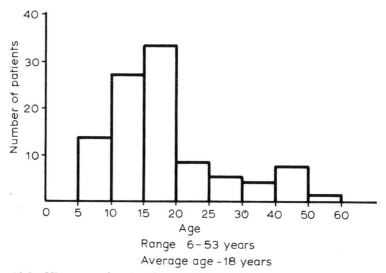

Fig. 10.2 Histogram showing the age of onset of symptoms. (Reproduced from Aichroth (1971) with permission.)

was present when initially seen. The majority of patients were between the ages of ten and twenty and in this series there was an age range from six to 53 years (Fig. 10.2).

In the survey described, 10% were considered to be acute osteochondral fractures but it is probable that more patients were affected by an injury than was first recognized and the lesion was only later called an osteochondritis dissecans.

10.2.1 TRAUMA AND ATHLETICS

In 46% of patients an injury of the knee joint was sustained which was severe enough for the patient to be taken to a doctor or to hospital for treatment. The others, however, did not admit to any trauma whatsoever. When the athletic ability of the patients was investigated most were found to be keen sportsmen. Sixty per cent were classified as excellent or good at their sports and most were involved in field games and athletics. It was thought that this was a remarkably high figure in any group of young people and was felt to be an aetiological factor.

The importance of trauma in the development of osteochondritis dissecans and the significance of osteochondral fractures will be fully discussed, but first two other aetiological factors will be considered.

10.2.2 ASSOCIATED MECHANICAL ABNORMALITIES

Genu valgum was present in 5% and genu varum in 9%. Those patients with some deformity of the knee were noted to have osteochondritic lesions which were bilateral and symmetrical. Many presented with ligamentous laxity which might be congenital or traumatic in origin. The patella dislocated in 7% but subluxed in a further 9%. In those patients with patellar instability, the lateral femoral condyle was usually affected, particularly on the anterior aspect. In a recent survey of patients with discoid menisci, an osteochondritis dissecans lesion was present on the lateral femoral condyle in 20% (Glasgow *et al.*, 1982).

10.2.3 EPIPHYSEAL ABNORMALITIES

Patients with epiphyseal dysplasia multiplex congenita and other similar conditions in which the joint surfaces are irregular may develop osteochondritis dissecans in various joints and frequently at the knee. It is important to consider all other joints in a patient affected with osteochondritis dissecans of the knee for in the series described additional asymptomatic lesions were found in 7%.

10.2.4 EXPERIMENTAL OSTEOCHONDRAL FRACTURES IN ANIMALS

In New Zealand White Rabbits an arthrotomy of the knee was undertaken under general anaesthesia and various osteochondral cuts were made into the medial femoral condyle (Fig. 10.3). The union and non-union rates in each group were noted and in group 1 (where the fragment was cut so that displacement was possible) most remained ununited. In group 2 there was a more stable fragment *in situ* and eight of the 13 fragments united. All those which were internally fixed, united rapidly and in group 4 the osteochondral cuts were made in such a way that the fragment was totally stabilized. As

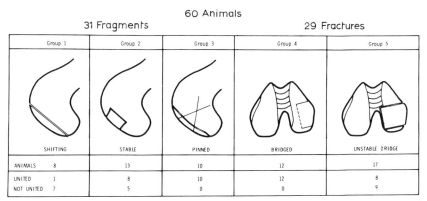

60 Animals

31 Fragments   **29 Fractures**

Group 1	Group 2	Group 3	Group 4	Group 5
SHIFTING	STABLE	PINNED	BRIDGED	UNSTABLE BRIDGE
ANIMALS 8	13	10	12	17
UNITED 1	8	10	12	8
NOT UNITED 7	5	0	0	9

Fig. 10.3 Diagram showing the types of osteochondral cuts made in 60 experimental rabbits. The figures below indicate whether or not bony union occurred. (Reproduced from Aichroth (1971) with permission.)

expected all united rapidly. In group 5 the medial femoral condylar cut was made leaving a minimal bridge which proved unstable and only eight of the 17 united.

Osteochondral fractures cut in such a way that displacement occurred were followed by non-union. Those which were adequately fixed united. Non-union of an osteochondral fragment was characterized by a necrotic osseous portion with viable articular cartilage. The zone between crater and fragment contained fibrous tissue and fibrocartilaginous material with appearances similar to that of osteochondritis dissecans in man.

10.2.5 CADAVERIC STUDIES

The typical site on the intercondylar region of the medial femoral condyle appears protected and placed away from areas which could be affected by direct trauma. This, however, is not so. A cadaveric demonstration with Bonney's blue painted on the medial articular facet of the patella showed the area of contact between the medial facet and the medial femoral condyle. In full flexion the typical site was coloured (Fig. 10.4). Osteochondral fractures may be caused by the impact of patella on the medial femoral condyle when the knee is in flexion for this area is the area stained by Bonney's blue. In full flexion, therefore, forces may be transmitted by way of the patella to the typical site.

10.2.6 OSTEOCHONDRAL FRACTURES

Osteochondral fractures of any part of the articular surface at the knee joint may be caused by an injury. Mathewson and Dandy (1978) showed that in both direct violence and in pivoting on the extended knee, avulsion of the articular cartilage and subchondral bone occurs particularly on the lateral femoral condyle. Osteochondral fractures of the patella have been recognized since the beginning of this century and a tangential osteochondral fracture is characteristic of patellar dislocation.

Landells (1957) and Rosenberg (1964) demonstrated that articular cartilage separates at the junction between the calcified and uncalcified zone in the mature person. The immature adolescent cartilage does not have this calcified zone and so shearing forces are transmitted to the subchondral layer. Osteochondral fractures, therefore, occur more readily in childhood and adolescence. O'Donoghue (1966) believed that there was no difference between an osteochondral fracture and osteochondritis dissecans and Kennedy et al. (1966) showed experimentally that all areas of the weight-bearing surfaces of the femoral condyles could be affected by osteochondral fracture with various axial compression and rotatory forces.

238

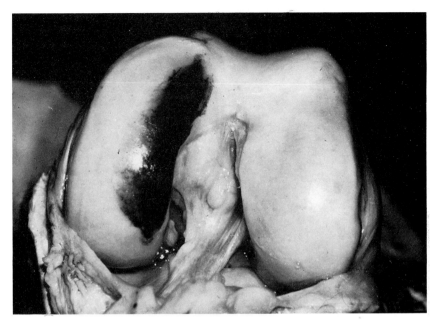

Fig. 10.4 When dye is applied to the medial patellar facet and the patella is then articulated, the medial femoral condyle is stained in the 'classical site'.

10.2.7 OSTEONECROSIS

Loose bodies in joints may develop from lesions resembling osteochondritis dissecans in multiple systemic disease processes. In the haemoglobinopathies bone infarcts develop from clumped red cells and peripheral embolisation may produce infarcts in many tissues including bone. In Caisson disease intravascular nitrogen bubbles embolise peripherally and bone may become infarcted. There are many other systemic abnormalities in which identical changes occur: such as Gaucher's disease, hyperuricaemia, alcoholism, steroid arthropathy and post-transplantation arthropathies. There is increasing evidence that fat emboli are responsible for alcoholic and post-transplantation arthropathies but the end result is the same with large areas of the femoral condyles developing bone necrosis. The post-mortem appearance of the knee joint of a patient who suffered from a post-renal transplantation arthropathy is seen in Fig. 10.5. Multiple loose bodies became detached from the periphery of infarcted necrotic bone. The fragments, therefore, separated through an avascular layer which is different from osteochondritis dissecans where the loose body separates from underlying normal vascularized bone. Once the fragment has become detached the crater in osteochondritis dissecans becomes covered with a layer of fibrous tissue and fibrocartilaginous material which, if removed, reveals normal bleeding bone.

239

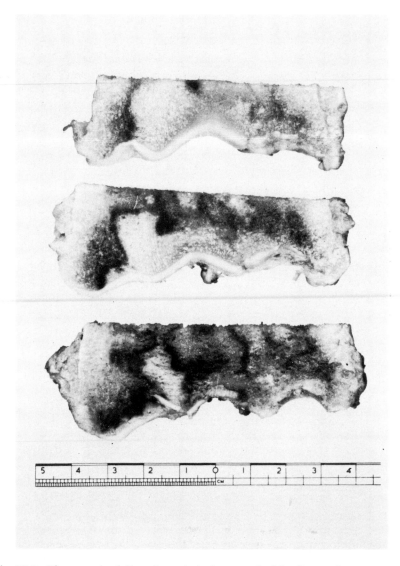

Fig. 10.5 Photograph of slices through the lower end of the femur of a patient with post-renal transplantation arthropathy.

Ahlbäck *et al.* (1968) initially described subchondral idiopathic avascular necrosis of the femoral condyle and the syndrome is characterized by the sudden onset of pain in an elderly patient. A pathological study of 28 patients was undertaken by Ahuja and Bullough (1978) and they classified the lesions into three types:

(1) Idiopathic primary osteonecrosis.

(2) Osteoarthrosis with associated osteonecrosis.

(3) Rheumatoid disease and osteonecrosis.

They demonstrated that isotope studies showed the lesion before radio-graphic changes became evident. They also found marked deformities of the articular surfaces resulting from fractures and fragmentation of necrotic bone and collapse of the overlying articular cartilage. Secondary arthritis usually occurs. Patients with rheumatoid arthritis who developed osteonecrosis frequently had a long history of steroid therapy. Rozing *et al.* (1980) found that the prognosis in this condition depended upon the size of the radiological lesion. They advocated conservative treatment with weight restriction and anti-inflammatory drugs. In two-thirds of their patients the symptoms resolved but one-third continued to have persistent and disabling symptoms frequently requiring surgical treatment. Osteotomy was preferred for the younger patient and total knee replacement was usually indicated in the elderly (see Chapter 15).

In summary, therefore, idiopathic osteonecrosis differs in several ways from true osteochondritis dissecans. The latter is present in the young athletic patient sometimes with a history of trauma. The typical site on the inter-condylar region of the medial femoral condyle is usually affected in osteo-chondritis dissecans but the weight-bearing surface of the medial femoral condyle is affected in patients with idiopathic osteonecrosis. In osteochon-dritis dissecans, the crater consists of fibrous tissue and fibrocartilaginous material which, if removed, reveals bleeding bone. In osteonecrosis the fragment separates from a bed of avascular bone which may be present through a large area of the femoral condyle. Osteonecrosis is also discussed in Chapters 3 and 13.

10.3 Clinical features

10.3.1 IN CHILDHOOD

Although osteochondritis dissecans most often occurs in adolescence, young children may be affected and the features may be different. The symptoms are likely to be intermittent pain, swelling and an occasional limp. There may be few, if any, physical signs; it is unusual to find an effusion or tenderness over the femoral condyle. At this age radiographs of the epiphysis of the femoral condyle show a rather irregular appearance which later develops into normal bone. When osteochondritis dissecans is present there is a definite crater containing a fragment of bone. The diagnosis may be confirmed by arthro-scopy. The most common site for the lesion is on the central area on the weight-bearing surface. The fragment is usually stable and heals spontan-eously.

10.3.2 IN ADOLESCENCE

The condition occurs most commonly in adolescents who are involved in sports of various kinds. The pain may be severe with associated swelling. There is a limp and the knee is externally rotated (Wilson, 1967). Instability may develop with episodes of 'giving way': this is probably the result of movement of a partly detached fragment in its crater. Intermittent locking can occur as the fragment moves, and when separation takes place there will be typical symptoms of a 'loose body' in the joint. Tenderness may be present over the affected area in the femoral condyle. In the later stages the loose body may be felt.

10.4 Radiographic appearances

The lesion will be seen in radiographs if correct views are taken. Antero-posterior, lateral, tunnel and skyline views must be requested routinely if the condition is suspected. Oblique views may be necessary to identify the position of a loose body or to recognize a recent osteochondral fracture. The characteristic feature of the 'fragment within a crater' is seen and this is differentiated from the ossification defect (Fig. 10.6). In osteochondritis dissecans with a well established pseudarthrosis there is a little sclerosis on

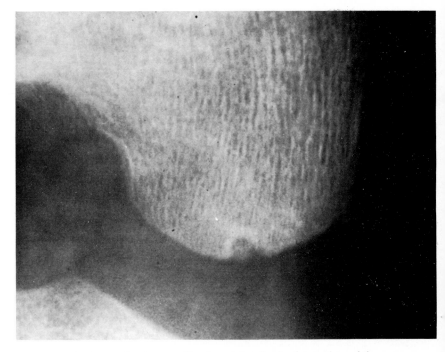

Fig. 10.6 Radiograph of an ossification defect in the femoral condyle.

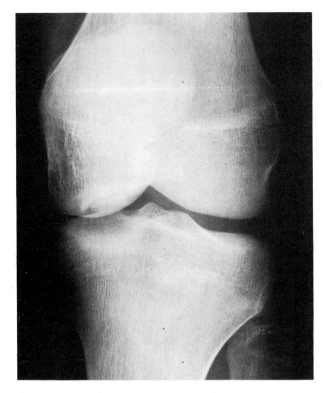

Fig. 10.7 Characteristic radiological appearance of well established osteochondritis dissecans.

the condylar side of the lesion (Fig. 10.7). The fragment may be hinged or if it has separated fully, a further fragment may become detached from the surrounding area. The loose body is nourished by articular synovial fluid and the articular hyaline cartilage on one side of the fragment may proliferate. Cartilage then surrounds the loose body which gradually grows in size (Fig. 10.8). Arthrography has little place in the diagnosis and management of osteochondritis dissecans but sometimes the dye may be seen to flow into the pseudarthrosis between fragment and condylar crater.

10.5 Management

10.5.1 THE LOOSE BODY

The loose fragment must be removed if pain, locking and swelling continue. If such locking occurs repeatedly secondary osteoarthritis changes in the knee joint are likely to develop.

Removal of the loose body by open operation should be immediately

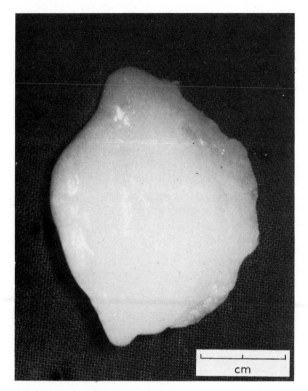

Fig. 10.8 Photograph showing a loose body which is completely surrounded by hyaline cartilage.

preceded by taking radiographs in the position in which the knee will be opened and after the tourniquet has been applied. An image intensifier may also be helpful. Most loose bodies will be found in the suprapatellar pouch but they also present in the anterior compartments or in the posteromedial and posterolateral recesses. An appropriate incision must be made and then the removal of loose fragments may either be exceedingly easy or most frustrating as the 'joint mouse' eludes one's grasp and skids away to another part of the joint cavity.

Arthroscopic removal of the loose body may similarly be the easiest or the most difficult and frustrating procedure. The arthroscopist must be conversant with all arthroscopic approaches in an attempt to identify, localize, hold and then remove the fragment through a small skin incision. This skin and capsule incision may need to be extended around the loose body. Arthroscopic removal of the fragment produces little disturbance to the joint and very rapid rehabilitation of the patient (see Chapter 11). The condylar defect should always be inspected in osteochondritis dissecans when the fragment has separated. In most instances the crater will be obvious and will

244

be characterized by bleeding bone if the lesion is recent or by a defect covered by a layer of fibrocartilaginous tissue if it has been present for some time. Frequently this defect fills in and appears absolutely smooth. The fibro-cartilaginous tissue may be of good weight-bearing quality. Both the quality and quantity of repair tissue depends on the depth of its crater and its area (Convery *et al.*, 1972). We have frequently seen knees with loose bodies of substantial size and no defect can be found both radiologically and arthro-scopically. It is likely that in these cases the fragment of osteochondritis dissecans separated completely from the joint surface and the condylar crater filled perfectly with fibrocartilaginous material which resurfaces the defect. Convery's experiments in large animals confirmed that articular cartilage has very limited capacity for repair if the separation is of partial thickness and for this reason it is always important to curette the cavity down to bleeding bone.

10.5.2 REPLACEMENT AND FIXATION OF THE ACUTE OSTEOCHONDRAL FRACTURE

An acute osteochondral fracture may displace a fragment which includes a substantial slice of bone. This may be replaced accurately into the crater from which it was detached and fixed with pins or wires. It is only the acute osteochondral fracture which may be treated this way for the chronic osteochondritis dissecans fragment is always covered by fibrous tissue or hyperplastic hyaline cartilage. When this tissue is removed bone apposition is poor and the fragment does not fit into its crater. The chance of successful fixation of the fragment with osseous healing is, therefore, very small. Fixation by Smillie's pins is not now much used because of the difficulty of removing them after healing has taken place.

It is recommended that the knee joint is immobilized for approximately six weeks after fixation of the fragment and the wires will have to be removed at a later stage (Fig. 10.9). If the wires have been passed through the fragment and the femoral condyle, and out into the subcutaneous tissues on the outer surface of one or other femoral condyles, then they may be removed without opening the joint. Excision of the loose body is recommended if it does not fit back into the crater with accuracy and stability.

10.5.3 TREATMENT OF THE UNSTABLE HINGED OSTEOCHONDRITIS DISSECANS FRAGMENT

Arthroscopic examination is recommended to assess the nature of the lesion. A hook or probe will help to determine whether or not the fragment is stable. Most commonly, the osteochondritis dissecans lesion has been unstable in its crater for a very long time, in which case there is much fibrous and fibro-cartilaginous tissue in the crater and on the surface of the fragment. It is then recommended that the fragment is removed and the crater is curetted to

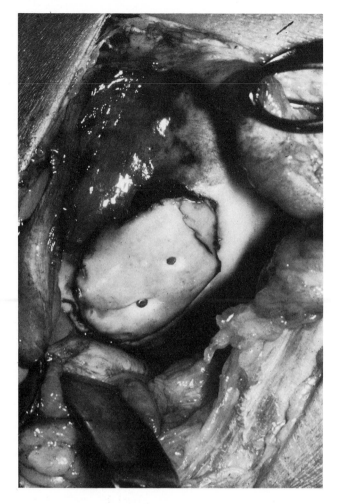

Fig. 10.9 The acute osteochondral fracture has been fixed back using wire.

bleeding bone. This may be undertaken either by arthrotomy or by arthroscopy. Satisfactory resurfacing of the crater will occur by fibrocartilage which grows from the bleeding surface and when this is inspected arthroscopically at a later stage, it is frequently found to be of good quality.

10.5.4 TREATMENT OF THE STABLE OSTEOCHONDRITIS DISSECANS FRAGMENT *IN SITU*

There is sometimes a breach in the hyaline cartilage but some lesions are totally subchondral and there is no abnormality visible on the articular surface. On probing the area, the articular cartilage may be soft or may indent. The stable fragment *in situ* may be drilled either from the condylar surface with the aid of an image-intensifier or from the hyaline articular surface by means of one or multiple drill holes. The articular cartilage is, therefore, disturbed as little as possible. Although this is a very attractive method of treating such a fragment *in situ*, there is little evidence that it is effective (Aichroth, 1971). It is probably better to leave the fragment alone and to review the patient regularly. If the fragment heals or no longer gives rise to symptoms, it should be left alone, but if it loosens or causes symptoms it should be removed.

There is frequently an area of synovitis in the intercondylar notch close to the lesion on the femoral condyle. The author usually removes this area of synovium and fibrous tissue which seems to allow an earlier return to athletic activities than would otherwise have been the case.

It would seem likely that the incomplete repair of large defects on the weight-bearing surfaces would result in osteoarthritis, but the surprising feature of osteochondritis dissecans at the knee is the large number of patients who when followed up show no evidence of osteoarthritis.

Bentley (1973) has shown that grafts of chondrocytes isolated from epiphyseal growth plates will allow rapid resurfacing of small defects with good quality hyaline cartilage and this important research continues. Much work has been undertaken in both small and large animals with shell allografts of articular hyaline cartilage and subchondral bone. In experimental animals allografts of this type show cartilage erosion and destruction in the long term due to immunological attack although the short-term results are excellent (Aichroth *et al.*, 1971).

References

Ahlbäck S, Bauer G C H, Bohne W H. Spontaneous osteonecrosis of the knee. *Arthr Rheum* 1968;11:705–33.

Ahuja S C, Bullough P G. Osteonecrosis of the knee. *J Bone Joint Surg [Am]* 1978;60–A:191–7.

Aichroth P M. Osteochondritis dissecans of the knee. *J Bone Joint Surg [Br]* 1971;53–B:440–7.

Aichroth P M. Osteochondral fracture and osteochondritis dissecans in sportsmen's knee injuries. *J Bone Joint Surg [Br]* 1977;59–B:108.

Aichroth P M, Burwell R G, Laurence M. An experimental study of osteoarticular grafts to replace articular surfaces. *J Bone Joint Surg [Br]* 1971;53–B:554.

Bentley G. Transplantation of isolated chondrocytes into joint surfaces. *J Bone Joint Surg [Br]* 1973;55–B:209–10.

Convery F R, Akeson W H, Keown G H. The repair of the large osteochondral defects. *Clin Orthop Rel Res* 1972;No. 82.

Fairbank H A T. Osteochondritis dissecans. *Br J Surg* 1933;21:67–82.

Glasgow M M S, Aichroth P M, Baird P R E. The discoid lateral meniscus: A clinical review. *J Bone Joint Surg [Br]* 1982;64–B:245.

Kennedy J C, Grainger R W, McGraw R W. Osteochondral fractures of the femoral condyles. *J Bone Joint Surg [Br]* 1966;48–B:436–40.

König F. Ueber freie Körper in den Gelenken. *Dtsch Zeitschr Chir* 1887;27:90.

Landells J W. The reactions of injured human articular cartilage. *J Bone Joint Surg [Br]* 1957;39–B:548–62.

Matthewson M H, Dandy D J. Osteochondral fractures of the lateral femoral condyle. *J Bone Joint Surg [Br]* 1978;60–B:199–202.

O'Donoghue D H. Chondral and osteochondral fractures. *J Trauma* 1966;6:469–81.

Paget J. On the production of some of the loose bodies in joints. *St Bartholomew Hosp Rep* 1870;6:1.

Rosenberg N J. Osteochondral fractures of the lateral femoral condyle. *J Bone Joint Surg [Am]* 1964;46–A:1013–26.

Rozing P M, Insall J, Bohne W H. Spontaneous osteonecrosis of the knee. *J Bone Joint Surg [Am]* 1980;62–A:2–7.

Smillie I S. *Osteochondritis dissecans*. Edinburgh and London: E & S Livingstone Ltd, 1960.

Watson-Jones R. *Fractures and joint injuries*. 4th ed. Edinburgh and London: E & S Livingstone Ltd, 1952; vol 1:97.

Wilson J N. A diagnostic sign in osteochondritis dissecans of the knee. *J Bone Joint Surg [Am]* 1967;49–A:477–80.

Arthroscopic Surgery

D. J. Dandy

Arthroscopic surgery is an extension of diagnostic arthroscopy, but the boundary between the two is ill-defined. The assessment of a hypermobile posterior horn of lateral meniscus, for example, requires more skill than a simple procedure such as synovial biopsy.

11.1 Advantages

The principal advantage of arthroscopic surgery for the patient is the dramatic reduction in the time taken for return to work and sport, and this advantage has led to very considerable public interest in arthroscopic surgery. Most patients are now able to return to heavy work within two weeks of operation, and those in light work within one week. If a patient is engaged in a sedentary occupation involving little more than sitting behind a desk, and the arrangements for his travel to and from work are uncomplicated, he will often be able to return to his normal work within 24 hours of meniscectomy (Dandy, 1978; Oretorp and Gillquist, 1979; Northmore-Ball et al., 1981).

A second advantage of arthroscopic surgery, which is perhaps more apparent to the patient than the surgeon, is the reduction in the size of the scars. Many patients, particularly young women, are reluctant to undergo surgery on the knee because of the scarring which will inevitably result but have no objection to the small puncture wounds of arthroscopic techniques.

A third advantage is that when the surgeon is adept at arthroscopic surgery, he will probably find that most operations can be performed more quickly than through an arthrotomy. Speed of operation is a somewhat dubious advantage, and one that may seem unattainable in the learning stages when the operations are difficult, tedious and protracted. Arthroscopic surgery can, however, reduce operating time and increase the number of patients who can be treated.

Another advantage, which cannot be measured precisely, is the greater accuracy in assessing the results of operation. With the older techniques, operation on the knee involved not only the correction of the intra-articular pathology itself but also a wound, a period of enforced rest, and a further period of rehabilitation. Critical analysis of patients undergoing such procedures would ideally include a control group of patients who had undergone arthrotomy alone leaving the intra-articular pathology untouched, a study that is clearly impossible for obvious ethical reasons. Arthroscopic surgery allows the intra-articular pathology to be corrected without an arthrotomy, which is helpful in analysing the effects of operation and in separating the effects of arthrotomy from those of the corrective procedure within the joint. Because of this, studies of the results of surgery are likely to be more reliable, and the selection of operation more accurate.

Less obvious advantages are that the operation within the knee can be performed more precisely than was previously possible and the meniscus cut more cleanly and neatly under the magnification of the arthroscope, which effectively functions as an operating microscope, than with the naked eye alone.

11.2   Disadvantages

The disadvantages of arthroscopic surgery are few, perhaps the greatest being the need to learn a new and difficult technique. The problems of learning arthroscopic surgery are simply an extension of those encountered in learning diagnostic arthroscopy, outlined in the Chapter 4. The techniques are not easy to learn, and proficiency can only be achieved slowly and painstakingly, starting with the basic skills of diagnostic arthroscopy. To believe that the most difficult step in embarking on arthroscopic surgery is the purchase of instruments is a trap into which many otherwise cautious surgeons have fallen and from which a graceful escape is difficult. As in other fields of surgery, if a surgeon is unable to use the instruments he has purchased, the reason is less likely to be that the instruments are faulty or the technique impossible but rather that the surgeon has overestimated his technical ability. In this respect, arthroscopic surgery is comparable to the internal fixation of fractures using the ASIF system, for which a thorough knowledge of the principles of fracture fixation is required before the instruments and equipment can be used correctly. In the case of ASIF fixation of fractures, however, the surgeon is still using the hammers, drills, screwdrivers and osteotomes to which he is accustomed, while in arthroscopic surgery he is using telescopes, light sources and fine cutting instruments alien to his previous training. Although the instruments and techniques of arthroscopic surgery are very different from those of conventional orthopaedic surgery, they are no less exacting and require more precision and attention to detail than conventional surgery if success is to be achieved. Arthroscopic surgery may appear deceptively simple when performed correctly, but the ease of operation depends on attention to many apparently trivial details.

A second, and somewhat philosophical, disadvantage of arthroscopic surgery is its disturbing impact on previous concepts of knee pathology. Assumptions which surgeons had previously taken for granted are disproved, while new disorders and sometimes even new anatomical structures are recognized. The unblinking gaze of the arthroscope has shown, for example, that the 'retained fragment' of meniscus is a rare condition indeed, and is seldom responsible for persistent symptoms following meniscectomy (Dandy and Jackson, 1975). The medial synovial shelf, one of four plicae in the knee, appears to have escaped general recognition until the advent of the arthroscope. This shelf is a normal structure present in some 75% of people, and is occasionally responsible for anterior knee pain. The characteristics of the 'synovial shelf syndrome' have yet to be defined accurately, but there is little doubt that the condition does exist and that it can be relieved by excision of the shelf (Fujisawa, 1976; Patel, 1978). With the experience that only the passage of time can give, the new thinking generated by arthroscopic surgery can be expected to take shape so that normal and abnormal arthroscopic findings can be more clearly defined. Until the results of the new procedures are precisely analysed and properly published, arthroscopic surgery will lack the signposts and landmarks needed to establish the precise indications for operation.

A further disadvantage is that arthroscopic surgery is not only difficult to learn, but also difficult to teach. For example, while a visitor to a centre for joint replacement will be able to watch the incision made, the joint exposed, the bone surfaces prepared and the prosthesis inserted and secured, on the other hand, those watching arthroscopic surgery without the help of endoscopic television will observe only the surgeon's back as he announces from time to time that various stages of the operation have been achieved, often without any visible sign of meaningful activity. In these circumstances, the scepticism of the visitor may quickly give way to incredulity. Indeed, if arthroscopic surgery did not bring such remarkable benefits to the patient that the patients themselves apply pressure to their surgeons to learn these new techniques, it is most unlikely that arthroscopic surgery would have reached its present stage of development.

11.3 Operations that are possible

Many operations are possible under arthroscopic control. Analysis of the author's first thousand arthroscopic procedures (Dandy and O'Carroll, 1982a) showed that a total of 26 different procedures had been performed.

Operations on the synovium included synovial biopsy, synovectomy, excision or division of the medial synovial shelf, division of the suprapatellar membrane, and division of isolated adhesions and fibrous bands following operation or other trauma.

Operations for meniscal lesions included partial and total meniscectomy, resection of the fibrous rim which forms after meniscectomy when these rims have become torn, debridement of torn segments of degenerate menisci, and excision of minor meniscal tears or splits not large enough to be called a partial meniscectomy. Foreign bodies and loose bodies were removed, and pedunculated 'loose' bodies mobilized and excised (Dandy and O'Carroll, 1982b).

Flap fractures of articular cartilage were levelled and the loose edges of osteochondral fractures excised to leave a clean and even edge. If chondral separations or osteochondral fractures resulted in exposed subchondral bone at the floor of the defect, the defects were drilled, as were the lesions of osteochondritis dissecans.

Chondromalacia patellae and irregular patches of degenerate articular cartilage were shaved or levelled with powered or hand instruments, and osteophytes debrided from the joint margin.

Long redundant stubs of ruptured anterior or posterior cruciate ligaments were excised and ruptured anterior cruciate ligaments replaced with a prosthetic substitute under arthroscopic control without arthrotomy.

Specimens of bony lesions at the lower end of the femur were excised arthroscopically for histological study, ganglia excised from the intercondylar notch, pedunculated lipomata removed, the fat pad excised and lateral release of the patellar mechanism performed.

This great variety of techniques makes arthroscopic surgery different from other types of endoscopic surgery, such as laparoscopy or urological endoscopy, in which only a few techniques are possible.

It must not be thought that all of the above conditions were performed with equal frequency; some procedures, such as bone biopsy, excision of ganglia from the base of the anterior cruciate ligament, and removal of foreign bodies were performed only once or twice, while the series included 475 partial meniscectomies.

11.3.1 INDICATIONS FOR ARTHROTOMY

At present, the only absolute indications for arthrotomy are joint replacement, meniscal reattachment and ligament reconstruction, but ligament reconstruction is now technically possible under arthroscopic control without arthrotomy (Dandy *et al.* 1981) and awaits only a suitable prosthetic material to become reality. Apart from these absolute indications for arthrotomy, relative indications include meniscectomy for complex meniscal lesions, particularly those of the lateral meniscus, and reattachment of osteochondral fragments resulting from recent injury. It must not be thought that every surgeon will immediately be able to limit his indications for arthrotomy in this way, but it is to be hoped that some operations, such as exploratory arthrotomy and open synovial biopsy, will quickly become obsolete.

11.3.2 ANAESTHESIA

Arthroscopic surgery under local anaesthesia is perfectly practicable but requires considerable confidence in the surgical technique (McGinty and Matza, 1978). Quite firm manipulation of the leg is sometimes required during arthroscopy. If local anaesthesia is used the patient may resist. General anaesthesia is preferred by most surgeons, but local anaesthesia is an accepted alternative in exceptional circumstances. Spinal anaesthesia is also practicable, and is preferred by some to general anaesthesia.

The choice of anaesthetic is dictated largely by local circumstances but it should be said that general anaesthesia is much to be preferred until the surgeon is sufficiently confident in his arthroscopic technique to allow the patient to be conscious and aware throughout his operation.

11.3.3 DAY CASE SURGERY

Day case arthroscopic surgery is practicable and is the standard technique in some centres. There is little to be said against this practice provided that the follow-up care after discharge is adequate. About 1% of patients develop an haemarthrosis and failure to recognize this complication and deal with it promptly will lead to pain, quadriceps inhibition and all the problems of arthrotomy that arthroscopic surgery is intended to avoid. Discharge of the patient to a distant place on the day of operation without proper follow-up arrangements by staff familiar with arthroscopic surgery may have disastrous consequences. It is preferable, for these reasons, to retain the patient in hospital until the day following operation to be certain that the knee is satisfactory before his discharge, and that the patient has been properly instructed by the physiotherapist in straight-leg raising and in walking.

11.3.4 SKILLS REQUIRED

It has already been said that the borderline between diagnostic and operative arthroscopy is hard to define. Examination of a doubtful meniscus lesion with a probing hook is a diagnostic procedure yet is technically more difficult than synovial biopsy in the suprapatellar pouch, which was first introduced by rheumatologists as an out-patient operation under local anaesthesia. In making the transition from diagnostic arthroscopy to arthroscopic surgery, the surgeon should be aware that he must progress gradually from the simple to the less simple procedures as experience is gained and skill in instrument handling improves.

Complete confidence in the use of the arthroscope for diagnosis is essential before attempting arthroscopic surgery and failure to appreciate this will create difficulties for both the patient and the surgeon. Familiarity with the probing hook is essential not only because of its value in diagnosis but because manipulation of the hook within the joint requires the same visuospatial skills as manipulation of a cutting instrument. If the surgeon cannot bring a blunt hook to the lesion he wishes to cut, he will not be able to reach it with a potentially dangerous cutting instrument either. 'Rehearsal' of the operation with the hook before inserting the instrument is good practice and makes it possible for the surgeon to assess his ability to accomplish the procedure that he is considering before he has become too deeply involved.

11.4 Approaches

Familiarity with several arthroscopic approaches is essential (Fig. 11.1). To attempt an arthroscopic operation knowing only one or perhaps two approaches is to introduce into the operation an element of chance that is best avoided. The anterolateral approach is probably the single most useful insertion for both diagnostic and operative arthroscopy but the central approach, which passes through the patellar tendon in the mid-line of the knee 1 cm below the lower pole of the patella, is an alternative preferred by some surgeons. The anteromedial approach is invaluable for inserting instruments when operating on the meniscus and the intercondylar notch, when the instrument and arthroscope may need to be transposed.

The exact point of entry for the anteromedial approach must be selected precisely. If the lesion to be dealt with is in the medial gutter, the incision should be made immediately above the meniscus so that the medial femoral condyle does not obstruct the movement of the instruments, but if the back of the intercondylar notch must be reached as, for example, when removing a locked bucket-handle fragment, the operation will be made impossible if this approach is used because the arthroscope, instrument and meniscal fragment will collide with each other since they all lie in the same horizontal plane. If the back of the notch is to be reached, the incision for the instruments must be made about 1 cm higher than the arthroscope so that they can reach over the top of the bucket-handle fragment to the back of the notch – one of the points of detail that makes the difference between difficulty and simplicity of operation.

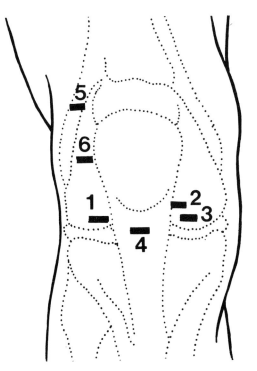

Fig. 11.1 The approaches most useful in athroscopic surgery. 1. The anterolateral approach; 2. the anteromedial approach to reach the back of the intercondylar notch; 3. the anteromedial approach to reach the medial gutter; 4. the central approach; 5. the lateral suprapatellar approach; 6. the lateral mid-patellar approach.

The posteromedial compartment, which can be entered either through the intercondylar notch from an anterior approach or directly from the postero-medial approach, is an important area of the knee because it is a frequent hiding place for loose bodies and meniscal debris. The posterior cruciate can also be seen in the lateral wall of this compartment, and its integrity assessed. Unless the posteromedial compartment can be entered easily, as it can in most patients, the surgeon must be prepared to abandon his attempts at arthro-scopic surgery and proceed to a posteromedial arthrotomy with depressing regularity.

The lateral suprapatellar approach, made about 1 cm above the supero-lateral corner of the patella, gives an excellent view of the inferior surface of the patella from above, the infrapatellar fat pad, the popliteus tendon, and the synovial plicae. If the arthroscope is inserted a little more distally, half-way down the length of the patella at its lateral edge (the lateral mid-patellar approach), the anterior horns of the menisci can be seen. With the help of a 70° telescope even the posterior part of the intercondylar notch can be seen from this approach, which is particularly helpful if there are abnormalities of the fat pad or the anterior horns of the menisci.

The straight-ahead 0° telescope is primarily for beginners and can be helpful in the learning stages when it is difficult to align the instrument and arthroscope correctly, but should be exchanged as soon as possible for the 30° telescope, which is the basic instrument for arthroscopic surgery. Correct use of the 30° arthroscope makes it possible to 'look round corners', and thus to keep the telescope away from the operating instruments.

The 70° telescope is useful enough to be kept sterile for occasional use but not so useful that it need be put out for every operation. The periphery of the view of the 70° telescope looks back towards the observer, making it particularly valuable for assessing the posterior recesses of the knee. Orientation is difficult with the 70° telescope and, although experience brings ease and familiarity with its use, it has no advantage over the 30° arthroscope for routine use. Nevertheless, use of the 70° telescope is a skill worth acquiring.

11.5 Equipment

The basic tools of arthroscopic surgery are simple hand instruments (Fig. 11.2). A trocar and cannula are useful for making the initial insertion for the

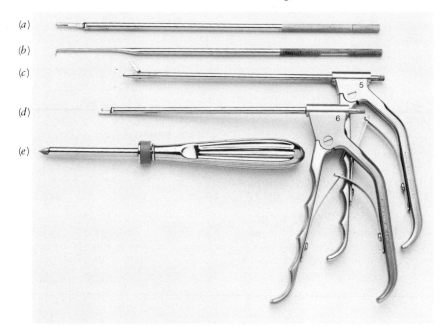

Fig. 11.2 Instruments for arthroscopic surgery. (*a*) Knife with disposable blade; (*b*) blunt probing hook; (*c*) straight meniscal scissors; (*d*) guillotine; (*e*) trocar and cannula.

operating instruments, as well as for inserting those with a circular cross-section, such as the blunt probing hook or a long-handled knife with disposable blades. A pair of scissors, punch or basket forceps, straight and curved rongeurs, grasping forceps and guillotine make up the basic set of instruments (Fig. 11.3). The instruments are designed so that their tips are smooth and rounded to minimize damage to the articular surface, with a hinge mechanism strong enough to stand up to heavy use without fracture, and cutting edges sharp enough to cut the meniscus.

Apart from these basic instruments, a number of other hand instruments are occasionally useful. A bone awl and a mounted Kirschner wire can be used for drilling the bases of bony defects, and a sharp curette for smoothing areas of irregular articular cartilage (Fig. 11.4). Powered instruments are occasionally useful. The shaver, for example, can be used to contour the edge of the meniscus after partial meniscectomy and to smooth areas of chondromalacia patellae but it will do little that is not accomplished as easily with hand instruments (Fig. 11.5). The shaver is, however, very useful for removing exuberant synovium, but a synovectomy performed in this way is essentially partial since it removes only the fronds and not the membrane itself. Powered instruments will not overcome any shortcomings in technique and will not make arthroscopic surgery any easier but are sometimes helpful if used cautiously; they are not an item of basic equipment, and should not be among the first instruments purchased by the surgeon embarking on arthroscopy.

The operating arthroscope is another useful accessory that makes some procedures a little easier but present designs of instruments do nothing that cannot be done with the basic set (Fig. 11.6). The limitations of the operating arthroscope are several. First, the instruments will move only in a straight line parallel with the telescope; this imposes considerable restrictions on the techniques that are possible because many structures need to be cut from the side. Secondly, the need for the arthroscope to carry the operating instruments as well as telescope, irrigation channel and light fibres, makes it much

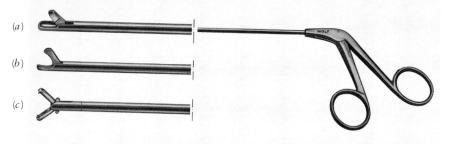

Fig. 11.3   Instruments for arthroscopic surgery. (*a*) Basket, or punch, forceps; (*b*) hook scissors; (*c*) toothed grasping forceps.

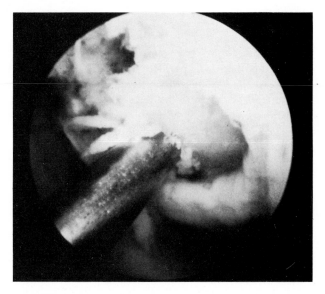

Fig. 11.4 Drilling the articular cartilage defect resulting from a chondral separation on the lateral femoral condyle using a Kirschner wire.

more bulky than the diagnostic arthroscope as well as limiting the size, and thus the strength, of the cutting instruments. The telescope in many operating arthroscopes is smaller than that of the diagnostic arthroscope, which in turn restricts the field of vision and makes orientation difficult. In short, although the operating arthroscope and powered shaver make several procedures a little easier, they are not essential for arthroscopic surgery and are not part of the basic set of instruments.

11.6   Techniques

Arthroscopic surgery can be performed by a variety of techniques but it must not be thought that the various techniques are in competition with each other. Rather than being in competition, the techniques are complementary one to another and every surgeon should be thoroughly familiar with each (Dandy, 1981).

The double-puncture technique, in which instruments are inserted through a second channel and manipulated under control of the arthroscope inserted separately, is the commonest and most versatile technique. The usual point of insertion of the arthroscope is anterolateral with instruments inserted from the anteromedial approach, but each and every combination of approaches will be needed at some time. A disadvantage of the double-puncture technique is the difficulty of applying traction to an object being divided, for example, a meniscus. The triple-puncture overcomes this shortcoming but

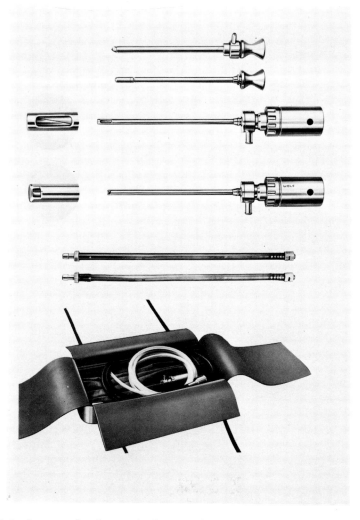

Fig. 11.5 A powered arthroscopic shaver and gouger.

requires a total of three incisions, one for the arthroscope, one for the grasping forceps and another for the cutting instruments. If the arthroscope is inserted from the central or lateral mid-patellar approach, the anterolateral and anteromedial approaches are available for operating instruments. While this technique is excellent in theory, difficulties arise in practice. There will be four objects in the joint to collide with each other – the meniscus, the arthroscope, grasping forceps and the cutting instrument. Secondly, the knee is not a particularly spacious joint even when distended with saline and precise manipulation of instruments is even more difficult if the synovial cavity is packed with metal. Finally, the technique requires three hands,

259

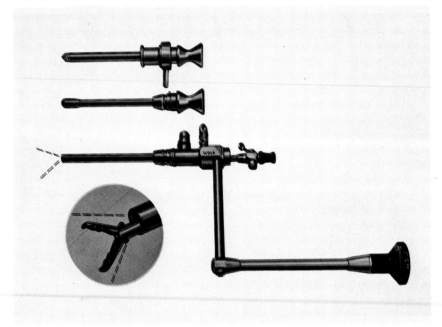

Fig. 11.6   An operating arthroscope.

making the help of an assistant necessary. The assistant will be unable to see what he is doing unless endoscopic television is available, and even then, orientation and co-ordination can be difficult.

The single-puncture technique using the operating arthroscope is superficially attractive, but is less than ideal for the reasons already mentioned. The operating arthroscope is best used when a grasping instrument has been applied to the object to be cut, and the operating arthroscope used to divide it at its base. This technique is particularly helpful when a synovial shelf or meniscal flap is being removed.

The surgeon should know all of these techniques and avoid the temptation to preach the merits of one technique over another. Although different surgeons are likely to prefer different techniques, there is no right or wrong way of performing an operation so long as the end result is satisfactory.

11.7   Complications

The complications of arthroscopic surgery are surprisingly few. Infection is a complication anticipated by most orthopaedic surgeons because they have been trained to maintain the highest standards of aseptic technique. Complete asepsis is impossible with arthroscopic surgery, which tends to be a 'semi-sterile' procedure; the eye-piece of the telescope is soon contaminated with the eye, the surgeon's glove touches the eye-piece and then the instruments, so that the total sterility is lost. Despite this, infection of the knee is exceptionally rare and the author has had no infections of the synovial cavity in over 3000 cases. The skin around the stitches occasionally becomes red, as it does after any procedure, but deep infection and stitch abscesses have not happened, although it is probable that an infection will eventually occur. Infections have been recorded by several surgeons after arthroscopic lateral release, when a large subcutaneous haematoma may form, and after arthroscopy through areas of infected or abraded skin. The very low incidence of infection after arthroscopic surgery is no excuse for poor technique and every effort should be made to avoid unnecessary contamination of the instruments that enter the knee, and to ensure that the tips are not touched at any stage after the arthroscope has been inserted.

Deep vein thrombosis can occur after any operation, and has an incidence of approximately 3 per 1000 after arthroscopic surgery. No serious pulmonary emboli have been reported after arthroscopy.

Although the 'traditional' complications of infection, deep vein thrombosis and quadriceps inhibition do not pose a problem after arthroscopic surgery, there are some new complications that do. Instruments break within the knee and the broken fragment may prove impossible to retrieve. The author has personally broken six instruments in the knee, and retrieved the broken fragments from four. The remaining two patients have small metallic fragments within the knee, one a small tenotomy blade embedded in the medial ligament (the use of tenotomy knives was rejected in the early stage of development of the technique because of this difficulty) and the other the jaw of a pair of basket forceps lying in the synovial sleeve that surrounds the posterior cruciate ligament. Although experience and careful handling of the instruments will reduce the incidence of instrument failure, it is unlikely to disappear completely and any surgeon who takes up arthroscopic surgery should work on the assumption that sooner or later he will break an instrument within the knee and be unable to retrieve the fragment.

Damage to the articular cartilage of the femoral condyle is easily inflicted by clumsy handling of the instruments and can be minimized by care and proper attention to the points of insertion, as well as by 'rehearsing' the operation with a blunt hook before inserting the cutting instrument. The appearance of the damaged cartilage is magnified by the arthroscope and can appear quite alarming. Repeat arthroscopy of the joint after a number of years will usually show that the articular surface has smoothed over without trace of injury, an observation that should not be taken as a licence to inflict unnecessary damage on healthy articular cartilage by clumsy instrument handling.

Haemarthrosis is a common complication after conventional arthrotomy and occurs after arthroscopic surgery in approximately 1% of patients. If a patient is unable to lift the leg straight within 24 hours of operation, it is very likely that a haemarthrosis has formed. If the blood is aspirated promptly, complete straight-leg raising will be restored immediately. If this is omitted, the haematoma may become organized and rehabilitation will be prolonged.

11.8 Methods of learning

It is not the purpose of this chapter to describe the practical details of arthroscopic surgery, which can only be learned by experience. The comments on learning diagnostic arthroscopy in Chapter 4 apply also to the learning of arthroscopic surgery. Although textbooks can describe the correct point of insertion of the instruments in the various approaches to different lesions, the skills of the technique can only be acquired by practice and experience.

Bringing the instrument in front of the arthroscope, referred to as triangulation, depends on the development of new visuospatial skills which some surgeons find easy to learn and others virtually impossible. Triangulation can be learned just as well on the knee model as on a live patient, although the models are never completely realistic. Models are also helpful in learning the correct sequence of the stages of the various operations, in the handling of the arthroscope, and in perceiving depth and perspective with monocular vision.

Video tapes and the observation of operations on a television monitor are also valuable in demonstrating the arthroscopic view, but no audiovisual aid can replace experience and practice. It has already been mentioned that arthroscopy is not a 'spectator sport', and that it is usual for the introduction of arthroscopic surgery to meet with the profound disapproval of operating theatre personnel of all grades. At first, it is advisable to limit the time spent on arthroscopy to, say, 20 minutes, and then to proceed to arthrotomy if progress is slow. In time, more and more can be accomplished in the period allotted, and the range of operations gradually extended. The alternative approach is to continue the arthroscopy without time limit, but this approach is more likely to lead to hostility and frustration than to success.

Learning arthroscopy has to be taken more conscientiously than the learning of other surgical techniques, and is perhaps best approached by reading an instructional book on the subject, attending a course, and even visiting a centre where the technique is regularly performed. Above all, it must be recognized that arthroscopic surgery is not only difficult, but that it is so radically different from other types of orthopaedic surgery that everyone learning the technique must start from basic principles. Skill with a hammer is no help when learning to triangulate.

11.9 Future of arthroscopy

The future of arthroscopy and arthroscopic surgery is a matter for speculation. In the USA there are now many surgeons whose practice is limited to arthroscopic surgery and who refer patients with knee conditions not amenable to arthroscopic techniques to other colleagues. Although this approach has some advantages in that it concentrates arthroscopic skills and may well provide us with the analysis of results that are so urgently needed a little more quickly than otherwise would be the case, the long-term future for arthroscopic surgery as an exclusive speciality is perhaps on less firm foundations. One does not hear of cystoscopic surgeons but of urologists, and of gynaecologists rather than laparoscopic surgeons. If a new speciality is to emerge as the result of the arthroscope, it is more likely to be that of knee surgery than of arthroscopic surgery. Only the future will determine if this surmise is correct.

References

Dandy D J. Early results of closed partial meniscectomy. *Br Med J* 1978;1:1099–100.

Dandy D J. *Arthroscopic surgery of the knee*. London and Edinburgh: Churchill Livingstone, 1981.

Dandy D J, Flanagan J P, Steenmeyer V. Arthroscopy and the management of the ruptured anterior cruciate ligament. *Clin Orthop Rel Res* 1982;167:43–9.

Dandy D J, Jackson R W. The diagnosis of problems after meniscectomy. *J Bone Joint Surg* [*Br*] 1975;57–B:349–52.

Dandy D J, O'Carroll P F. Arthroscopic surgery of the knee. General experience of the first 1000 cases. *Br Med J* 1982a;285:1256–8.

Dandy D J, O'Carroll P F. Removal of loose bodies from the knee under arthroscopic control *J Bone Joint Surg* [*Br*] 1982b;64–B:473–4.

Fujisawa J. Problems caused by the medial and lateral synovial folds of the patella. *Kanstetsukyo* 1976;1:40–4.

McGinty J B, Matza R A. Arthroscopy of the knee. Evaluation of an out-patient procedure under local anaesthesia. *J Bone Joint Surg* [*Am*] 1978;60–A:787–9.

Northmore-Ball M D, Dandy D J, Jackson R W. A comparative study of the results of arthroscopic and open partial meniscectomy. *Br. Orthop Assoc* April, 1981.

Oretorp N, Gillquist J. Transcutaneous meniscectomy under arthroscopic control. *Internat Orthop* 1979;3:19–25.

Patel D. Arthroscopy of the plica-synovial folds and their significance. *Am J Sports Med* 1978;6:217–25.

CHAPTER 12

Restoration
of Flexion

William Waugh

It is not often necessary to carry out operations to restore flexion of the knee joint, but the fact that quadricepsplasty is such a satisfactory procedure justifies a description of the technique and management afterwards. First, it seems reasonable to discuss briefly an entirely separate cause of loss of flexion.

12.1 Quadriceps contracture following injections

Progressive fibrosis of the vastus intermedius in children was first described by Fairbank and Barrett (1961) and Hněvkovsky (1961). The cause was considered to be repeated intramuscular injections in infancy and the result was loss of flexion of varying degree. Further series of cases were reported (Karlen, 1964; Gunn, 1964; Lloyd-Roberts and Thomas, 1964). Williams (1968) demonstrated that habitual dislocation of the patella was a related condition which occurred when the contracture was in vastus lateralis. In this case, if the patella is held in the midline then the knee cannot be flexed.

Bose and Ching (1976) described 38 Asian children and adolescents who presented with either stiffness of the knee, genu recurvatum, habitual dislocation or dislocation of the patella. These conditions were all considered to be manifestations of a contracture of the extensor mechanism. In the first group the main components involved were in the mid-line of the limb and in the second group the vastus lateralis and the iliotibial band were affected. It was recommended that operation be undertaken as early as possible in order to avoid secondary adaptive changes and the results were reported to be satisfactory.

When there is loss of flexion from this cause the extensor mechanism should be explored through a mid-line incision. The rectus femoris tendon is isolated from vastus medialis and vastus lateralis. The vastus intermedius (which is the commonest site of the contracture) is divided. If the knee cannot then be flexed past a right angle it may be necessary to lengthen the rectus femoris tendon. This operation is thus similar, but rather more limited, to the technique of surgical mobilization of the knee which will now be considered in rather more detail.

12.2 Loss of flexion due to injury

Better methods of treatment have led to a decreased risk of stiffness of the knee following fractures of the shaft of the femur. Adequate internal fixation can be followed by early mobilization and the use of cast bracing results in rapid restoration of function in patients treated without operation (Wardlaw *et al.*, 1981; Thomas and Meggit, 1981; Roper, 1981). Delayed union, infection and repeated operations can, however, still result in loss of flexion. Furthermore, the violence producing the fracture may also cause direct bony or soft-tissue damage to the knee itself and this will be an important factor: intra-articular adhesions may be responsible for the limitation of flexion as well as adhesions in the quadriceps muscle.

Although lengthening of quadriceps tendon to restore flexion was described many years ago (Bennett, 1922), the first account in the English literature of the modern quadricepsplasty operation was by Campbell Thompson in 1944. Judet (1959) described a different technique which he claimed gave better results. Intra-articular adhesions were first divided through a short anteromedial incision. A long posterolateral incision was used through which the vastus lateralis was detached from the linea aspera and the vastus intermedius freed from its attachment on the lateral and anterior surfaces of the femur. This method not only restored flexion satisfactorily in the 53 operations which were reported, but reduced the incidence of an extensor lag.

Daoud *et al.* (1982) used the Judet operation in 6 patients and concluded from their results that it was superior to the Thompson operation.

Nicoll (1964) made a most important contribution in describing his experience with the Thompson type of quadricepsplasty and at this time he gave a rational description of the mechanisms which produced limitation of flexion. He emphasized not only the part played by fibrosis of the vastus intermedius, but he stressed the importance of retropatellar adhesions (Fig. 12.1) and of fibrosis in the lateral expansions of the vasti, which he called the 'check-rein' effect (Fig. 12.2). This together with adhesions in the paracondylar gutters, will fix the patella and prevent the normal excursion which takes place during flexion (Fig. 12.3). His good results were due not only to the operative technique, but to meticulous attention to a regime of management after the operation. Subsequently, he had a series of more than 80 operations (Nicoll, 1982). The average gain in flexion was 70°. Only five patients had a residual extension lag and this was compatible with excellent function since full passive extension was maintained.

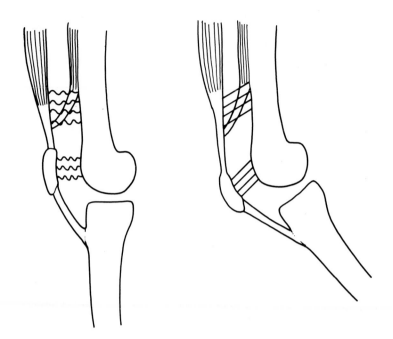

Fig. 12.1 Diagram showing retropatellar adhesions and adhesions between rectus femoris and vastus intermedius.

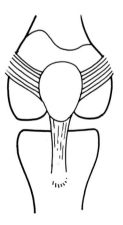

Fig. 12.2 Diagram showing site of fibrosis in the capsule which anchors the patella.

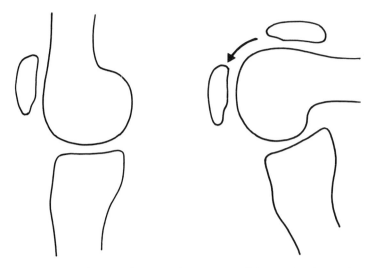

Fig. 12.3 Diagram showing the normal excursion of the patella during flexion.

A paper by Hesketh (1963) also reported good results in ten patients. Further accounts of experience with the operation have been published by Jeffrey (1972) seven cases, Thomas (1972) nine cases and Pick (1976) three cases.

The author was particularly fortunate in being able to work with Nicoll in the 1960s, and so learnt detailed operative technique and management. The following description follows Nicoll's method and is based on experience of 12 operations.

12.2.1 CAUSES OF STIFFNESS

In this series ten patients had sustained a fracture of the femur; in four there was also a fracture of the patella and in two an associated fracture of the tibia. There were two other unusual cases which illustrate that the operation can be done when the damage is confined to the knee joint: in one patient, loss of flexion occurred after a repair of a medial ligament tear which was followed by new bone formation in the soft tissue; in the other, adhesions followed infection after a meniscectomy which had been carried out abroad.

12.2.2 REQUIREMENTS FOR A SUCCESSFUL OUTCOME

(1) The loss of flexion should be sufficient to produce disability in each individual patient. In the author's series every patient had less than 50° of flexion. There may, however, be special circumstances when the operation may be considered; if, for example, 90° of flexion is not enough to allow a

particular job to be carried out. It is important to have a realistic aim and the patient must understand the possible risks and consequences of failure.

(2) It is, of course, essential that the patient must have made determined efforts to regain movement by persistent vigorous exercises. The quadriceps must be strong and full, active and passive extension must be possible. The operation can be successful even when the patella has been removed.

(3) The articular surfaces should be reasonably smooth. This is difficult to define, but it is usually possible to reach a decision before operation. Correctly centred radiographs are necessary to demonstrate that the 'cartilage space' is preserved. Clearly, gross irregularity and destruction of the articular surfaces will be a contraindication, but it is possible to restore movement when there is some degree of cartilage damage.

(4) The skin on the front of the knee should be in a good condition. The presence of scarring will increase the risk of necrosis which will inevitably prevent vigorous exercises in the early stages and so prejudice the result.

(5) There should be no sign of residual infection in or around the knee joint.

(6) Once it is clear that the knee is completely 'stuck' the operation should not be delayed. However, it is possible to restore movement after many years of stiffness. In one patient who was operated on six years after injury the range of flexion was increased from 40° to 135°.

(7) As might be expected the best results are achieved in young active people and it is probably wise not to operate on those over the age of 50 years.

12.2.3   OPERATIVE TECHNIQUE

The operation is not difficult, but it needs to be carried out meticulously and with confidence. It will be seen that the procedure is more than a quadricepsplasty and it might better be called *surgical mobilization of the stiff knee.*

(1) A tourniquet is used.

(2) The skin incision should be straight and precisely in the mid-line extending from distal to the tibial tuberosity to at least mid-way between the knee and hip (Fig. 12.4). A transverse scar over the knee can be safely crossed at a right angle. It is, however, wrong to be parallel to another longitudinal scar. If the earlier scar is near to the mid-line it can be used again, but it is important to avoid raising skin flaps for more than 2 or 3 cm.

(3) Incisions through the soft tissues and capsule are made on each side of the patellar tendon and extended proximally on each side of the patella so that the knee joint is opened. The parallel incisions are then continued so that the tendon of rectus femoris is completely isolated from vastus medialis and lateralis (Fig. 12.5).

(4) The next step is to explore the knee and whatever the cause of the stiffness, there will be almost certainly intra-articular adhesions to a greater or lesser extent. The patella may be stuck to the lower end of the femur and

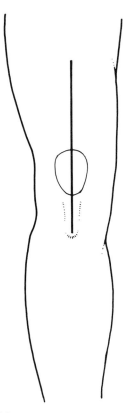

Fig. 12.4 The skin incision.

must be separated from it by sharp dissection. This will allow the patella and its tendon to be lifted up freely. Dissection is then carried out on first the medial and then the lateral side of the knee, so that adhesions in the para-condylar gutters are widely divided. This is an essential step after which it may be possible to bend the knee with controlled force past a right angle.

(5) There may, of course, be dense adhesions in the thigh muscles. Rectus femoris must be completely separated from vastus intermedius by dissection with scissors (Fig. 12.6). This can be extended proximally as far as is necessary.

(6) It is usually now possible to flex the knee sufficiently, say to 120° or 130°. The author has never found it necessary to lengthen the rectus femoris tendon and this certainly should be avoided unless it is clearly the only obstruction to regaining what seems to be a reasonable degree of flexion.

(7) Once maximum flexion has been achieved the tourniquet can be removed and most of the bleeding will stop when the knee is flexed. No deep stitches are needed and no attempt is made to suture the vasti back to the

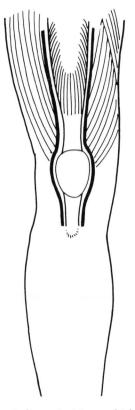

Fig. 12.5 The thick lines indicate incisions which are made through the deeper tissues and which allow the patellar tendon, the patella and the rectus femoris to be isolated.

rectus tendon. The skin must be closed meticulously and it is essential to obtain primary healing.

(8) It is now necessary to decide the angle of flexion at which the knee is to be immobilized. This is a matter of judgement, but the knee is to be flexed to the maximum which can be achieved without undue force and then extended 20° or 30°. This means that in most cases the angle will be in the region of 90°. It is important to be sure that there is adequate circulation to the skin edges before applying dressings.

(9) A plaster cast is applied over a thick dressing with the knee at about a right angle. The case must be split through its length. The foot need not be included.

12.2.4 TREATMENT AFTER OPERATION

The leg is elevated on pillows with the hip at a right angle.

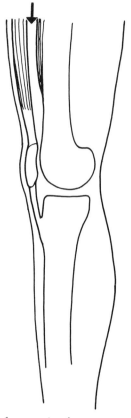

Fig. 12.6 Shows the plane of separation between rectus femoris and vastus inter-medius.

After 48 hours, the surgeon should remove the cast, the knee is then allowed to extend slowly. This can be painful and sedation should be used. The patient may be apprehensive and the surgeon should hold the leg himself and not delegate this task to others. The reasons for this are psychological rather than physical, but there is no doubt that it is important to maintain the patient's confidence. When the knee is straight a plaster back splint is made in this position. The knee is then gently flexed and a second splint is made on the front of the leg with the knee in the flexed position. The knee is kept straight at night and flexed during the day.

The splint should be removed for exercise every hour during the day. The physiotherapist needs to be gentle, but firm, if the range of movement is to be maintained. Efforts must also be made to restore quadriceps function.

The patient's progress dictates the pace of treatment and the splints usually discarded after three weeks. It may be that a powered exercise machine might be useful in some instances.

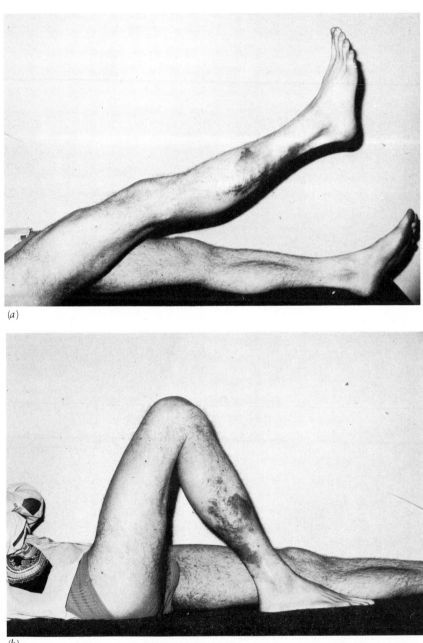

(a)

(b)

Fig. 12.7 Shows the result in a patient in whom the operation was carried out six years after a fracture of the femur, of the patella and of the tibia in the same leg. The range of movement was 0–40° and flexion has been improved by 120°. (a) shows full action extension and (b) the range of flexion; both after operation.

If progress is slow, manipulation should be carried out early when only a little force is necessary. Indecision and delay make manipulation difficult and often ineffective. If considerable force is used there is a risk of rupturing the patellar tendon or of producing a supracondylar fracture.

12.2.5 RESULTS

The range of movement before and after operation on 12 patients is shown in Table 12.1.

A useful improvement was usually achieved, but three patients did not maintain flexion to a right angle. In one, movement was lost as a result of a complication which will be described below. An example of a successful outcome is shown in Fig. 12.7(a) and (b).

12.2.6 COMPLICATIONS

(a) Skin necrosis

Any delay in healing is likely to result in loss of movement and skin necrosis which occurred in one patient was particularly disastrous. Immobilizing the knee in too much flexion at the end of the operation is a possible cause and the importance of attention to this has already been emphasized. This occurred in the one patient in the series who lost movement and is recorded at the end of Table 12.1. Figure 12.8(a) and (b) show the area the necrosis at three weeks and the more extensive skin loss at three months. Poor skin over the patella and associated scarring are a contraindication to the operation.

Table 12.1

Before	After
10	80
50	115
45	110
15	70
20	150
40	120
25	110
25	100
45	120
30	90
45	110
35	20

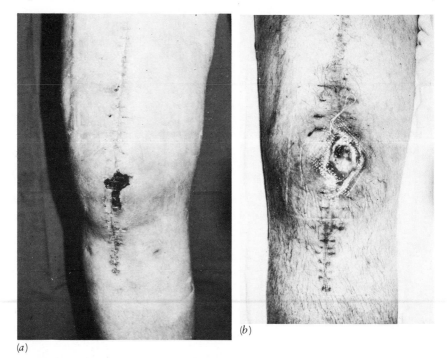

(a)

(b)

Fig. 12.8 (a) Shows an area of skin necrosis over the patella three weeks after operation. (b) shows the area of skin loss at three months. The knee flexed to 35°, but the movement gained at operation was lost and flexion was only possible to 20° one year later.

(b) Haematoma

One patient developed a large haematoma. After some delay the wound was reopened, but nevertheless she had 110° of flexion after one year. It is clear that a haematoma should be evacuated without delay and the wound sutured. This does not necessarily prejudice the result.

(c) Extension lag

It is usual to find an extension lag for 2–3 months after the operation. In some patients it may persist for longer and it may take up to a year before full extension is achieved. The only patient in this series of 12 operations who had a persistent extensor lag was the man whose operation was complicated by skin necrosis. A lag is only likely to persist if the rectus femoris has been lengthened and even then it may not produce too much functional disability (except on steps and stairs) provided full passive extension is possible.

274

12.2.7 CONCLUSION

Surgical mobilization of the stiff knee will give excellent results provided the requirements for success, which have been outlined, are understood. The operation can be carried out with confidence and the patient must be capable of taking part in the programme of exercises which is necessary afterwards. Patience and determination are needed by all concerned, but the gradual restoration of flexion is an adequate reward.

ACKNOWLEDGEMENT

The author is grateful to Mr E. A. Nicoll for his instruction about all aspects of the operation. Mr Nicoll was also good enough to read this paper in typescript and to make helpful suggestions.

References

Bennett G E. Lengthening of the quadriceps tendon. *J Bone Joint Surg* [*Br*] 1922;4–B:593–9.

Bose K, Ching K C. The clinical manifestations and pathomechanics of contracture of the extensor mechanism of the knee. *J Bone Joint Surg* [*Br*] 1976;58–B:478–84.

Daoud H, O'Farrell T, Cruess R L. Quadricepsplasty. *J Bone Joint Surg* [*Br*] 1982;64–B:194–7.

Fairbank T J, Barrett A M. Vastus intermedius contracture in early childhood. *J Bone Joint Surg* [*Br*] 1961;43–B:326–34.

Gunn D R. Contracture of the quadriceps muscle. *J Bone Joint Surg* [*Br*] 1964;46:492.

Hesketh K T. Experiences with the Thompson quadricepsplasty. *J Bone Joint Surg* [*Br*] 1963; 45–B:91–5.

Hněvkovsky O. Progressive fibrosis of the vastus intermedius muscle in children. *J Bone Joint Surg* [*Br*] 1961;43–B:318–25.

Jeffrey C C. Quadricepsplasty. *Injury* 1972;4:131–36.

Judet R. Mobilisation of the stiff knee. *J Bone Joint Surg* [*Br*] 1959;41–B:856–7,

Karlen A. Congenital fibrosis of the vastus intermedius muscle. *J Bone Joint Surg* [*Br*] 1964;46–B:488–91.

Lloyd-Roberts G C, Thomas T G. The aetiology of quadriceps contracture in children. *J Bone Joint Surg* [*Br*] 1964;46–B:498–502.

Nicoll E A. Quadricepsplasty. *J Bone Joint Surg* [*Br*] 1963;45–B:483–90.

Nicoll E A. Quadricepsplasty. *Postgrad Med J* 1964;40:521–6.

Nicoll E A. Personal communication, 1982.

Roper B A. Functional bracing of femoral fractures (editorial). *J Bone Joint Surg* [*Br*] 1981; 63:1–2.

Pick R Y. Quadricepsplasty. *Clin Orthop Rel Res* 1976;120:138–41.

Thomas F B. Quadricepsplasty. *Injury* 1972;4:137–41.

Thomas F B, Meggit B F. A comparative study of methods for treating fractures of the distal half of the femur. *J Bone Joint Surg* [*Br*] 1981;63–B:3–22.

Thompson T C. Quadricepsplasty to improve knee function. *J Bone Joint Surg* [Br] 1944;26–B:366–79.

Wardlaw D, McLauchlan J, Pratt D J, Bowker P. A biomechanical study of cast-brace treatment of femoral shaft fractures. *J Bone Joint Surg* [*Br*] 1981;63–B:7–11.

Williams P F. Quadriceps contracture. *J Bone Joint Surg* [*Br*] 1968;50–B:278–84.

PART THREE

Chronic Arthritis

CHAPTER 13

Osteoarthritis
of the Knee

J. P. Jackson and
W. Waugh

13.1   Introduction

Pain in the knee is a common complaint and one of the most frequent causes is osteoarthritis. Radiographic signs of this condition are often present, but not all individuals with these changes have symptoms. Lawrence *et al.* (1966) reported a survey of male industrial workers, of whom 24% had 'degenerative' joint changes and complained of pain, whereas 8% of those examined had pain without radiographic evidence of osteoarthritis or other disease. Environmental conditions, such as cold and wet, were associated with more frequent complaints; whereas workers in a warmer atmosphere had less incapacity despite a high incidence of radiographic changes.

The incidence of osteoarthritis of the knee may depend on a number of factors. In those occupations involving trauma to the joint, such as footballing or coal mining, the condition is frequent (Kellgren *et al.*, 1953). Fat

279

people suffer from osteoarthritis of the knees and not of the hip preferentially (Lawrence *et al.*, 1966), though the reason for this not obvious.

13.2   Osteoarthritis or osteoarthrosis?

Medical terminology is constantly changing and the reasons given are sometimes, but not always, good; however, should we be writing about osteoarthritis or osteoarthrosis or 'degenerative changes'?

First, we must ask whether it is right to consider osteoarthritis as a purely degenerative condition with the implication that its occurrence is part of the normal ageing process? This matter has been succinctly reviewed by Meachim (1980). It is difficult not to agree that osteoarthritic articular cartilage breakdown should be distinguished from age-related cartilage breakdown. The concept that osteoarthritis is a progressive condition (Byers *et al.*, 1970) should be acceptable to orthopaedic surgeons who are able to observe deterioration is untreated osteoarthritic knees. The argument can be extended by suggesting that osteophyte formation could be regarded as a teleological response which is part of a repair mechanism intended to increase the articular load-bearing surface which has become diminished as a result of a mechanical derangement. Repair takes place by an inflammatory process and this in itself may seem to justify the suffix '. . . itis' rather than '. . .osis', although Radin (1976) specifically disagrees with this point. Perhaps the hypervascularization demonstrated by Harrison *et al.* (1953) is also part of an inflammatory response. Those who see the inside of osteoarthritic joints also know that there is frequently an associated synovitis.

If this argument seems a little thin to those with other views, the argument against '. . .osis' can be put on firm etymological grounds. Adams (1981) points out that in ancient Greek '. . .itis' implies any disease of the part affected and it has been misapplied in recent years to denote inflammatory disease. The suffix '. . .osis', on the other hand, had a meaning quite unrelated to disease and implied a process or activity (as in metamorphosis).

Osteoarthrosis has had its vogue; its introduction was not universally accepted and now rapidly seems to be in decline. The *British Journal of Bone and Joint Surgery* has always preferred osteoarthritis (Catterall, 1982) and those of us who never adopted the new fashion of osteoarthrosis are not only in good company, but have both semantic and etymological justification for our prejudice. Orthopaedic surgeons all know what they mean when they speak of osteoarthritis and it might be best if we stopped talking about degeneration when we mean the osteoarthritis which affects our patients.

The earliest radiographic signs of osteoarthritis are loss of articular cartilage and subchondral sclerosis (Fig. 13.1). The sclerosis represents trabecular hypertrophy which is the response of bone to increased load per unit area. With time trabecular microfractures follow and this will result in bony collapse (Fig. 13.2). Consequently, there are areas of very hard bone and also,

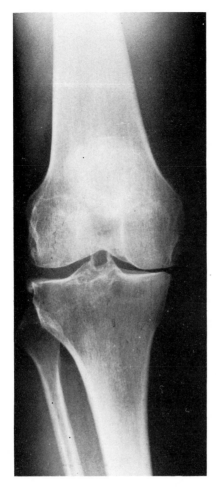

Fig. 13.1 This radiograph shows early medial compartment osteoarthritis with partial loss of articular cartilage (Ahlbäck type 1).

(often on the opposite side of the joint) areas of very soft bone as a result of lack of pressure. For example, in medial compartment osteoarthritis the bone in the medial femoral and tibial condyles will be hard and that in the lateral femoral and tibial condyles will be relatively soft.

It is relevant at this point to refer to the potential for repair which exists in osteoarthritic joints. This is of particular interest in relation to tibial osteotomy and Coventry (1979) has produced histological evidence which confirms that regeneration can occur after this operation. Maquet (1980a) bases his assumptions of repair on detailed radiological studies which are convincing. More direct evidence from arthroscopy has come from Japan (Fujisawa *et al.*, 1979). Bauer (1982) concludes that 'osteotomy performed at

281

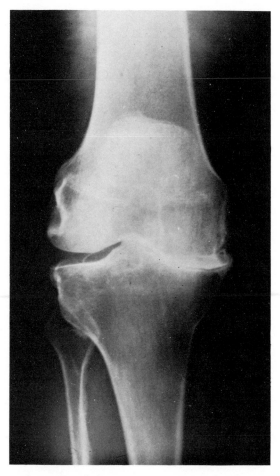

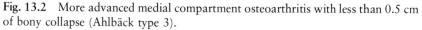

Fig. 13.2 More advanced medial compartment osteoarthritis with less than 0.5 cm of bony collapse (Ahlbäck type 3).

a reasonably early stage may not only arrest the condition, but also even produce permanent improvement of the articular cartilage'.

13.3 Some causal factors

Underlying mechanical factors may be obvious in many knees affected by osteoarthritis. For example, disorders which produce irregularities of the surface of the joint (such as osteochondritis dissecans, inflammatory disease or trauma) are frequently followed by osteoarthritic changes which are tempting to describe as 'abnormal wear'. This phrase may be useful in explaining the condition to patients, but it does not do justice to the complexities of the developing osteoarthritic lesion. Changes in the mechanisms of joint loading within the knee have been shown to follow meniscectomy (Chapter 5, page 138) and may explain the occurrence of osteoarthritis. Changes at a distance from the joint (for example, following varus malunion of a femoral or tibial fracture) may have similar consequences.

However, in many patients there may well be no obvious aetiological factor which can explain the cause of their osteoarthritis. Helfet (1974) suggested that in most instances there was likely to be an undiscovered meniscal tear which was responsible. In contradiction to this, Noble and Hamblen (1975) found that 'meniscal tears are common in joints with no sign of osteoarthritis'.

The primary cause of osteoarthritis is likely to lie in disorders of proteoglycan synthesis and related disintegration of the collagen framework, but there are two theories which have been put forward and need to be considered since they can be used to provide a rational explanation for the success of an operation such as a tibial osteotomy.

13.3.1 INTRAOSSEOUS HYPERTENSION

Brookes and Helal (1968) demonstrated that the subchondral medullary sinusoids were distended in primary osteoarthritis and that injected Hypaque cleared more slowly than in normal knees. All these patients gave a history of diffuse aching pain. Pain was relieved after tibial osteotomy in 14 patients and it was demonstrated that the distended subchondral vessels returned to normal. Sinusoidal engorgement produced experimentally in rats resulted in the formation of a thicker subchondral bone plate and stouter trabeculation both in the tibia and femur.

Arnoldi *et al.* (1975) were not able to show such a clear relationship between osteoarthritis and venous hypertension. Although some patients with a raised intraosseous pressure (above 40 mm Hg) suffered from rest pain, this was not always associated with osteoarthritis. Patients with painful osteoarthritis often had a low intramedullary pressure in the tibia, although that in the femur was high. Their conclusion was that there was an association between pain and intraosseous hypertension, but not between increased intraosseous pressure and the presence of osteoarthritis.

13.3.2 MECHANICAL ASPECTS

Radin (1976) suggested that the initiating cause of osteoarthritis (he prefers 'osteoarthrosis') is increased stress on articular cartilage which may follow 'low magnitude, poorly prepared for, impulsive loading'. Consequent trabecular microfractures heal and so the subchondral bone becomes stiffer which results in further progressive damage to articular cartilage. It is not clear whether the cartilage changes precede the bony changes or vice versa, but there appears to be an intimate relationship between the changes in these two tissues. Radin concluded his review by suggesting that further clarification of the interrelationship between mechanical stress and cellular metabolism should allow an entirely new approach to treatment.

Whatever the initial cause of osteoarthritis, it is inevitable that once the changes have begun the joint stresses are altered so that the condition progresses. Correction of these stresses would, therefore, seem logical and provide a rationale for such procedures as osteotomy.

13.4   The natural history of osteoarthritis of the knee

Although osteoarthritis is common, our knowledge of its evolution in the knee joint is limited. Hernberg and Nilsson (1977) reviewed a series of patients who presented in Malmo between 1950 and 1958. Their criteria for diagnosis were that juxta-articular sclerosis should be visible in the radiographs of the femorotibial joint and, secondly, that there was no history of trauma, infection, rheumatoid arthritis or congenital deformity.

A total of 71 untreated patients were reviewed (94 knees), 56 were female and the age at diagnosis was 63 ± 8 years. Follow-up was from 10 to 18 years. In 49 patients (69%) the symptoms had become worse; 23 were unchanged but 15 had improved. Instability was worse in those knees that were unstable at the time of diagnosis. The osteoarthritis in most cases had remained confined to one compartment. They were unable to point to any poor prognostic factors except that the outlook was unfavourable if symptoms were first noticed when there were only early radiographic changes. Their observations suggested that some patients improved spontaneously, so it is wise to be sure that osteoarthritis is progressive before undertaking operative treatment.

At first, an ache is most often noticed after exercise; later pain and stiffness may develop after prolonged rest and improve rapidly with movement. As the condition worsens the pain occurs at rest and may be troublesome at night. The onset in most cases is slow, but occasionally it may be sudden and a haemarthrosis may occur without any apparent injury: this is probably due to trabecular microfractures. Many patients will attribute the onset of symptoms to an injury, either to a direct blow or a twist of the joint (page 285).

The site of the pain is often ill-defined, but it may occur on either side of the joint. Sometimes the pain seems to be in the affected tibiofemoral compartment, but at other times it is felt on the opposite side where the soft tissues are stretched (for example, the inner side of a valgus knee). When the patellofemoral compartment is most seriously affected the pain is felt around or just below the patella and is increased by walking up or down hills or stairs.

The pain of osteoarthritis comes and goes over the years; perhaps because patients tend to rest as the pain gets worse and in this way obtain temporary relief from their symptoms.

'Giving way' of the joint may be related to weakness of the quadriceps muscle or to ligamentous laxity. Those patients who develop a flexion contracture are more likely to complain of this symptom, since there is usually marked loss of quadriceps power.

13.5 Medico-legal implications

Many people who injure their knee (or any other joint) find it difficult to accept that osteoarthritis had been present previously, even when radiographs taken immediately after the accident show advanced changes. After all, they feel their knee did not hurt them before (and this is quite likely to be true), but it has been very painful since the incident. A doctor who is called on to write a report for solicitors or an insurance company can, to some extent at any rate, choose one of two explanations. It may be possible to suggest that if this particular joint had been normal at the time of the accident, the symptoms would have worn off in, say, six months. Alternatively, if the injury had not occurred then the joint would anyway have become painful within, say, the next five years. Unfortunately, there are no hard facts on which to base these surmises and in any individual cases it is necessary to try to be as fair as possible to all concerned. Sometimes, a compromise may be reached by putting forward the opinion that, in view of the minor nature of the violence (which is often the case), the effect of the injury could be said to have worn off after a 'reasonable time' and any subsequent disability attributed to the presence of the pre-existing osteoarthritis. The whole situation is made more difficult since it is impossible to relate the severity of the symptoms in osteoarthritis to the stage of radiographic changes. Lawyers are, of course, asking unanswerable questions, but provided doctors are reasonable there should not really be any difficulty in reaching an agreed settlement.

13.6 Clinical examination

It is helpful to have an examination room in which the patient can be watched while walking at least ten strides. This will give an indication of the patient's disability and will allow assessment of alignment of the leg in both the stance and swing phases of gait. Most patients seeking advice will already have significant loss of articular cartilage in one or other tibiofemoral compartment and as load is put on to the knee either lateral or medial thrust (Fig. 13.3) can be seen as the affected side is compressed, allowing either increasing valgus or varus angulation to develop. Further information about the degree of disability can be gained by allowing the patient to walk with and without the aid which he normally uses. He should also be observed going up and down steps and sitting down and getting up from a chair.

Careful examination of the whole locomotor system should be carried out. Disease of the spine or hips may well be an additional cause of disability and may even be a factor in producing the osteoarthritis of the affected knee.

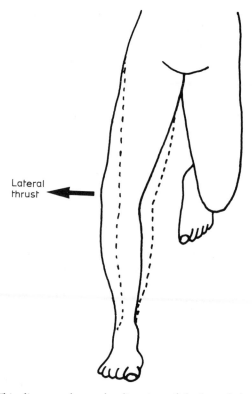

Fig. 13.3 This diagram shows the direction of the lateral thrust during the stance phase in a varus knee.

Measurement of the coronal tibiofemoral angle should be attempted with an much accuracy as possible. Our method using a goniometer with extendable arms (Fig. 13.4) has been described (Tew and Waugh, 1980). The accuracy and reproducibility of this and other techniques has been reviewed by Johnson (1982).

13.7   Radiographic assessment

13.7.1   ANGULAR MEASUREMENTS

Measurement of the coronal knee angle is an essential requirement in the radiographic assessment of the osteoarthritic knee, particularly when an operation is being planned (see page 295). For many years we have used long films (Fig. 13.5) which include the whole of the leg (from hip to ankle). We were recently able to compare measurements of the coronal tibiofemoral angle made on these films with similar measurements on films 43 cm long and found that there was no significant difference (Lawrence, 1980). There are

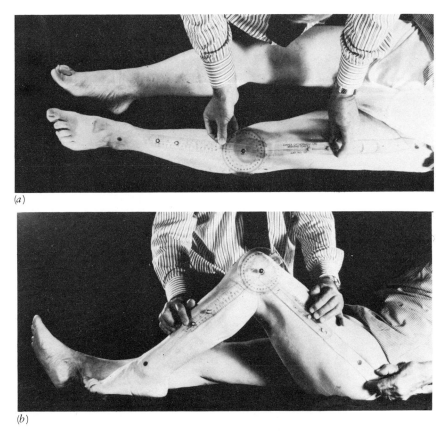

(a)

(b)

Fig. 13.4 Photographs demonstrating the use of a goniometer with extendable arms to measure the coronal tibiofemoral angle (*a*) and the angle of maximum flexion (*b*).

practical difficulties (including cost) in obtaining what may be ideal, so we now use 43 cm films routinely. Films of the hip, knee and ankle are requested only if there is a special indication: for example, when medial compartment osteoarthritis is secondary to varus malunion of a fracture of the femoral shaft. It is important that radiographs should be taken with the patient standing, but this is not always easy for the elderly person with a painful knee. It, therefore, becomes difficult to be sure of obtaining reproducible views on which reliable precise measurements can be made. The technique devised in Lund (Hagstedt *et al.*, 1980) uses the posterior surface of the femoral condyles as a reference point and seems to be the best method at the present time. The patient stands on the affected leg and the knee is screened from the lateral side. The position of the leg is adjusted until the back of the medial and lateral femoral condyles are seen precisely to overlap. When this is achieved an anteroposterior view is taken at right angles to the first beam. This provides a reproducible method which allows standard measurements of the angle of deviation of the mechanical axis to be made. The technique of stereophotogrammetry which involves the implantation of tantalum pellets into the bone (Tjornstrand *et al.*, 1981) allows even more accurate measurements.

Unfortunately these sophisticated techniques are not available to us, but

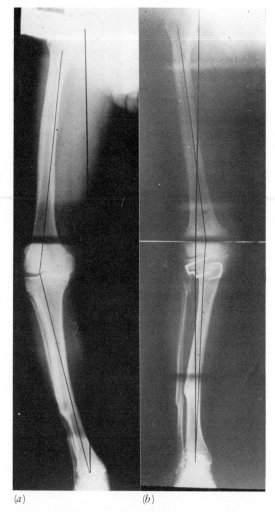

(a)   (b)

Fig. 13.5 These are two examples of standing long leg radiographs. In (a) there is medial compartment osteoarthritis and malunion of a fracture of the tibial shaft. The mechanical axis and the axes of the femoral and tibial shafts have been drawn, but the femoral line does not correspond exactly with the shaft. (b) Shows the correction achieved by tibial osteotomy and the mechanical axis now passes through the lateral side of the joint. The femoral head is more clearly seen in the original radiographs, but it is often difficult to identify its centre accurately, particularly in fat patients.

we believe it is important to attempt to make estimations of angular deformity as accurately as possible. It is, however, very important to recognize the limitations of the method which is being used. The relation of the fibular shaft to the tibia in the anteroposterior view will give some guide. It is clearly useless to compare measurements of, say, a standing and a lying film of the same knee, when in one view the gap between the two bones in very narrow and in the other it is very wide (Fig. 13.6). In the first the knee will be facing

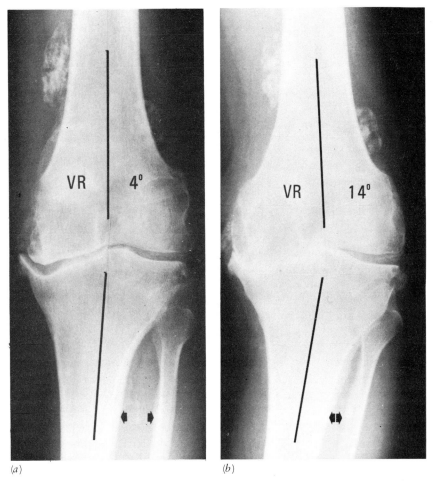

(a)   (b)

Fig. 13.6 These two radiographs demonstrate the difficulty in taking comparable films. (a) Shows a coronal tibiofemoral angle of 4° of varus when non-weight bearing and on standing (b) this appears to increase to 14°. The cartilage space in the medial compartment has closed on weight bearing (b), but this angle is exaggerated because of the externally rotated posture of the leg which is indicated by the approximation of the shafts of the fibula and tibia. The presence of a flexion contracture of 15° further increases the angle.

'outwards' and in the second 'inwards'. Errors will be compounded when there is a flexion contracture and where there is a coronal deformity of any magnitude (Lawrence, 1980; Johnson, 1982).

It may be important to know whether a particular knee joint extends fully or not, so we always take a lateral view on a 43 cm film with the heel on a pad and measure the angle between the shafts of the femur and tibia in the sagittal plane.

13.7.2   SEVERITY OF THE OSTEOARTHRITIS

This is not the place to recount in detail the radiographic appearance of osteoarthritis, but it is appropriate to put forward a plea to orthopaedic surgeons to use a system of grading which provides an objective assessment of the severity of the changes. Ählback (1968) has proposed a classification into 5 grades:

(1) Narrow joint line (loss of 50% of the articular cartilage) (Fig. 13.1)
(2) Absent joint line.
(3) Minor bone attrition (Fig. 13.2).
(4) Moderate bone attrition (bone loss of 0.5–1 cm).
(5) Gross bone attrition, often subluxation (Fig. 13.7).

It is not difficult to place a knee affected by medial compartment osteoarthritis into the appropriate grade. This, together with the angular measurement gives a good description of the joint before operation and this is essential in order to evaluate any procedure and to make appropriate comparisons.

13.8   Medial compartment osteoarthritis and tibial osteotomy

13.8.1   HISTORICAL BACKGROUND

Orthopaedic surgeons had very little effective treatment to offer patients with osteoarthritis of the knee before the 1960s. Physiotherapy, weight reduction and the use of a stick might be followed by arthrodesis in those knees which deteriorated inexorably. Debridement or 'house-cleaning' (Magnuson, 1946; Isserlin, 1950) had a vogue and is still used by some surgeons, but it was only after tibial osteotomy became accepted that effective surgical management was possible.

The operation itself was not new and had been practised in Liverpool for many years, mainly to straighten bow legs and knock knees caused by rickets. In 1961 we published the results of tibial osteotomy which we used to correct deformities in osteoarthritic knees and we demonstrated that pain was often relieved (Jackson and Waugh, 1961). Many of our colleagues were sceptical about the procedure and felt that it was unlikely that knee movement would recover after operation. There was also a fear of vascular complications which might be followed by amputation. To avoid this risk, Wardle (1962) carried out the osteotomy more distally than we did. We also came to recognize that loss of articular cartilage occurred mainly in the medial compartment in varus knees and in the lateral compartment in valgus knees. The unicompartmental nature of the disease, which is the case in the majority of patients, was illustrated in a paper published sometime later (Jackson et al., 1969). We were using standing anteroposterior radiographs of the knee at this time and we also tried to assess the state of the articular cartilage in the more normal compartment by stress films and by contrast arthrography. The review of the results of 70 operations showed that 50 patients were completely relieved of pain, 17 had partial relief and only three were no better. We used the operation in both valgus and varus knees and, although we knew that others (Bouillet and van Gaver, 1961) were advocating a supracondylar osteotomy for valgus deformities, the direction of the original deformity did not appear to affect our clinical results. We accepted that in valgus knees a tibial osteotomy left the coronal plane of the joint oblique to the horizontal, but we thought that this did not seem to matter. However, we subsequently were impressed with the review of tibial osteotomies at Oxford (Harding, 1976) and we accepted that the operation was less likely to be successful for valgus deformities: the treatment of lateral compartment osteoarthritis is discussed in Section 13.9.4.

Over the years we had used a number of different operative techniques, each of which had its own advantages and disadvantages, and we thought it would be of interest to relate the incidence of complications to the method used (Jackson and Waugh, 1974). Between 1956 and 1973 we had done 226 consecutive operations in 206 patients, carrying out the operation by the techniques described in Table 13.1.

In our first operations a curved 'ball-and-socket' osteotomy was carried

Table 13.1

Site and type of osteotomy	Number of operations	
Below the tuberosity	92	
Curved and plaster immobilization		47
Curved and external fixation		45
Above the tuberosity	83	
Wedge and staples and plaster		67
Curved and staples and plaster		16
Through the tuberosity	51	
Wedge and plaster		21
Wedge, transposition and plaster		30

out as high as possible below the tibial tuberosity (the fibula having been first divided through a separate incision) and the leg was immobilized in a plaster cast for about six weeks. Union was sometimes slow and a bone graft was needed in three patients. The position of the proximal fragment was difficult to control, particularly when the patient was fat. In an effort to overcome this in one particular patient, immobilization was obtained by using external compression with Steinmann's nails and a Charnley clamp. The result was satisfactory so we designed a special device using two nails above and two nails below the osteotomy. Rigid fixation was achieved so that plaster immobilization was not necessary and early movements were allowed. Unfortunately infection occurred in the nail tracks in 19 out of 45 operations. The sinuses healed on removal of the nails in all but two cases.

In 1964 Gariepy published his method of osteotomy using a lateral approach to the tibia after removal of the head of the fibula. The tibia was divided above the tuberosity and correction of deformity obtained by a removal of a laterally based wedge of bone. The wider area of vascular cancellous bone in the upper part of the tibia appeared to offer the likelihood of more certain bony union. We found it difficult to estimate the size of the wedge from the lateral approach and we therefore preferred an anterior incision (dividing the fibula separately). Union occurred readily and only one patient in our group of 83 high osteotomies needed a bone graft.

We next modified our technique by removing the tibial tuberosity and carrying out the osteotomy through its base. This gave an excellent exposure and the operation was easier to do, but in nine out of 30 cases the tuberosity (which we fixed with a screw) became detached.

We also did a small number of curved osteotomies above the tuberosity and wedge osteotomies below, but these methods did not seem to us to have any special advantages.

Our experience of rigid internal fixation is very small, but this method is advocated by some surgeons (for example, Lemaire, 1982) and it has the advantage of allowing early movement of the knee.

We concluded from our review that the simplest and safest technique was a wedge osteotomy above the tuberosity, but that the proximal cut should be at least 2 cm below the lowest point of the articular surface. This is necessary to avoid intra-articular fracture. We used staples and plaster fixation for 4 weeks. Our present operative technique is described on page 295.

13.8.2 INDICATIONS FOR TIBIAL OSTEOTOMY

Some of the difficulties and complications of this operation have already been discussed and before going on to describe the technique which we now use, it is important to consider the indications for the procedure.

Although there may be instances where correction of a varus deformity may seem to be indicated for cosmetic reasons and to prevent osteoarthritis, this is always a difficult decision because of the potential risks involved. It is not possible to give precise guidance, but every patient must be considered as an individual problem, and it is wise to be cautious.

Tibial osteotomy will be indicated when medial compartment osteoarthritis is clearly the cause of disabling pain and loss of function. Whether it is preferred to other possible operations (such as arthrodesis or total knee replacement) will depend on several factors which now need to be discussed:

(a) The age of the patient

The younger the patient the more likely is tibial osteotomy to be the operation of choice. Over the age of 65, particularly when both knees are affected, knee replacement should be considered (Chapter 15).

(b) The degree of deformity

(1) In medial compartment osteoarthritis a varus deformity (to a greater or lesser degree) will invariably be present, but there is a limit to the degree of angular deformity which can be corrected, particularly by an osteotomy carried out proximal to the tibial tuberosity. This limit may be a coronal tibiofemoral angle of 5° varus. If the angulation is greater than this it may be impossible to 'fit in' a wedge of sufficient size below the articular surface. It may then be necessary to consider using a curved osteotomy above and around the tuberosity (Maquet, 1980a) which will probably allow greater correction with less risk of articular fracture. A large correction can certainly be achieved by an osteotomy below the tuberosity, but the potential hazards will be discussed later.

(2) The knee must be able to flex to 90° or more and there should not be a flexion contracture greater than 10° before operation.

(3) The operation should not be carried out if there are more than a few degrees of abnormal mobility in the sagittal or coronal plane.

(c) The pathological condition of the knee

This is, of course, related to the clinical findings: the greater the deformity, the greater will be the damage to the joint. Radiographs provide valuable information and should always be taken with the patient bearing weight on the affected leg. There will be loss in height of articular cartilage in the affected compartment and in the later stages there will be bony collapse and ultimately lateral subluxation of the tibia. It seems too much to hope that osteotomy will benefit a severely disorganized joint and it is probably best not to do the operation if there is bony collapse of more than 0.5 cm (Fig. 13.7).

The condition of the lateral compartment is of importance since the osteotomy is designed to transfer load to it. The state of the articular cartilage can be assessed to some extent by taking a radiograph with valgus stress;

293

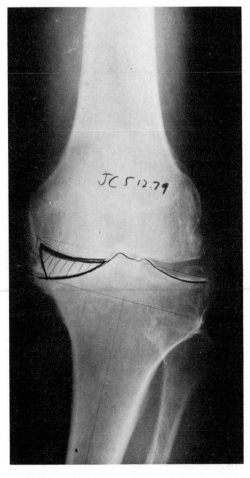

Fig. 13.7 Radiograph showing medial compartment osteoarthritis with the extent of bony collapse delineated and shaded (Ahlbäck type 5). This knee is too severely damaged for tibial osteotomy to be successful.

arthrography may be of value and arthroscopy should be carried out if there is any doubt.

The foregoing assumes that the best results are likely to be achieved at an early stage of osteoarthritis, but this does not mean that patients should be persuaded to have the operation when their symptoms are not bad enough. Although most surgeons have reported satisfactory results in about four out of five patients, it is difficult to predict the outcome in the individual case.

In general terms it seems reasonable to make the following propositions:

(1) Tibial osteotomy is the operation of choice at any age (and certainly below 65 years) in medial compartment osteoarthritis with articular cartilage

loss, but with little bony collapse (Fig. 13.1).

(2) The operation will still be indicated in younger patients with more advanced disease since the long-term results of knee replacement are not sufficiently reliable.

(3) There are a number of factors any one of which can be considered as being so unfavourable as to contraindicate tibial osteotomy: for example, a coronal tibiofemoral angle of more than 5° varus, 10° of fixed flexion, flexion movement of 90° or less, gross abnormal lateral or anteroposterior mobility, bony collapse of more than 0.5 cm or lateral subluxation of the tibia. In these situations arthrodesis will be best for the young and knee replacement for the elderly.

13.8.3 PLANNING BEFORE OPERATION (SEE PAGE 286)

The size of wedge to be removed can be estimated by measuring the coronal tibiofemoral angle and allowing for slight over-correction. For example, in a knee with a coronal tibiofemoral angle of 4° varus, a 14° laterally based wedge will be planned to achieve the desired 10° valgus (Fig. 13.8(a) and (b)). This corresponds to an angle of deviation of the mechanical axis of 10° varus corrected to 3° or 4° valgus.

Alternatively, if hip/knee/ankle films are available, the mechanical axis can be drawn and a wedge calculated which will overcorrect the deformity by from 2–4 degrees.

Rotation

Rotational deformity is frequently present to some degree in association with osteoarthritis of the knee. Whether this is primary or secondary is difficult to know. Turner and Smillie (1981) and Blaimont and Schoon (1977) have emphasized the importance of torsional deformities in osteoarthritis and when carrying out a tibial osteotomy, a rotational deformity may also need to be corrected. Some correction may be achieved with the usual techniques of tibial osteotomy, but Brunelli (1969) advocated a Z-osteotomy for correction of both rotational and varus deformities. Melere described on oblique osteotomy which not only corrects internal rotation and varus deformity, but also allows forward displacement of the distal fragment.

13.8.4 OPERATIVE TECHNIQUE

Many different operative techniques have been described, but the details are not really important provided correction is achieved and complications are avoided. In our standard procedure we excise a laterally-based wedge above the tuberosity and use temporary compression with Steinmann's nails and a Charnley clamp during the operation since this gives good control of the short

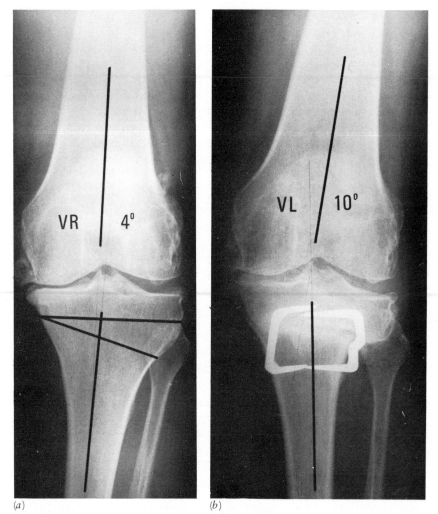

(a)   (b)

Fig. 13.8 Shows radiographs before and after tibial osteotomy. (a) Shows medial compartment arthritis with a coronal tibiofemoral angle of 4° varus; a laterally based wedge of 14° is drawn on the film. The radiograph after operation (b) shows a 10° valgus angle which is adequate correction, although the films are not strictly comparable.

proximal fragment and achieves firm apposition of the bony surfaces. Relatively early knee movement and weight-bearing is allowed in a cast brace. The details are as follows:

(a) Osteotomy of the fibula

The fibula is divided through a separate incision which is made along the intermuscular septum behind the peroneal muscles. The osteotomy should be carried out in the middle third of the bone in order to decrease the risk of damaging the anterior tibial or peroneal vessels (page 302). A small portion of bone is removed by two parallel oblique cuts. This will allow the fibular ends to slide on each other and still maintain contact when the tibial alignment is corrected.

(b) Osteotomy of the tibia

(i) Exposure

A transverse incision is made, centred on the upper part of the tibial tuberosity. The exposure can be extended by curving it upwards at the lateral and downwards at the medial end. The incision should not be extended downwards at the lateral end as this may damage branches of the lateral cutaneous nerves of the calf.

The patellar tendon is defined and isolated by two vertical incisions. The periosteum is then reflected medially as far as the posteromedial border of the tibia and laterally to the posterolateral border.

(ii) Insertion of Steinmann's nails

The next step is to insert two Steinmann's nails, parallel to the proposed surfaces of the wedge to be removed (Fig. 13.9(a)). The proximal nail should be parallel to the articular surface. The position of the nails and the relation of the proximal nail to the joint surface should be checked by a radiograph. The upper of the two nails should be at a sufficient distance above the wedge to be removed so that it will not cut out. The upper surface of the wedge must be planned to allow a depth of at least 2 cm of bone in the proximal fragment. When the wedge is removed and compression applied the nails should be parallel.

(iii) Division of the tibia

The patellar tendon must be held forward by a retractor to give space and, if further room is required, part of the tibial tuberosity may be elevated by a cut downwards into the angle between the tendon and bone. Care should be taken not to separate completely the patellar insertion from the tibia. A wedge of bone is then removed from the tibia using a small keyhole handsaw (Fig. 13.9(b)). Division of the posterior cortex may be difficult, but once the front part of the wedge is removed, the cancellous bone can be curetted away so that the posterior cortex can easily be seen: it can then be nibbled away or cut with an osteotome. Failure to remove the posterior cortex fully may make it impossible to appose the two cut surfaces accurately.

(iv) Fixation

Compression is produced by means of two Charnley clamps applied to the

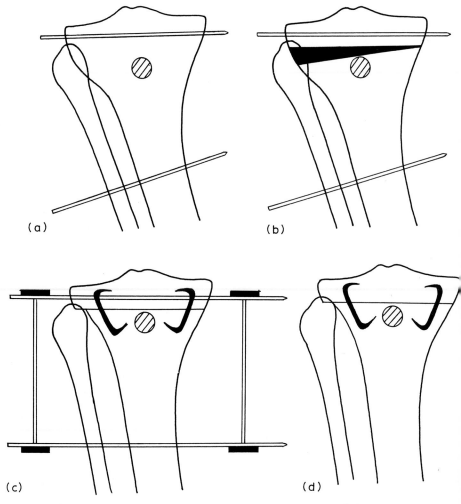

Fig. 13.9 These diagrams illustrate the steps in our technique of tibial osteotomy. In (a) the Steinmann's nails have been inserted at the angle of the wedge to be excised. A radiograph at this stage will check the level of the proximal cut. The wedge is defined and removed (b). The gap left is then closed and after the bone ends have been compressed, two staples are inserted (c). Finally, the nails and clamps are removed (d).

Steinmann's nails (Fig. 13.9(c). The osteotomy should then feel solid as the knee is flexed and extended. Two staples are inserted, one on each side of the patellar tendon. A stepped Coventry staple will fit on the anterolateral surface, but an oblique staple may be better on the medial side. When the staples are firmly in position the nails are withdrawn (Fig. 13.9(d)). The wound is closed and suction drainage is used. A well-padded plaster including the foot is then applied. The plaster is split and the leg is elevated for 24 hours.

As soon as possible during the first week the patient is got up with crutches and partial weight bearing. When he is walking comfortably, the plaster can be removed and a cast brace applied (Fig. 13.10(a) and (b)). The advantage of using a brace is that it will allow early knee movement without sacrificing stability and in addition the position of the knee can be controlled so that full correction is maintained. Patients will need crutches at first, but by the end of the second week should be walking with a reasonably normal gait.

Union will usually be firm after about six weeks. The brace is then removed and the patient encouraged to walk normally.

13.8.5 FAILURE TO OBTAIN CORRECTION

There is now considerable evidence that slight overcorrection is essential to obtain a good lasting result (Kettelkamp *et al.*, 1976; Maquet, 1976; Tjornstrand, 1981; Coventry and Bowman, 1982). The results produced by these authors are convincing and must challenge the casual attitude of some surgeons. It is not good enough simply to aim 'to get it about right'. Those who take this line will often say 'they are satisfied with their results', but are usually unable to quote chapter and verse. We are well aware that it is not easy to operate to within one degree of accuracy, but the published papers

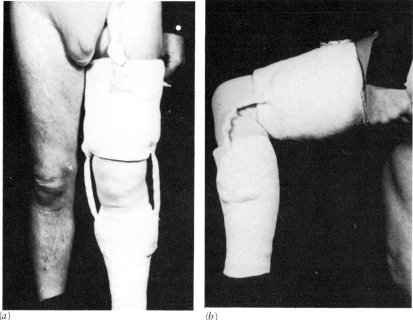

(a) (b)

Fig. 13.10 Photographs of the knee in cast brace from the front (a) and side (b). (a) demonstrates that the valgus correction is controlled in the brace.

already quoted provide overwhelming evidence to support the need for slight overcorrection. This is not always easy to achieve (Bauer, 1982), but we firmly believe that a careful and calculated approach is essential.

The first step is to calculate the size of the wedge which must be removed in order to obtain a satisfactory realignment of the mechanical axis, so that after operation the axis falls through the centre of the knee or just to the lateral side.

Theoretically, there are three reasons why adequate correction may not be achieved.

(a) Miscalculation of the degree of correction needed

The problems of radiographic measurement are discussed elsewhere (page 286), but every attempt must be made to obtain standard films taken with the patient bearing weight on the affected leg. Many surgeons use the tibio-femoral angle in order to calculate the degree of correction (Bauer *et al.*, 1969; Hagstedt, 1974; Insall *et al.*, 1974; Harding, 1976; Kettelkamp *et al.*, 1976); but Maquet (1976), Harris and Kostuik (1970) and Tjornstrand (1981) prefer the angle of deviation of the mechanical axis.

Kettelkamp *et al.* (1976) advised aiming at '5° or more of genu valgum', Coventry (1973) 5° overcorrection beyond the normal angle of 5–8°, and Tjornstrand (1981) recommended a tibiofemoral angle of 170° (10° valgus). Recording angular measurements around 180° rather than 0° has some merit, but it is not familiar to many orthopaedic surgeons (including ourselves).

Maquet (1976) measures the angle of deviation of the mechanical axis and then adds 3–5°. Harris and Kostuik (1970) aim to restore the mechanical axis to the centre of the joint.

It does not matter whether the coronal tibiofemoral angle (which we prefer) or the angle of deviation of the mechanical axis is used for calculation provided the method is understood. It is necessary to achieve 2–4° of over-correction: this means a coronal tibiofemoral angle of 9–10° of valgus or a deviation from the angle of the mechanical axis of 2–4° of valgus.

(b) Failure to remove the correct amount of bone

This is a technical problem depending to some extent on the skill of the operator. One method of measuring the wedge is to estimate the height of the lateral border and assume that 1 mm = 1°. This is, however, an approxi-mation and leads to errors. A direct measurement with some form of template is to be preferred. The use of Steinmann's nails also helps.

Although difficulties of measurement and surgical technique may make a high degree of precision seem unrealistic, it is better to have a clear aim when carrying out the operation rather than relying on a visual assessment.

(c) Displacement after operation

This should not occur if the surfaces have been accurately cut and apposed. It is, however, important to use well-fitting plaster casts or cast-braces when weight bearing is allowed.

13.8.6 ASSOCIATED PATELLOFEMORAL OSTEOARTHRITIS

Patellofemoral osteoarthritis, which may or may not cause symptoms, may occur together with medial compartment osteoarthritis. Maquet (1976) advised advancing the patellar tendon to reduce the stresses on the patella and displace the distal tibia forwards at the osteotomy by as much as 1.5 cm. Many surgeons believe that the presence of patellofemoral osteoarthritis does not affect the results of tibial osteotomy (Coventry, 1965; Hagstedt, 1974; Harding, 1976; Engel and Lippert, 1981); but Insall *et al.* (1974) suggested that night pain persisting after operation frequently arose in the patello-femoral compartment. He did not, however, advocate excision of the patella at the same time as tibial osteotomy and most surgeons, including the authors, would agree. Should it later be considered that symptoms are continuing as a result of patellofemoral osteoarthritis, the patella may be removed or the tibia tuberosity may be advanced. In our 226 operations patellectomy was only once carried out and this was done three years after the tibial osteotomy.

13.8.7 COMPLICATIONS

(a) Delayed union and non-union

Union occurs readily when the osteotomy is carried out above the tuberosity and we had only one case of non-union in 83 osteotomies at this level. Tjornstrand *et al.* (1978) reported 10 cases in 280 high tibial and in all these patients union was finally obtained by external compression or a combination of compression and excision of the pseudarthrosis (a bone graft was only used in one case). They advised that the soft tissues on the medial side of the osteotomy should be preserved and allowed to act as a hinge. With this technique there were no non-unions in 60 osteotomies.

MacIntosh and Welsh (1977) had delayed union in 3% of their cases which had been treated with two nail-compression and a staple. The osteotomies had been done through rather than above the tuberosity. Bauer *et al.* (1969) and Harris and Kostuik (1970) reported one case each – the first was thought to be due to a diabetic neuropathy, but in Harris's case the osteotomy was considered to be too low.

(b) Fracture into the knee joint

This is an unusual complication, but may on occasion give rise to unfortunate results. It is most likely to occur if the osteotomy is carried out too close to the tibial articular surface. There is general agreement that the proximal fragment needs to be at least 2 cm in thickness and if thinner than this there is an increased risk of a fracture occurring. The site of the fracture is usually where the hard bone underlying the compressed side of the joint joins the area of softer bone under the opposite compartment. The fracture splits the tibial plateau vertically in the region of the tibial spines. Bauer *et al.* (1969) reported six fractures in 63 osteotomies and regarded them as of no consequence. We noted fractures in nine out of 67 wedge osteomies and three out of 16 curved osteotomies carried out above the tuberosity. The consequences may be serious, as shown in Fig. 13.11.

(c) Neurovascular complications

The most puzzling and potentially dangerous symptom after tibial osteotomy is weakness of dorsiflexion of the big toe or foot. We drew attention to this when we reported weakness of one or more muscles supplied by the common peroneal nerve in eight out of 70 cases (Jackson *et al.*, 1969). Coventry (1965) had one case in 30 osteotomies and suggested that the cause was damage to the peroneal nerve. Judet (1969) reported eight 'complications nerveuse' in 176 osteotomies.

MacIntosh and Welsh (1977) found weakness of the foot and toe dorsiflexors in 14 out of 105 operations and they referred to the complication as 'peroneal weakness'.

In a further review we found that 27 patients in our 226 operations had some weakness of dorsiflexion (Jackson and Waugh, 1974). In most cases recovery was complete and when it was not, there was no significant disability. One patient developed a contracture of the extensor hallucis longus muscle, and in retrospect we considered that this was evidence of a mild compartment compression syndrome.

The popliteal vessels are in no immediate danger if the knee is flexed during division of the tibia (Benjamin, 1969) and pressure on the popliteal fossa is avoided. The anterior tibial artery is at risk as it passes over the upper edge of the interosseous membrane. A bone lever should never be placed around the posterolateral border of the tibia at the level of the tuberosity.

We have recently appreciated the possibility of injury to the peroneal and anterior tibial vessels during osteotomy of the fibula and believe that this might cause a compartment syndrome after operation. If the fibular head is resected (Bauer *et al.*, 1969; Harris and Kostuik, 1970; Coventry, 1973; Tjornstrand, 1981) there seems no likelihood of vascular injury although the peroneal nerve may be at risk.

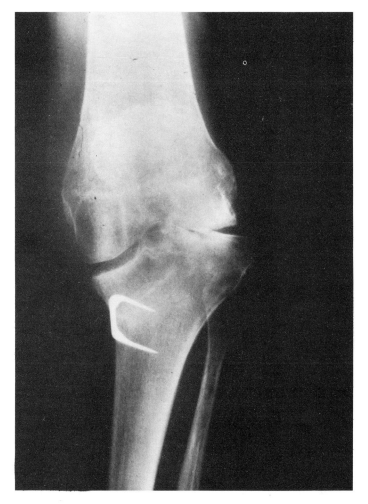

Fig. 13.11 Radiograph showing a severe deformity of the upper tibia which has followed an intra-articular fracture during the operation.

Allen *et al.* (1982) reviewed 36 patients who had a tibial osteotomy for medial compartment osteoarthritis at Harlow Wood Orthopaedic Hospital and found that 13 had some weakness of dorsiflexion when this complication was looked for after operation. In nine the extensor hallucis was affected alone and in another five there was also weakness of the tibialis anterior muscle. The fibula had been divided at different levels and, although the numbers were too small to allow statistical evaluation, weakness seemed to occur more often when the fibula was divided below the head and above the midshaft. Half the patients who had an osteotomy of the fibula between 8–11 cm from its proximal tip developed some degree of weakness. It is important

303

to stress that recovery always followed, although three patients had weakness of extensor hallucis longus which lasted from six months to a year.

The peroneal veins and the anterior tibial vessels are close to the fibula in the upper half of its shaft (Fig. 13.12). It may be that damage to these vessels could cause a compartment syndrome. Although it is not possible to draw definite conclusions, it seems safest to divide the fibula either through its head or below the midpoint of the shaft. Alternatively, Bauer's suggestion of mobilizing the superior tibiofibular joint and allowing the fibula to slide upwards should be safe (Bauer *et al.*, 1969).

Measurement of anterior tibial compartment pressure in a small number of cases suggests that it becomes higher when a complete plaster is applied (rather than a back splint) and if the foot is allowed to become plantarflexed (Allen, 1982). It therefore seems best to immobilize the leg in a cast which includes the foot and which should be split.

We know of one patient who had an above-knee amputation as a result of ischaemia of the muscles in the anterior and lateral compartments. Although this must be a rare occurrence its possibility cannot be disregarded. It is, therefore, essential to observe the foot carefully after operation and severe pain in the lower leg is a warning symptom which must not be ignored. It should, however, be emphasized that the compartment syndrome can appear and lead to serious consequences without loss of arterial pulsation in the foot. Once a vascular disaster is suspected, immediate action must be taken. The first step is to remove the plaster and inspect the whole leg carefully. If the

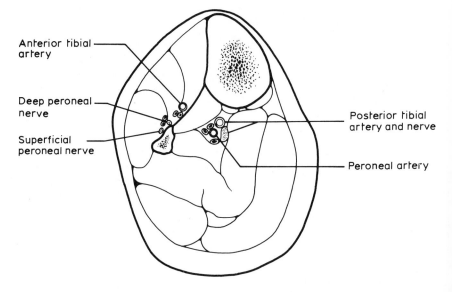

Fig. 13.12 Diagram showing the close relationship between the vessels and nerves to the shaft of the upper half of the fibula. This cross-section is 10 cm below the knee.

signs suggest a major arterial injury, arteriography may be indicated, but exploration of the popliteal fossa should not be delayed. If there is any evidence of a compartment syndrome, urgent decompression is needed. The fact that many surgeons will be fortunate enough never to see this sort of disaster does not excuse delay in diagnosis or treatment. All concerned must be aware of the potential hazards which do not only happen to 'other people'.

13.8.8 CONCLUSIONS

It is our experience that tibial osteotomy will give substantial and lasting relief of pain in patients with medial compartment osteoarthritis. The selection of patients is important and it is essential to achieve adequate correction. This is in keeping with all the most recent reports in the literature (Tjornstrand, 1981; Bauer, 1982; Coventry and Bowman, 1982; Maquet *et al.* 1982).

Many surgeons are concerned with the disappointing results of knee replacement operations and at the present time tibial osteotomy still has an important place in the treatment of patients with osteoarthritis of the knee. Figure 13.13 shows that the numbers of tibial osteotomies done each year at

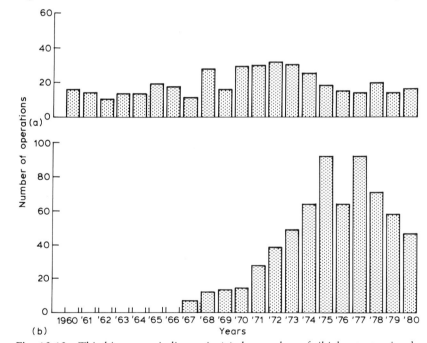

Fig. 13.13 This histogram indicates in (*a*) the number of tibial osteotomies done each year at Harlow Wood Orthopaedic Hospital between 1960 and 1980. (*b*) Shows the number of knee replacements carried out for osteoarthritis and rheumatoid arthritis during the same period.

Harlow Wood Orthopaedic Hospital has remained between 15 and 30 over the last 20 years, whereas the dramatic rise in the annual numbers of knee replacements is now beginning to decline.

13.9   Lateral compartment osteoarthritis

Although this chapter has been largely concerned with medial compartment osteoarthritis and its treatment by tibial osteotomy, osteoarthritis of the lateral compartment needs special consideration. The incidence and aetiology may be different for the two conditions, and treatment certainly presents different problems.

13.9.1   INCIDENCE AND AETIOLOGY

It is difficult to know the relative incidence of medial and lateral compartment osteoarthritis in the population at large because studies of the prevalence of osteoarthritis do not distinguish between these two forms of the disease (Lawrence *et al.*, 1966). This is perhaps due to a failure to recognize the two types of osteoarthritis in the past, together with the difficulties of making angular measurements. A review from Malmo (Hernborg and Nilsson, 1977) describes a series of osteoarthritic knees which were not selected for operation. Surgeons carrying out tibial osteotomy or knee replacement also have some information, but the groups of patients they are dealing with are specially selected for a number of reasons. Some idea of the incidence of varus and valgus deformities (medial and lateral compartment osteoarthritis) can be obtained from our own and Coventry's series (1973) of osteotomies for osteoarthritis. Our cases were done at a time when we used tibial osteotomy to correct valgus as well as varus deformities and Coventry also included some supracondylar osteotomies. In a much larger series of osteotomies for all types of osteoarthritis collected from several centres in Belgium there were 464 knees with medial compartment (and also patello-femoral) osteoarthritis and 116 with lateral compartment osteoarthritis. There is also our own and Freeman's series (1980) of knee replacement for osteoarthritis. These figures are summarized in Table 13.2. Varus deformities are clearly a good deal more common than valgus, except at the London Hospital where the incidence is almost equal.

The sex distribution is not always given, but in the 50 valgus knees operated on at Harlow Wood all were in women. Furthermore, in the Malmo series, there were 18 men and 42 women with medial compartment osteoarthritis, but the six knees with lateral compartment osteoarthritis were all in women. Freeman's figures again are at variance since the distribution of deformities between the sexes in his series was almost equal. Clearly men do develop lateral compartment osteoarthritis, particularly following lateral meniscectomy, but they probably do so less frequently than women (certainly

Table 13.2 Varus and valgus deformity in osteoarthritic knees

	Varus	Valgus	Source and reference
Malmo (1977)	60	6	Unselected (Hernborg and Nilsson, 1977)
Mayo Clinic (before 1973)	70	16	Tibial osteotomy and some supracondylar osteotomies (Coventry, 1973)
Harlow Wood (before 1975)	75	25	Tibial osteotomy (Waugh, 1981)
Belgium (1982)	464	116	Tibial and femoral osteotomies (Maquet et al., 1982)
Harlow Wood (1981)	66	25	Knee replacements (Waugh, 1981)
London Hospital (1980)	32	33	Knee replacements (Freeman, 1980)

as far as our experience is concerned). These matters may seem to be philosophical rather than practical and, although nowadays no-one cares how many angels can dance on the point of a pin, two interesting questions arise:

(a) Why should lateral compartment osteoarthritis be less common than medial compartment osteoarthritis?

It has already been pointed out that the primary cause of the articular cartilage lesion in osteoarthritis is not known, but mechanical factors in the subsequent progress of the condition are accepted to be important. Some studies, using dynamic gait analysis, have suggested that during walking more load is transmitted through the medial tibial plateau than the lateral (Morrison, 1970; Johnson et al., 1980). A simple explanation of the higher medial load might be that the area of the articulating surface of the medial tibial condyle is greater than that of the lateral. This, of course, is not to say that in the normal knee the load per unit area is different on each side of the knee, although the experimental evidence on this point is not conclusive (Kettelkamp and Jacobs, 1972; Maquet, 1976). The dilemma is not yet fully resolved and needs further investigation (Johnson et al. 1981). It might, however be reasonable to suppose that a derangement (such as a meniscectomy) on the medial side of the knee would reduce the area of contact so that the higher medial load would operate over a smaller area. This might be effectively responsible for aggravating, if not actually producing osteoarthritic changes, on that side of the joint. The fact that lesions of the medial

307

menisci are more common than lateral might be an additional reason for the higher incidence of medial compartment osteoarthritis. Furthermore, we have been able to produce some evidence that patients with a valgus deformity are able to develop a compensatory gait which will tend to decrease the load on the lateral compartment (Johnson and Waugh, 1980) and this mechanism may provide some protection to the lateral side of the joint which might account for the relative rarity of lateral compartment osteoarthritis.

(b) Why is lateral compartment osteoarthritis apparently more common in women than men?

The answer to this question is even more uncertain. It is facile to suggest that the increased pelvic width of the female might be a factor. If the femoral heads were further apart there might always be a higher valgus angle at the knee in women than in men. The evidence is not entirely conclusive (Johnson, 1982), but the slightly higher valgus angle in women could not explain the clinical occurrence of lateral compartment osteoarthritis which is often unilateral (Fig. 13.14(a)) with the opposite knee being completely normal. Severe bilateral valgus deformities also occur, or the opposite knee may have a varus deformity. With the pelvic theory rejected, it is only possible to make totally

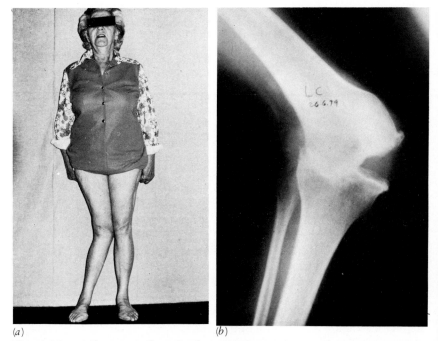

(a)   (b)

Fig. 13.14 (a) Shows a unilateral valgus deformity (coronal tibiofemoral angle 16° valgus) and (b) is a radiograph of an even more severe deformity in another patient.

hypothetical suggestions: perhaps there is a difference in bone structure between male and female knees; or even more far-fetched, perhaps some social custom like the different way men and women get out of a chair may have a part to play. The mechanisms involved in the development of lateral compartment osteoarthritis may be unique, and certainly they deserve further thought and investigation.

13.9.2 CLINICAL PRESENTATION

Pain and loss of function are the main symptoms, and it is noticeable that the angular deformity is often greater (together with the degree of bony collapse) than the corresponding varus deformity which is seen in patients with medial compartment osteoarthritis who present themselves for treatment. Hagstedt (1974) has given a mechanical explanation to account for his observation that 'valgus deformity causes less pain than varus deformity'. It may be that the 'ability to compensate' for a valgus deformity during walking is also relevant.

It certainly is true that in our practice most patients with lateral compartment osteoarthritis are not only elderly, but have severe deformities with badly disorganized knees (Fig. 13.14(b)). In these circumstances, knee replacement has often seemed the best solution. There are, however, a few younger patients (and these are often men or women who have had a lateral meniscectomy) in whom a less radical solution is needed.

13.9.3 INDICATIONS FOR SUPRACONDYLAR OSTEOTOMY

If the patient is under 65 years of age and if the coronal tibiofemoral angle is less than 15° (with correspondingly less than 0.5 cm of bony collapse), corrective osteotomy will be indicated. There must, of course, be less than 10° of flexion deformity, 90° of flexion movement must be present and there should not be more than a few degrees of abnormal mobility in the coronal or sagittal planes. If these strict criteria are observed, then the number of patients needing a supracondylar osteotomy is small and our experience of this operation is limited. We do, however, fully accept that the correction must be carried out through the femur and not through the tibia.

13.9.4 TECHNIQUES OF SUPRACONDYLAR OSTEOTOMY

There are three principle methods, each of which will have its strong advocates. Our clinical experience is such that we cannot present comparative results for each technique.

(a) Internal fixation (Fig. 13.15(a))

Coventry (1973) described a method of carrying out a lower femoral osteotomy using a blade-plate for fixation which he had done in eight patients with valgus deformities. AO instrumentation can also be used (Muller *et al.*, 1979) and provides accurate and sound fixation so that the knee need not be immobilized subsequently.

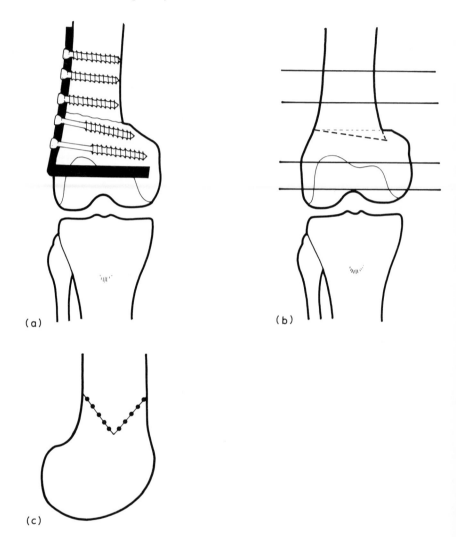

(a)

(b)

(c)

Fig. 13.15 These three diagrams illustrate different techniques of supracondylar osteotomy using *(a)* internal fixation and *(b)* external fixation (after Maquet). *(c)* shows the line of the osteotomy in the sagittal plane which provides some inherent stability.

(b) External fixation (Fig. 13.15(b))

Maquet (1980b) uses a wedge excision with external fixation using two nails above and two below the osteotomy. He reported at that time the results in 20 knees: 14 were excellent or good and four fair or poor (two had died at the time of review). Technically this seems a sound procedure which should achieve and maintain the desired alignment. It is interesting to note that these 20 supracondylar osteotomies were included in a series with 141 tibial osteotomies which indicates the relative rarity of the former operation.

(c) Plaster immobilization

Through a medial incision a 'V' shaped osteotomy is performed at the junction of the shaft and the flare of femoral condyles (Fig. 13.15(c)). The apex of the 'V' points distally. The osteotomy is held with staples and weight bearing is allowed seven days after operation is a plaster cylinder. The cylinder is changed to a cast brace at about four weeks and this is maintained until union has occurred (Tasker, 1982).

13.10 Patellofemoral osteoarthritis

Age-related surface degeneration in the patellar articular cartilage becomes almost universal after the age of 25 years and this should not be regarded as a precursor of osteoarthritis. Meachim (1975) does, however, exclude the patellofemoral joint in women from this generalization. Abernethy *et al.* (1978) also demonstrated a high incidence (85%) of cartilage fibrillation in the medial facet at necropsy and considered that this should be regarded as an 'incidental' finding which should not be related to symptoms.

Certainly it is our experience that progressive patellofemoral osteoarthritis is rather uncommon in the absence of tibiofemoral osteoarthritis. When the former does occur it usually has followed injury, recurrent subluxation or dislocation, or is associated with abnormal movement of the patella during flexion and extension of the knee (this latter condition can be conveniently, but inelegantly, referred to as 'maltracking').

If retropatellar pain is not relieved by rest or physiotherapy (or does not subside spontaneously) operative treatment should be considered. One of the following procedures may be indicated:

13.10.1 REALIGNMENT OF THE PATELLA

This operation theoretically requires an exactitude which is almost impossible, particularly as there will already be significant loss of articular cartilage (Fig. 13.16). It is probably best restricted to patients in whom there is 'maltracking' or subluxation, visible clinically and in patellar views, but

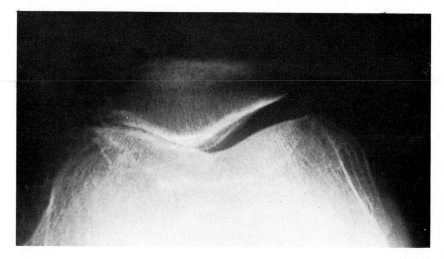

Fig. 13.16 A tangential radiograph of the patella showing lateral subluxation and severe loss of articular cartilage of the lateral facet. Such advanced patellofemoral osteoarthritis would not be suitable for a realignment procedure.

where the cartilage loss is not too severe. In these cases a release of the lateral capsule, including detachment of the vastus lateralis insertion, should be carried out together with reefing of the medial capsule. More radical surgery to displace the tibial tendon insertion, such as the Hauser operation, is not indicated in this condition. Crosby and Insall (1976) found that distal realignment carried out for patellar subluxation may actually increase the incidence of osteoarthritis. They did not find any clinical evidence of progressive osteoarthritic changes in knees treated by soft-tissue release alone. A conservative approach was advocated, but when operation is indicated, proximal realignment (advancement of vastus medialis with lateral release and medial capsule repair) is the best choice since it does not 'anatomically disturb the patellar mechanism'.

13.10.2 PATELLAR ADVANCEMENT

Maquet (1982) has shown that advancement of the tibial tuberosity reduces stress on the patella and so relieves symptoms. The effect is mainly related to the lower pole and could result in increased stress on the upper part of the patella. However, the regions of patellar contact with the femur become progressively larger and migrate superiorly as the knee flexes (Goodfellow *et al.*, 1976) so that the stress is distributed over a wider area of the patella. Ferguson (1982) showed that there is a diminishing return as the tuberosity is increasingly elevated since there will be an increase in the proximal stress; there may be difficulties of skin closure and there are also cosmetic

312

considerations. The optimum amount of elevation was considered to be 1.25 cm.

Technique

A transverse incision is made over the tibial tuberosity (this is easier to close than a vertical incision). The tendon is exposed and isolated. The tuberosity is brought forward by means of an osteotome driven downwards into the angle between the tendon and the bone for a distance of about 5 cm. The tuberosity is then raised; care being taken not to divide the bone completely. A small graft is taken from the medial surface of the tibia. This should be of sufficient size to hold the tuberosity forwards, when it is placed beneath it by 1.25 cm (Fig. 13.17).

13.10.3 PATELLECTOMY

This may be indicated when it is clear that symptoms are caused by patellofemoral osteoarthritis. A disadvantage which follows removal of the patella is loss of extensor power of the knee (Stougard, 1970; Kaufer, 1971; Sutton *et al.*, 1976). Kaufer estimated that, after the patella has been excised, full active extension required 15–30% increase in quadriceps strength. In the normal knee this increase is well within the functional reserve of the muscle,

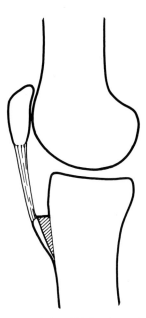

Fig. 13.17 Advancement of the tibial tuberosity by the technique described by Ferguson (1980).

but it may not always be possible in the elderly patient with rheumatoid or osteoarthritis, and an extensor lag may follow operation. Nonetheless, the relief of pain resulting from patellectomy may lead to an improvement in function.

Some authors report good results after patellectomy carried out for osteoarthritis (O'Donoghue *et al.*, 1952; Sewell, 1952). Geckeler and Quaranta (1962) in a long-term follow-up ranging from 5 to 16 years (average 9 years) found no evidence of progression of the osteoarthritis and out of 27 patients 74% had good or excellent results. A more recent paper (Ackroyd and Polyzoides, 1978) is less optimistic since only 53% of patients had a good result in a series of 81 operations followed for a mean of 6.5 years. A poor result was likely if osteoarthritis was present in the tibiofemoral joint. It was also concluded that immobilization for 3 or 4 weeks afterwards was of benefit.

There seems every reason to be cautious in advising excision of the patella in osteoarthritis and in our experience the operation is rarely indicated since associated changes are nearly always present. In isolated patellofemoral osteoarthritis the patella is nearly always laterally displaced and steps have to be taken to ensure that the remaining tendon stays in the trochlear groove during flexion and extension (see below).

Technique

Various methods have been described and there is still some debate as to whether a longitudinal or transverse repair of the tendon should be carried out. Kaufer (1971) argued that, if a longitudinal repair was used, the pull of the quadriceps is diverted to the medial and lateral patellar retinacula. Since the course of the retinacula is closer to the flexion axis they act on a shorter moment arm and produce less extensor torque. At the same time the quadriceps muscle mass is shortened, which puts the muscle at a physiological disadvantage. Transverse repair would therefore seem the better choice. In cases in which it is thought likely that extensor lag will develop, advancement of the tibial tuberosity using a bone block should be carried out at the same time (Kaufer, 1971).

Whether the repair is transverse or longitudinal the vastus medialis insertion should be advanced (Compere *et al.*, 1979) in order to prevent the lateral subluxation of the quadriceps tendon.

13.11 Osteonecrosis

Although osteonecrosis has been discussed in Chapter 10 in relation to osteochondritis dissecans, it seems worthwhile giving further consideration to the condition here. The lesion has been described as occurring after lupus erythematosus (Ruderman and MacCarthy, 1964) and Ahlbäck *et al.* (1968) recognized that the osteonecrosis also occurs spontaneously.

13.11.1 AETIOLOGY

In Muheim and Bohne's (1970) series of 51 patients the mean age at onset of symptoms was 67 years: 38 were women and 13 were men.

The mechanism of development and evolution of the lesion is by no means certain. The site affected is invariably the weight bearing surface of the medial femoral condyle. The pathological appearances are of an area of bone infarction which might be traumatic in origin (Lotke *et al.*, 1977).

13.11.2 SYMPTOMS AND SIGNS

The characteristic features are a sudden onset of intense pain and tenderness over the medial femoral condyle. The pain is worse during walking and at night. There may be swelling and pain on flexion of the knee, but movement is not usually restricted.

13.11.3 RADIOGRAPHIC APPEARANCES

The lesion is shown by an area of subchondral radiolucence with a margin of sclerosis (Fig. 13.18). The defect may contain a small fragment of dense bone. An important feature which helps to establish the diagnosis is the increased uptake of strontium-85 or technetium-99m in the affected area in the medial femoral condyle.

In a paper on 'Painful knees in older patients' Lotke *et al.* (1977) have demonstrated that the diagnosis can be made from the history and from the bone scan, even when there are no radiographic changes.

13.11.4 PROGNOSIS

This type of surface osteochondral defect would seem likely to lead to osteoarthritis and sometimes osteoarthritic changes are already present when the diagnosis is made. The prognosis, however, depends on the size of the lesion when it is first seen and on the degree of radioactive uptake. This has been demonstrated by Muheim and Bohne (1970) who concluded that a small lesion had a better chance for repair and less risk of collapse of the overlying cartilage. Nevertheless, 13 out of 15 of their patients who were examined more than two years after the acute episode had evidence of osteoarthritis. Where the lesion was not seen in the radiographs, or was scarcely visible, as in the 12 cases described by Lotke *et al.* (1977) complete recovery invariably occurred, although symptoms might persist (although becoming less severe) for as long as 15 months.

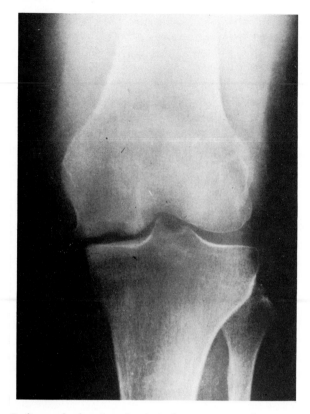

Fig. 13.18 Radiograph showing the typical appearance of osteonecrosis of the medial femoral condyle.

13.11.5 TREATMENT

There appears to be no indication for arthrotomy and decompression or excision of the lesion. Analgesics and protection from weight bearing by using crutches will usually be followed by gradual improvement. Where medial compartment osteoarthritis develops, tibial osteotomy is considered to give satisfactory results (Bauer *et al.* 1969). There is now evidence that better results can be obtained if osteotomy is combined with drilling and bone grafting the local defect (Koshino, 1982). In a small number of cases a later arthrotomy showed that the site of the lesion was covered by fibrocartilage.

13.12 Allografting in osteoarthritis

In 1968 Dr Volkov from Moscow read a paper at the British Orthopaedic Association Meeting in Nottingham on the transplantation of whole joints (Volkov, 1970). The results seemed remarkable, but there were not sufficient details to allow an assessment to be made of the potential value of the treatment in chronic arthritis.

Lawrence (1970) reported allografting in seven patients with 'advanced degenerative arthritis', but this reference is to an abstract of a paper and consequently presents only an outline of the results.

Gross *et al.* (1975) gave an account of nine allografts replacing parts of the knee in eight patients with osteoarthritis. A graft which consisted of a relatively thin slice of bone and articular cartilage was used to replace one or other tibial plateau (usually medial). Case histories of four of the patients were given. All nine allografts became incorporated and in one case histological examination at 14 months revealed 'cartilage viability'. These 'two years interim observations' were considered to be encouraging enough for the authors to continue using this technique in knees with 'disease severe enough not to be helped by osteotomy, but not so diffusely damaged as to require total knee arthroplasty'.

This would seem to open a new field of treatment, but, although we have reason to believe that work is continuing in some centres, the method does not appear to be in general use. A computerized world literature search, using the words 'articular cartilage grafting' and 'allografting', did not reveal any relevant publications in 1980, 1981 or 1982 (up till November). At the Combined Meeting of the Orthopaedic Associations of the English-Speaking World held in Capetown in 1982, Gross and his colleagues (1982) reported their further experience of 100 fresh allografts. Thirty-six grafts had been performed for unicompartmental osteoarthritis with an average follow-up of 48 months. Two-thirds of the patients were judged to have obtained 'good results'. No doubt details will be published in due course.

Most surgeons are continuing to use tibial osteotomy and knee replacement operations for their patients. Allografting may, or may not, be shown to be a practical method of treatment in future, but at present there is insufficient evidence to encourage its use outside special centres dedicated to research into the subject.

References

Abernethy P J, Townsend P R, Rose R M, Radin E L. Is chondromalacia a separate clinical entity? *J Bone Joint Surg* [*Br*] 1978;60–B:205–10.

Akroyd C E A, Polyzoides A J. Patellectomy for osteoarthritis. *J Bone Joint Surg* [*Br*] 1978;60–B:535–7.

Adams J C. *Outline of orthopaedics*. Edinburgh: Churchill Livingstone, 1981;55.

Ahlbäck S. Osteoarthrosis of the knee: a radiographic investigation. *Acta Radiol (Diagn)* 1968;Suppl No. 227.

Ahlbäck S, Bauer G C H, Bohne W H. Spontaneous osteonecrosis of the knee. *Arthr Rheum* 1968;11:705.

Allen T. Personal communication, 1982.

Allen T, Jackson J P, Waugh W. Neuromuscular complications of high tibial osteotomy. *Internal publication Harlow Wood Orthopaedic Hospital* 1982.

Arnoldi C C, Lemperg R K, Linderholm H. Interosseous hypertension and pain in the knee. *J Bone Joint Surg [Br]* 1975;**57-B**:360–3.

Bauer G C H. Treatment of gonarthrosis. *Am Acad Orthop Surg Instr Course Lect* 1982; 31:152–66.

Bauer G C H, Insall J, Koshino T. Tibial osteotomy in gonarthrosis (osteoarthritis of the knee). *J Bone Joint Surg [Am]* 1969;**51-A**:1545–63.

Benjamin A. Double osteotomy for the painful knee in rheumatoid arthritis and osteoarthritis. *J Bone Joint Surg [Br]* 1969;**51-B**:694–9.

Blaimont P, Schoon R. A propos de 2 cas de gonarthrose associée à un vicé de torsion interne du tibia. *Acta Orthop Belg* 1977;**43**:476–81.

Bouillet R, van Gaver P. L'arthrose du genou; étude pathogenique et traitment. *Act Orthop Belg* 1961;**27**:1.

Brookes M, Helal B. Primary osteoarthritis. Venous engorgement and osteogenesis. *J Bone Joint Surg [Br]* 1968;**50-B**:493–504.

Brunelli G. La osteotomia en z desrotadora y valgizante en las artrosis. Estaticas de la rodilla. *Excerpta Medica* 1969;**192**:32.

Byers P D, Contemponi C A, Farkas T A. A postmortem study of the hip joint. *Ann Rheum Dis* 1970;**29**:15–31.

Catterall R C F. Personal communication, 1982.

Compere C L, Hill J A, Lewinnek G E, Thompson R C. Patellectomy for patello-femoral arthritis. *J Bone Joint Surg [Am]* 1979;**61-A**:714–19.

Coventry M B. Osteotomy of the upper portion of the tibia for degenerative arthritis of the knee. *J Bone Joint Surg [Am]* 1965;**47-A**:984–90.

Coventry M B. Osteotomy about the knee for degenerative and rheumatoid arthritis. *J Bone Joint Surg [Am]* 1973:55-B:23–48.

Coventry M B. Upper tibial osteotomy for gonarthrosis. *Orth Clin North Am* 1979;**3**:586.

Coventry M B, Bowman P W. Long-term results of upper tibial osteotomy for degenerative arthritis of the knee. *Acta Med Belg* 1982;**48**:139–56.

Crosby E B, Insall J. Recurrent dislocation of the patella. *J Bone Joint Surg [Am]* 1976; 58-A:9–13.

Engel G M, Lippert F G. Valgus tibial osteotomy. *Clin Orthop Rel Res* 1981;**160**:137–43.

Ferguson A B. Elevation of the insertion of the patellar ligament. *J Bone Joint Surg [Am]* 1982;**64-A**::766–71.

Freeman M A R. Surgical anatomy and pathology of the arthritic knee. In: Freeman M A R ed. *Arthritis of the knee.* Berlin, Heidelberg, New York: Springer-Verlag, 1980;38–9.

Fujisawa Y, Masuhara K, Shiomi S. The effect of high tibial osteotomy on osteoarthritis of the knee. *Orth Clin North Am* 1979;**3**:586.

Gariepy R. Genu varum treated by high tibial osteotomy. *J Bone Joint Surg [Br]* 1964; **46-B**:783–4.

Geckeler E O, Quaranta A V. Patellectomy for degenerative arthritis of the knee. Late results. *J Bone Joint Surg [Am]* 1962;**44-A**:1109–14.

Goodfellow J W, Hungerford D S, Zindel M. Patello-femoral mechanics and pathology I. Functional anatomy of the patello-femoral joint. *J Bone Joint Surg [Br]* 1976;**58-B**:287–90.

Gross A E, Silverstein E A, Falk R, Langer F. The allotransplantation of partial joints in the treatment of osteoarthritis of the knee. *Clin Orthop Rel Res* 1975;**108**:7–14.

Gross A E, McKee N, Lotem N, Locht R, Langer F. The role of allografts in orthopaedic surgery. *J Bone Joint Surg [Br]* 1982;**64-B**:619.

Hagstedt B. High tibial osteotomy for gonarthrosis. Thesis (Lund, Sweden) 1974.

Hagstedt B, Norman O, Olsson T H, Tjornstrand B. Technical accuracy in high tibial osteotomy for gonarthrosis. *Acta Orthop Scand* 1980;**51**:963–70.

Harding M L. A fresh appraisal of tibial osteotomy for osteoarthritis of the knee. *Clin Orthop Rel Res* 1976;114:223–234.

Harris W R, Kostuik J P. High tibial osteotomy for osteoarthritis of the knee. *J Bone Joint Surg [Am]* 1970;52–A:330–6.

Harrison M H M, Schajowicz F, Trueta J. Osteoarthritis of the hip. A study of the nature and the evolution of the disease. *J Bone Joint Surg [Br]* 1953;35–B:598–626.

Helfet A. *Disorders of the knee.* Philadelphia, Toronto: J B Lippincott Co., 1974.

Hernberg J S, Nilsson B E. The natural course of osteoarthritis of the knee. *Clin Orthop Rel Res* 1977;123:130–7.

Insall J, Shoji H, Mayer V. High tibial osteotomy. *J Bone Joint Surg [Am]* 1974;56–A:1397–1405.

Isserlin B. Joint debridement for osteoarthritis of the knee. *J Bone Joint Surg [Br]* 1950;32–B:302.

Jackson J P, Waugh W. Tibial osteotomy for osteoarthritis of the knee. *J Bone Joint Surg [Br]* 1961;43–B:746–51.

Jackson J P, Waugh W. The technique and complications of upper tibial osteotomy. *J Bone Joint Surg [Br]* 1974;56–B:236–45.

Jackson J P, Waugh W, Green J P. High tibial osteotomy for osteoarthritis for the knee. *J Bone Joint Surg [Br]* 1969;51–B:88–94.

Johnson F. The knee. *Clin Rheum Dis* 1982;8:677–70.

Johnson F, Leite S, Waugh W. Distribution of load across the knee. *J Bone Joint Surg [Br]* 1980;62:346–9.

Johnson F, Scarrow, P, Waugh W. Assessments of loads in the knee joint. *Med Biol Eng Comp* 1981;19:237–43.

Johnson F, Waugh W. Evidence for compensatory gait in patients with a valgus knee deformity. *Acta Orthop Belg* 1980;46:558–65.

Judet J. *Traitement de gonarthroses.* 11e Congress de la Societe Internationale de Chirurgie Orthopedique at de Traumatologie. Brussels: Imprimerie des Sciences, 1969;405–7.

Kaufer H. Mechanical function of the patella. *J Bone Joint Surg [Am]* 1971;53–A:1551–60.

Kellgren J S, Lawrence J S, Aitken-Swan J. Rheumatic complaints in an urban population. *Ann Rheum Dis* 1953;12:5–15.

Kettelkamp D B, Jacobs A W. Tibiofemoral contact area – determination and implications. *J Bone Joint Surg [Am]* 1972;54–A:349–56.

Kettelkamp D B, Wenger D R, Chao E Y S, Thompson C. Results of proximal tibial osteotomy. *J Bone Joint Surg [Am]* 1976;58–A:952–60.

Koshino T. The treatment of spontaneous osteonecrosis of the knee by high tibial osteotomy with and without bone grafting and drilling of the lesion. *J Bone Joint Surg [Am]* 1982;64–A:47–58.

Laurence M. Allograft arthroplasty of the knee. *J Bone Joint Surg [Br]* 1970;52–B:781.

Lawrence J S, Bremner J M, Bier F. Osteoarthrosis: prevalence in the population and relationship between symptoms and X-ray changes. *Ann Rheum Dis* 1966;25:1–23.

Lawrence M R. The role of goniometry and radiography in the assessment of tibio-femoral alignment and knee joint mobility. Br Med Sci Thesis (Nottingham University) 1980.

Lemaire R. Etude Comparative de deux series d'osteotomies tibiales fixation par lame – plaque ou par cadre de compression. *Acta Orthop Bel* 1982;48:157–171.

Lotke P A, Ecker M L, Alavi A. Painful knees in older patients. *J Bone Joint Surg [Am]* 1977;59–A:617–21.

MacIntosh D L, Welsh R P. Joint débridement. A complement to high tibial osteotomy in the treatment of degenerative arthritis of the knee. *J Bone Joint Surg [Am]* 1977;59–A:1094–7.

Magnuson P B. Technique of debridement of the knee joint for arthritis. *Surg Clin North Am* 1946;26:249.

Maquet P. *Biomechanics of the knee with application to pathogenesis and the surgical treatment of osteoarthritis.* Berlin: Springer-Verlag, 1976.

319

Maquet P. The biomechanics of the knee and surgical possibilities of healing osteoarthritic joints. *Clin Orthop Rel Res* 1980a;**146**:102.

Maquet P. Osteotomy. In: Freeman M A R. ed. *Arthritis of the knee*. Berlin, Heidelberg, New York: Springer-Verlag, 1980b;**149–83**.

Maquet P. Traitement chirurgical de l'arthrose patello-femorale. *Acta Med Belg* 1982;**48**:172–89.

Maquet P, Watillon M, Burny F, Andrianne Y, Quinfin J, Rasquin C, Donkenvolcke M. Traitement chirurgical de l'arthrose du genou. *Acta Orthop Bel* 1982;**48**:204–60.

Meachim G. Articular cartilage lesions in the Liverpool population. *Ann Rheum Dis* 1975;**2**:122–4.

Meachim G. Cartilage breakdown. In: Owen R. ed. *Scientific foundations of orthopaedics and traumatology*. London: Heinemann, 1980;290–6.

Melere G. Traitement de l'arthrose fémoro-tibiale interne par osteotomie de valgisation.

Morrison J B. The mechanics of the knee joint in relation to normal walking. *J Biomech* 1970;**3**:51–61.

Muheim G, Bohne W H. Prognosis in spontaneous osteonecrosis of the knee. *J Bone Joint Surg [Br]* 1970;**52–B**:605–12.

Muller M E, Allgower M, Schneiser R, Willenegger H. *Manual of internal fixation*. Berlin: Springer-Verlag, 1979:376–7.

Noble J, Hamblen D L. The pathology of the degenerate meniscus lesion. *J Bone Joint Surg [Br]* 1975:**57–B**:180–6.

O'Donoghue D H, Tompkins F, Hays M B. Strength of the quadriceps function after patellectomy. *Western J Surg Obstet Gynecol* 1952;**60**:159–67.

Radin E L. Mechanical aspects of osteoarthrosis. *Bull Rheum Dis* 1976;**26**:862–4.

Ruderman M, MacCarthy D G. Aseptic necrosis in lupus erythematosus. *Arth Rheum* 1964;**7**:709.

Sewell R H. Excision of the patella. *J Bone Joint Surg [Br]* 1952;**34–B**:516,

Sutton F S, Thompson C H, Lipke J, Kettelkamp D B. The effect of patellectomy on knee function. *J Bone Joint Surg [Am]* 1976;**58–A**:537–40.

Stougard J. Patellectomy. *Acta Orthop Scand* 1970;**41**:110–21.

Tasker T. Personal communication, 1982.

Tew M, Waugh W. Guide to recording information about knee replacements. *A manual for use in outpatient clinics and hospitals*. University of Nottingham 1980.

Tjornstrand B. *Tibial osteotomy for medial gonarthrosis*. Lund, Sweden: Dept Orthop Surg, University Hospital, 1981;**S–221**:85.

Tjornstrand B, Hagstedt B, Persson B M. Results of surgical treatment for non-union after high tibial osteotomy in osteoarthritis of the knee. *J Bone Joint Surg [Am]* 1978;**60–A**:973–7.

Tjornstrand B, Selvik G, Egund N, Liundstrand A. Roentgen stereophotogrammetry in high tibial osteotomy for gonarthrosis *Arch Orthop Traumat Surg* 1981;**99**:73–81.

Turner M S, Smillie L S. The effect of tibial torsion in the pathology of the knee. *J Bone Joint Surg [Br]* 1981;**63–B**:396–8.

Volkov M. Allotransplantation of joints. *J Bone Joint Surg [Br]* 1970;**52–B**:49–53.

Wardle E N. Osteotomy of the tibia and fibula. *Surg Gynecol Obstet* 1962;**115**:61–4.

Waugh W. The clinical consequences of deformities about the knee joint. In: Stokes I A F ed. *Mechanical factors and the skeleton*. London: John Libbey, 1981;163–70.

CHAPTER 14

Inflammatory Arthritis

J.K. Lloyd Jones

14.1 Monoarticular synovitis of the knee

The pattern of onset and the distribution of the affected joints are important factors in the differential diagnosis of polyarthritis. The diagnosis of monoarticular synovitis presents an additional challenge with significant therapeutic implications. In our own series of monoarticular synovitis the knee has been the most commonly affected joint. This was so also in the series of 151 patients reviewed by Fletcher and Scott (1975) of whom 112 had involvement of one knee. Monoarticular synovitis in children follows the same trend with the knee affected in 23 out of a series of 33 children reviewed by Bywaters and Ansell (1965). When the knee is involved as part of a generalized inflammatory polyarthritis the diagnostic possibilities are fewer but the general principles of management are similar.

14.1.1 HISTORY AND EXAMINATION

Patients will often relate accurately their experience of pain and stiffness. Swelling is easily seen and felt by the patient; nevertheless it is wise to question carefully a history of swelling unless corroborated by an independent observer. The mode of onset is important. Patients are prone to attribute their symptoms to injury even when some weeks have passed between injury and onset. It is important to know whether the symptoms are constant or variable and what factors ease or aggravate them. Minor repetitive trauma may be overlooked, as may the history of being pricked by a thorn some weeks before the synovitis began. Morning stiffness, which is suggestive of inflammatory arthritis, is an important symptom and should be asked about.

There is a wide spectrum of possible diagnoses and a detailed medical history is needed. In addition a careful systemic enquiry should be made for associated symptoms such as inflammation in the eye (iritis, scleritis or conjunctivitis), rash including the scalp and fingernails, mucosal ulceration, cough, abdominal symptoms or diarrhoea, urethritis, malaise, rigors or shivering bouts and change in weight.

A history of previous self-limiting episodes suggests gout or other crystal synovitis though episodic inflammation also occurs in other conditions including intermittent hydrarthrosis, palindromic rheumatism, familial Mediterranean fever and occasionally in psoriatic arthropathy.

A family history of iritis, psoriasis, inflammatory bowel disease, gout or specific types of inflammatory arthritis may also be helpful.

A full general medical examination is essential as is a careful examination of the spine and all the joints. Unsuspected involvement of more than one joint may be found which alters the diagnostic probabilities. Children, in particular, frequently do not complain spontaneously of pain in all the affected joints.

14.1.2 INVESTIGATION OF SYNOVITIS OF THE KNEE – INFLAMMATION

Much of the synovial cavity of the knee lies close to the skin and both synovial thickening and effusion can usually be detected by clinical examination. Hyperaemia accompanying inflammatory synovitis causes increased warmth of the overlying skin and this can be quantified by thermography (Bacon et al., 1976). The severity of inflammation can also be measured by radio-isotope scanning (Dick et al., 1970) and by clearance from the knee joint of radioactive sodium (Harris et al., 1958) or radioactive xenon (St Onge et al., 1968). In rheumatoid arthritis and in similar types of inflammatory disease the hyperaemia seldom causes redness of the skin and an inflamed red joint should always arouse suspicion of intra-articular infection. Acute gout and other crystal synovitis may also result in a red joint.

14.1.3 SYNOVIAL FLUID

When an effusion is present aspiration of synovial fluid from the knee is usually a simple procedure which, using a strict aseptic technique, can be carried out quickly in the patient's home, in the consulting room or out-patient clinic. Despite this, joint aspiration is frequently overlooked or avoided by physicians who lack special experience of joint disease. In contrast orthopaedic surgeons are usually quick to aspirate joint effusions, though examination of the fluid may be incomplete. As well as routine culture and microscopy, the fluid should be examined under polarized light to detect the presence of crystals (Phelps *et al.*, 1968). A Gram-stained specimen may reveal the presence of bacteria which sometimes grow slowly or not at all on culture, particularly when the patient has previously received inadequate antibiotic therapy. The culture of tubercle bacilli or the finding of acid-alcohol fast bacilli on Ziehl–Nielson staining provide useful confirmation of the presence of tuberculous arthritis; but failure to detect tubercle bacilli in the synovial fluid does not exclude tuberculosis.

A total and a differential white cell count are seldom diagnostic but give useful information which can be assessed together with other features in making a diagnosis (Hollander *et al.*, 1961). About 2–4 ml of fluid should be put directly into a tube containing EDTA and mixed thoroughly to prevent clotting – the tubes provided for routine blood counts are usually satisfactory but precise arrangements should be agreed with the staff of the local laboratory. In uncomplicated osteoarthritis the cells are predominantly monocytic and the count is usually less than 2×10^9 cells l^{-1} (2000 cells mm^{-3}). In rheumatoid and other inflammatory arthritides 60–90% of the cells present will be polymorphonuclear leucocytes and the count may vary between 4×10^9 and 60×10^9 cells l^{-1}. Very high cell counts, predominantly polymorphs, are characteristic of bacterial infection. Inclusion-body cells are seen in the fluid in a number of conditions but are of no diagnostic importance unless the components of the inclusions can be identified by immunofluorescent staining (Zvaifler, 1973).

Rheumatoid factors can be detected in synovial fluid, but few laboratories do this routinely. The interpretation of such tests is difficult. False positive results are common, and the finding of rheumatoid factors in synovial fluid but not in the serum of the same patient is of doubtful diagnostic significance (Seward and Osterland, 1973).

Synovial fluid complement levels are of more value but are rarely estimated outside research laboratories. Complement activity is usually normal in osteoarthritis, low in rheumatoid arthritis and in systemic lupus erythematosus, high in acute gout and very high in Reiter's disease (Pekin and Zvaifler, 1964).

Healthy synovial fluid is highly viscous and does not clot on standing. In the presence of inflammation both viscosity and lubricating power are impaired, the total protein content is increased and there is a tendency to form a spontaneous clot. The alteration in viscosity is paralleled by a change in the quality of the mucin clot formed when a few drops of synovial fluid are added to 2% acetic acid in a test tube (Ropes and Bauer, 1953). The mucin clot formed by normal fluid and by non-inflammatory effusion is tight and strong. Highly inflammatory effusions form a poor clot which fragments readily. It has been our experience that this test may give an equivocal result when there is a doubt clinically whether or not the effusion is inflammatory.

14.1.4 RHEUMATOID FACTORS AND OTHER BLOOD TESTS

In the differential diagnosis of monoarthritis the single most useful blood test is the erythrocyte sedimentation rate (ESR) carried out by the Westergren method. An ESR within the normal range makes serious inflammatory disease unlikely, although infrequently cases are seen of active rheumatoid arthritis without a raised ESR, and the same is seen rather more often in ankylosing spondylitis. Most cases of tuberculous synovitis have a slightly raised ESR. The ESR is raised during a gouty attack. In an elderly patient a mildly or moderately raised ESR has less significance because values greater than 20 mm in the first hour are found in one-third of subjects over the age of 65 without any apparent underlying abnormality (Boyd and Hoffbrand, 1966). The ESR is not a test for arthritis but establishes the presence of inflammation: it is raised also in the presence of tissue ischaemia (such as pulmonary or myocardial infarction), infection, blood dyscrasia, malignancy, dysproteinaemia, hyperthyroidism and liver disease (Zacharski, 1976). High values are found in pregnancy. When there is polycythaemia or congestive heart failure normal values may be found even in the presence of overt inflammation.

Rheumatoid factors are proteins in the serum which act as antibodies against IgG immunoglobulins. As detected by the RA Latex test or by the Rose–Waaler test (SCAT), rheumatoid factors are themselves IgM immunoglobulins reacting respectively with human IgG (Latex test) or with rabbit IgG (Rose–Waaler test). As with all biological tests a balance must be sought between sensitivity and specificity. Acceptable techniques for IgM rheumatoid factors should give up to 4% positive results in the adult population. Random testing will therefore yield a number of positive results in subjects with no evidence of rheumatoid disease (Ball and Lawrence, 1961); while about 30% of adult patients with undoubted rheumatoid arthritis have persistently negative tests. The tests are also positive in a proportion of patients suffering from illnesses other than rheumatoid arthritis, particularly other multisystem inflammatory connective tissue diseases and some chronic infections (Dresner and Trombly, 1959). The RA Latex test is more sensitive but less specific while the Rose–Waaler test is slightly more specific but less sensitive. It follows that the presence or absence of IgM rheumatoid factors in the serum is not a diagnostic test for rheumatoid arthritis but merely another factor to be taken into account when trying to arrive at a diagnosis. It is seldom helpful to test for rheumatoid factors in a patient in whom the ESR is normal.

It has been suggested that rheumatoid factors belonging to the IgG class of immunoglobulins may have greater specificity and greater diagnostic significance. At the time of writing this lacks confirmation. IgG rheumatoid factors and rheumatoid factors belonging to other immunoglobulin classes are not detected by the RA Latex or Rose–Waaler tests and their presence can be shown only by more sophisticated techniques.

C-reactive protein is an abnormal serum constituent which appears in response to infection, tissue damage or inflammation. In general terms its appearance parallels a rise in ESR though it may appear earlier or later in certain diseases (McConkey *et al.*, 1972). Increased plasma concentrations of alpha-two globulins and of gamma-globulins usually have a similar significance.

A high or rising antistreptolysin-0 titre implies recent infection with Group A beta-haemolytic streptococci. The significance of this test is that rheumatic fever is almost excluded by titres persistently below 200 units. It is not a relevant test in the investigation of chronic monoarthritis and is of little value in the diagnosis of active streptococcal infection.

Serum uric acid results should be interpreted with considerable caution. High values occur in the absence of gout. Patients occasionally have a normal value at the time of an acute gouty episode; and in such patients serial estimations over a period of weeks may be needed in order to confirm hyperuricaemia. In acute gout the clinical diagnosis is best confirmed by the demonstration in the synovial fluid of birefringent crystals of sodium monourate.

14.1.5 HISTOCOMPATIBILITY ANTIGENS

Histocompatability antigens are carried on the surface of cells throughout the body and are inherited in a similar manner to ABO blood groups. They are most easily determined in blood leucocytes and are known as human leucocyte antigens (HLA antigens).

A very close relationship has been established between the antigen HLA B27 and the tendency to develop ankylosing spondylitis (Brewerton *et al.* 1973; Schlosstein *et al.*, 1973). There is also an association between HLA B27 and certain related conditions such as Reiter's disease, arthritis following intestinal infection and acute anterior uveitis. The HLA B27 antigen is present in 90–96% of patients with classical ankylosing spondylitis but is also found in between 5% and 10% of the normal European population. It has been calculated that of subjects who are B27 positive only 5% of men and 1% of women will develop clinical ankylosing spondylitis (Brewerton *et al.*, 1974). Although studies on B27 positive blood donors have suggested more frequent involvement (Calin and Fries, 1975) this means that seeking the HLA B27 antigen is of little help in reaching a diagnosis in any individual patient, although it is of great importance in research studies as a genetic marker.

At present typing sera for HLA antigens are scarce and the tests are expensive. If simpler methods could be found for detecting the presence of a range of HLA and related antigens, including HLA antigens of the D series, then in future it might be that tissue typing would become more valuable in the diagnosis and prognosis of individual patients.

14.1.6 RADIOLOGY

In addition to films of the knee to demonstrate any local abnormality, every adult patient with otherwise unexplained synovitis of one or both knees should have a single plain radiograph of the sacroiliac joints and an anteroposterior view of the feet. Of patients with ankylosing spondylitis 10% are said to seek medical advice first because of symptoms in a peripheral joint, and rheumatoid erosions are sometimes seen in the foot in the absence of symptoms. Radiographs of the sacroiliac joints in children and adolescents are unhelpful because of difficulty in interpretation.

14.1.7 SYNOVIAL BIOPSY

Many types of synovitis are self-limiting and biopsy is seldom indicated until synovitis has been present for three months or more. Samples of synovium for histology can be obtained by blind needle biopsy (Schumacher and Kulka, 1972), during arthroscopy or at arthrotomy. Synovial involvement is rarely uniform throughout the joint (Cruickshank, 1952; Fassbender, 1975) and it is better to take biopsies under direct vision. This is now most commonly done by arthroscopy (Yates and Scott, 1975) which avoids the delayed convalescence and morbidity of open operation.

Characteristic histological changes are seen in typical cases of gout and pseudogout, malignant synovioma, pigmented villonodular synovitis, sarcoidosis, synovial chondromatosis and osteochondromatosis and tuberculosis. In monoarticular rheumatoid arthritis the synovium may show the typical changes specified in the American Rheumatism Association diagnostic criteria (Ropes *et al.*, 1959). These require the presence of three or more of the following:

(1) Marked villous hypertrophy.
(2) Proliferation of superficial synovial cells, often with palisading.
(3) Marked infiltration of chronic inflammatory cells (lymphocytes and plasma cells predominating) with a tendency to form lymphoid follicles.
(4) Deposition of compact fibrin, either on the surface or interstitially.
(5) Foci of cell necrosis.

Using these criteria it is sometimes possible to identify cases of monoarticular rheumatoid arthritis (Fletcher and Scott, 1975) many of whom later develop rheumatoid involvement of other joints. Similar but less severe abnormalities may be seen in mild or early rheumatoid arthritis, in synovitis due to other inflammatory arthritides, sometimes in tuberculosis, and also in the synovitis sometimes associated with osteoarthritis or secondary to a mechanical derangement. There may be difficulty in distinguishing between late proliferative rheumatoid synovitis with haemosiderin deposition and pigmented villonodular synovitis. The interpretation of synovial histology is seldom easy and several authors stress the non-specificity of the histological appearance in synovitis due to different causes (Gardner, 1972; Fassbender, 1975; Revell and Mayston, 1982). Soren (1978) tabulates the frequency of various histopathological changes (including plasmacytic and other cellular infiltrates and fibrin deposition) in several different categories of synovitis among which he lists osteoarthritis, chronic post-traumatic synovitis and unclassified synovitis. Fassbender has suggested that in rheumatoid synovitis the only truly specific feature is the finding of rheumatoid nodular necrosis with a surrounding cellular palisade.

In summary, cellular proliferation, exudate formation and plasmacyte and lymphocyte infiltration are part of any sterile synovitis, and synovial histology alone often fails to distinguish with certainty between the common causes of monoarticular synovitis. The histological appearance of such biopsies is often reported as being 'compatible with a diagnosis of rheumatoid arthritis', but such a report should not be taken as indicating that the diagnosis is necessarily one of rheumatoid arthritis. Even tuberculous synovitis may not show pathognomonic changes and it is essential to send to the laboratory specimens of synovium both for histology and for culture. The purpose of the biopsy and the sites from which samples were taken should be clearly stated and the laboratory should be asked to seek evidence of tuberculous infection both by direct microscopic examination and by culture.

14.2   Rheumatoid arthritis

Typical rheumatoid arthritis affects 1–2% of the adult population of Europe and Northern America. When mild and probable disease is included the overall prevalence of rheumatoid arthritis is of the order of 2–5% (Lawrence et al., 1966). The disease is twice as common in women as men.

Rheumatoid arthritis usually starts in the fingers, wrists and feet spreading later to involve other joints, so that in late and severe cases nearly every joint in the body may be involved. The knees are often involved early. The pattern of onset is not constant and the disease may appear first in almost any joint. Presentation with apparent capsulitis of the shoulder or with synovitis in one or other knee is not uncommon.

14.2.1   PROGNOSIS

Rheumatoid arthritis is characterized by spontaneous and unpredictable episodes of exacerbation and remission. This increases the difficulty of assessing the benefits of different management regimes and carefully controlled studies are always needed in the evaluation of new treatments.

The long-term prognosis in rheumatoid arthritis is especially unpredictable. Nearly half the patients seen during the first year from onset may be expected eventually to go into remission with no or only minor permanent sequelae, while only between 5–15% will develop progressive joint damage and severe crippling (Ragan, 1949; Duthie *et al.*, 1964). The remainder will run a fluctuating course, often with periods of long remission, but probably with slowly deteriorating function. In any individual patient there are no consistent pointers to prognosis, although there is an increased tendency to severe disease among patients who have persisting high titres of rheumatoid factors, rheumatoid nodules or very high ESR (over 100 mm h^{-1}), in those who develop marginal joint erosions early and in those with a family history of severe disease. The possession of certain HLA antigens of the D series may also influence prognosis. Patients with asymmetrical and scanty joint involvement fare better overall than those with symmetrical disease though they may still suffer severe damage to individual joints. Younger patients and those with disease of acute onset requiring early hospitalization do slightly better as a group. Patients in whom the onset is insidious may do badly in the end.

14.2.2 AETIOLOGY

The cause, or causes, of rheumatoid arthritis remain unknown. Current theories postulate a genetically determined susceptibility and that in such subjects a chronic inflammatory response may be provoked by a suitable trigger, which may be a persisting antigen (possibly an infecting organism) or a transient antigen which resembles antigenetically some constituent of the human body. It is not known whether this hypothetical antigen is located in the joints or not, but the histological appearance of rheumatoid synovium suggests that it is the site of intense immunological activity. Rheumatoid synovial fluid is usually rich in white blood cells with neutrophil polymorphs predominating over lymphocytes. The fluid itself contains not only inflammatory mediators but also phosphatases and a variety of proteolytic enzymes.

14.2.3 CONSERVATIVE MANAGEMENT OF RHEUMATOID ARTHRITIS

The basis of sound management is an accurate diagnosis coupled with a full discussion with the patient of the nature of the disease, the probable prognosis and the proposed plan of action. The objectives are to relieve pain and stiffness, to minimize damage to the joints, to prevent deformity and at all costs in the knee to avoid the development of flexion contracture.

In any but the earliest disease, and in particular if any operative treatment is likely to be needed, close co-operation between the orthopaedic surgeon and a physician experienced in the natural history of the disease is of great importance. Where crippling and permanent deformity have already occurred team management by the physician, surgeon, family doctor, hospital and community-based remedial therapists and community agencies will be needed. The general principles of management are similar whether the knee is involved alone or as part of a generalized polyarthritis.

(a) Simple analgesic drugs

A few patients with mild disease can be managed with simple analgesics alone taken intermittently as required. These drugs (see Table 14.1) are non-narcotic analgesic drugs acting centrally with no effect on the local inflammation.

The great majority of patients will need non-steroid anti-inflammatory drugs and the simple analgesics are most useful when used to supplement anti-inflammatory therapy.

(b) Non-steroid anti-inflammatory drugs

Non-steroid anti-inflammatory drugs (see Table 14.1) in general do not affect the course of the disease but provide symptomatic treatment only. They seldom produce complete remission of symptoms though in some patients the response may be gratifying. In patients with early disease and without permanent joint damage non-steroid anti-inflammatory drugs have been shown to reduce the diameter of swollen proximal interphalangeal joints (Boardman and Hart, 1967), reduce skin temperatures over inflamed joints, reduce the uptake of technetium by inflamed synovium (Dick, 1972) and shorten the duration of morning stiffness. This latter is a valuable clinical indicator of the severity of disease activity. They do not affect the ESR or titres of rheumatoid factor.

The mode of action of the non-steroid anti-inflammatory drugs is unknown. Members of this group of drugs have been shown to have a variety of biological actions including effects on cell membrane and lysosomal membrane function and on a number of intracellular enzyme systems. Many of these drugs have a powerful inhibitory effect on prostaglandin synthesis while others may inhibit the migration into the synovium of acute and chronic inflammatory cells. There is no overall unifying hypothesis and it is likely that several mechanisms are involved.

(c) Choice of non-steroid anti-inflammatory drugs

Aspirin is a potent anti-inflammatory drug but only when used in doses greater than 3.6 g daily. There is a high incidence of side effects and less than 50% of patients will be able to tolerate doses of this order for more than three months. Aspirin is now seldom regarded as the drug of first choice for symptomatic relief in rheumatoid arthritis.

Phenylbutazone is associated with an unacceptable risk of serious toxicity including fluid retention, gastrointestinal bleeding, bone marrow aplasia and

Table 14.1 Drugs used in the management of rheumatoid arthritis

Simple analgesic drugs without anti-inflammatory activity
Paracetamol (acetaminophen)
Codeine
Dihydrocodeine (DF 118)
Dextropropoxyphene (with Paracetamol in Distalgesic)
Aspirin in small doses

Drugs with analgesic and anti-inflammatory activity (NSAID)
(1) Ibuprofen (Brufen, Motrin)   Diclofenac (Voltarol)
    Naproxen (Naprosyn)   Fenclofenac (Flenac)
    Ketoprofen (Alrheumat, Orudis)
    Fenoprofen (Fenopron)   Azapropazone (Rheumox)
    Flurbiprofen (Froben)   Feprazone (Methrazone)
    Fenbufen (Lederfen)
                                        Flufenamic acid (Meralen, Arlef)
                                        Mefenamic acid (Ponstan)
    Sulindac (Clinoril)
    Tolmetin (Tolectin)
                                        Piroxicam (Feldene)
    Diflunisal (Dolobid)
    Benorylate (Benoral)   Tiaprofenic acid (Surgam)
(2) Possibly more powerful but more toxic:
    Aspirin in full dosage (greater than 3.6 g daily)
    Indomethacin (Indocid, Indocin)
    Phenylbutazone (Butazolidin)
    Oxyphenbutazone (Tanderil)

Powerful anti-inflammatory drugs without analgesic action
Corticosteroids (e.g. Prednisolone)
Corticotrophin (ACTH)

Slow-acting (remission-inducing) drugs
Gold – sodium aurothiomalate (Myocrisin)
        Auranofin
Penicillamine (Distamine)
Antimalarials – Hydroxychloroquine (Plaquenil)
                Chloroquine
Immunosuppressives – Azathioprine
                     Chlorambucil
                     Cyclophosphamide
Immunostimulants – Levamisole

dyscrasia and chromosome abnormalities.

We should use the minimum effective dose of the drug likely to have the least toxicity. Doctors and patients have their favourite preparations but it is usual to start with one of the proprionic acid derivatives such as ibuprofen (Brufen) 800 mg morning and evening with an additional 400 mg or 800 mg midday if necessary, or naproxen (Naprosyn) 500 mg morning and evening. The newer preparations differ from each other not so much in effectiveness as in duration of action. Patient response to each of these drugs is very variable both in terms of unwanted and of therapeutic effects; it may be necessary to try several before one is found which suits the individual. Except in mild or intermittent disease the chosen drug should be taken regularly, used at the recommended frequency and at maximum dose for 7–10 days before concluding that it is ineffective. Dyspepsia may be troublesome but is not necessarily dangerous: none of these drugs, however, is entirely free from the risk of gastrointestinal bleeding. Care should be taken if the patient is concurrently taking oral anticoagulants, hypoglycaemic agents or other drugs which are highly protein-bound in the plasma. When it is not possible to find a preparation that is tolerated orally several of these drugs can be administered in the form of suppositories.

In general, mixtures of anti-inflammatory drugs should be avoided, but when the regime outlined above does not control morning stiffness adequately it may be useful to add a night-time dose of indomethacin. Indomethacin may be associated with headaches, light-headedness, giddiness or nightmares as well as with gastrointestinal symptoms. These side effects can often be eliminated by reducing the dose.

(d) Physical measures

Physical treatments are frequently needed as an adjunct to the anti-inflammatory drug regime. The most important are exercises to maintain muscle power and splinting to protect the inflamed joint from stress and to prevent deformity.

Ice packs help to reduce pain and ease muscle spasm (Kirk and Kersley, 1968). They are particularly useful during episodes of acute inflammation. Moist heat in the form of hot packs or in the hydrotherapy pool is comforting and also helps to relax muscle spasm; but many rheumatoid patients find that their pain is made worse by radiant heat and electrical treatments such as short-wave diathermy. There is seldom justification for using heat except as a preliminary to exercise.

Normal gait, on the level, requires full extension in the knee joint and free painless flexion to at least 70°. In the presence of an effusion the knee lies in greatest comfort at about 30° of flexion and a tense effusion will prevent full extension. If extension is inhibited by pain or by an effusion, a fixed flexion deformity will occur due to contracture and adhesions affecting the

331

hamstring muscles, the posterior capsule and possibly the anterior cruciate ligament. In late disease, articular cartilage loss and collapse of the weight-bearing surfaces lead to deformity. In early disease, it seems that flexion contracture precedes the development of the typical rheumatoid knee deformities of valgus and external rotation as well as posterior subluxation of the tibia. Fixed flexion may develop quite rapidly even in the absence of an effusion and in children flexion contractures may develop within a few days. The regime of management should include a programme of exercises and splinting designed to prevent or overcome this deformity. Loss of flexion range is less common and is easier to overcome.

The exercise programme should be supervised by a physiotherapist experienced in the management of inflammatory joint disease. Isometric exercises (static quadriceps drill) are essential in order to maintain and increase quadriceps power but injudicious flexion and extension exercises may aggravate the inflammation. The physiotherapist needs to gain the patient's confidence and the treatment should not be painful.

(e) Rest and splinting

The patient is whom there is active synovitis in many joints, severe morning stiffness, fatigue, anaemia and a high ESR should, if possible, be admitted for a period of rest in hospital either under the care of a rheumatologist or of a rheumatologist and an orthopaedic surgeon working together. We have also found it helpful on occasions to admit patients in whom there is severe synovitis in one or both knees without generalized disease.

The use of rest in the management of pain and inflammation was advocated by Hilton in 1863. The dangers of indiscriminate bed rest were graphically described by Asher (1947). Unsupervised rest in bed at home is particularly harmful for rheumatoid patients because of the additional risk of developing fixed joint deformities, especially flexion contracture of the knee, and rapid loss of muscle tone and power. Unsupervised bed rest in hospital during the treatment of an acute intercurrent illness may be equally harmful. The posture of the rheumatoid patient in bed should be carefully supervised by nurses and physiotherapists familiar with the management of the disease.

The knees should be kept in full extension and, if necessary, supported either by a posterior gutter splint or by a plaster cylinder split down each side and held in place by a firm bandage. For longer term use at home, a light-weight plastic splint may be provided.

Controlled studies have shown that immobilization of an inflamed knee in a plaster cylinder for up to four weeks has a beneficial effect on pain, swelling and ultimate range of movement, though physiotherapy was necessary after removal of the cast in order to regain movement (Harris and Copp, 1962; Partridge and Duthie, 1963). Where damage to the joint surfaces has already occurred, such immobilization may lead to permanent stiffness and it is our practice to compromise by removing the splint for washing and once a day for movement within the pain-free range supervised by the physiotherapist. Isometric quadriceps exercises are instituted from the outset.

If the patient is unable to tolerate splinting of the knee in full extension, aspiration of the joint is indicated.

(f) Flexion contracture

Once a flexion contracture has occurred there is a high risk of recurrence and the patient will need to continue to use a back splint at night at home for as long as active synovitis persists.

Fixed flexion due to muscle spasm can be overcome by serial splinting. Improvement can often be obtained also by skin traction applied to the leg.

Any but the earliest degree of flexion contracture is accompanied by posterior subluxation of the tibia on the femur. When this is present attempts to overcome the contracture by serial plaster casts or wedging a plaster cylinder will fail because the tibia will not slide forward normally on the femur during the last 30° of extension. Consequently the anterior border of the tibial condyles impacts on the femoral condyles and further extension of the tibia on the femur is achieved only by the posterior half of the joint becoming wedged open. Weight bearing in this situation is painful and early recurrence of the flexion contracture is probable. Furthermore, abnormal stresses are imposed on the joint surfaces resulting in increased articular cartilage damage and collapse of the underlying bone. Prevention of flexion deformity before posterior subluxation has occurred is therefore vital.

Attempts have been made to overcome the problem of posterior subluxation by using three-pin traction to reduce the flexion contracture: a posterior force is applied by a pin through the lower end of the femur, an anterior force by a pin through the upper tibia, and distraction by a pin in the lower tibia. This combination of forces will overcome even severe flexion contractures, but the method cannot be recommended because the result will be a painful stiff extended knee instead of a painful stiff flexed knee. Furthermore posterior subluxation recurs when the correcting force is removed. If injudicious traction is applied there is also a risk to the viability of the tissues behind the knee.

It has not been our practice to carry out soft-tissue operations to overcome flexion contracture. This topic is well reviewed by Goldie (1980).

(g) Intra-articular corticosteroids

Aspiration and intra-articular injection can safely be carried out in the consulting room or ward treatment room using pre-sterilized disposable needles and syringes with strict asepsis and a meticulous no-touch technique.

In the presence of continuing active synovial inflammation such an effusion will recur within a few days of aspiration and it is often helpful to inject corticosteroid into the joint through the needle which was inserted for aspiration. This has the advantage of delivering a powerful anti-inflammatory drug close to the site of the inflammation and obviates many of the hazards of systemic corticosteroid administration. There is, however, some absorption of the injected steroid into the general circulation and patients will often comment on the improvement in non-injected joints and a reduction in morning stiffness for a few days after the injection. Transient impairment of pituitary–adrenal function can be demonstrated following intra-articular steroid injection.

The steroid injected should be one which is active locally without needing first to be metabolized in the liver. An insoluble preparation should be used: soluble preparations such as hydrocortisone succinate or prednisolone phosphate are ineffective because they are rapidly absorbed from the knee joint into the circulation.

Occasionally patients experience an acute increase in pain and inflammation in the injected joint lasting from a few hours to a day or so. This appears to be due to an acute crystal synovitis, akin to gout, induced by the injected steroid (McCarty and Hogan, 1964); this reaction has become much less common now that manufacturers are aware of the importance of crystal size. Poor distribution of the steroid within the knee may occur if a small volume is injected into a joint in which there is considerable synovial proliferation but only a small effusion. When injecting the knee the steroid suspension should either be washed in and out of syringe with synovial fluid or, better, diluted with 10 ml of sterile normal saline before injection.

Aspiration and injection of the knee joint anteriorly may be indicated in the management of a tense or large popliteal cyst (see page 347).

When the injection is part of a general regime to which the patient is responding, the improvement in the injected joint may last for several months. More commonly the injection may need to be repeated in 1–3 weeks. Hollander (1972) advocates repeated injections into the same joint over a number of years. Most clinicians, however, reserve intra-articular steroid injections for occasional use and as an adjunct to general measures. There have been infrequent reports of avascular necrosis and, in joints submitted to frequent injections, of damage similar to that seen in neuropathic joints.

The rheumatoid joint, especially in long-standing disease, is very susceptible to secondary bacterial infection. This may present as obvious septic arthritis, but commonly the infection is subacute or indolent and may not be detected unless the synovial fluid is carefully examined. It is just such a joint, which may be a little more hot and painful than the others, that is often selected for steroid injection. We have seen cases in which Gram-positive cocci were seen on direct microscopic examination of the synovial fluid but where the organism did not grow on culture until after two or three days. Each time a joint is injected the synovial fluid must be sent for microscopy and culture, and it is helpful to send a small volume with anticoagulant for total and differential white cell count. If there is doubt, the fluid should be cultured in broth as well as on a plate. Unless there is a strong suspicion of infection, it is not necessary to withhold the steroid injection while awaiting the results of culture. If bacteria are present in the joint, appropriate treatment can be started after the bacteriological report has been received.

14.2.4 SLOW-ACTING (REMISSION-INDUCING) DRUGS IN RHEUMATOID ARTHRITIS

All the drugs in this group in use at present (see Table 14.2) are potentially dangerous and the decision to prescribe them should only be made by an experienced clinician. Careful monitoring for side-effects is mandatory.

The mechanisms by which these drugs act remain unknown. The clinical response does not appear for several weeks or even months after the treatment has started and the response in an individual patient is unpredictable. Recently it has been claimed that some of the anti-inflammatory drugs may have a secondary slow-acting effect. If these claims can be confirmed this will be a valuable advance, for they are less likely to be associated with dangerous side-effects.

Table 14.2 Side-effects and toxicity of slow-acting drugs in rheumatoid arthritis

Gold	Rashes
	Oral ulceration
	Diarrhoea
	Proteinuria
	Thrombocytopaenia, neutropaenia, aplastic anaemia
Penicillamine	Rashes (some potentially serious such as pemphigus)
	Proteinuria
	Thrombocytopaenia, neutropaenia, aplastic anaemia
	Myasthenia
Antimalarials	Retinal damage
	Dermatitis
	Neuropathy, myopathy
Immunosuppressives	Infection
	Bone marrow suppression
	Cystitis with cyclophosphamide
	Cirrhosis with chlorambucil
	Long term risk of neoplasia, especially lymphoma
Levamisole	Bone marrow suppression
	Oral ulceration

Because of the dangers involved, slow-acting drugs are at present reserved for:

(1) Patients with generalized disease in whom there is clear evidence of progressive joint damage.

(2) Patients whose synovitis cannot be adequately controlled by the regime outlined above.

(3) For systemic complications of rheumatoid disease.

(4) For those patients with continuing active synovitis for more than twelve months from the onset, when spontaneous remission is becoming less likely.

Where only one or a few joints are affected then local measures are to be preferred.

14.2.5 SYSTEMIC CORTICOSTEROID THERAPY

Corticosteroids are powerful anti-inflammatory agents but have no intrinsic analgesic effects nor do they modify the disease process in the long term. They are the only group of drugs that will predictably suppress rheumatoid inflammation. This effect is only achieved at a high cost in undesirable effects, with the possibility of dangerous and life-threatening complications. Systemic use is, therefore, rarely justified unless other measures, including a trial of the slow-acting drugs, have failed. If the use of corticosteroids is unavoidable, they should be used in the smallest possible dose, while continuing with a full non-steroid anti-inflammatory regime. Prednisolone is the drug usually used and in the long term in rheumatoid arthritis the daily dose should not exceed 7.5 mg. Even at this level there is a significant risk of complications. In order to reduce pituitary–adrenal suppression the drug should be taken in a single morning dose. In children, an alternate day regime helps to reduce the disturbance of growth.

ACTH is associated with the same hazards as prednisolone and some of the side-effects are more troublesome.

As with the slow-acting drugs systemic corticosteroids should be used only for generalized disease.

The hazards of corticosteroid therapy in relation to surgical treatment are discussed on page 340.

14.3 Management of other types of inflammatory synovitis

In general, the conservative management of sterile inflammatory synovitis in the knee due to causes other than rheumatoid arthritis is similar to that outlined under the conservative management of the knee joint in rheumatoid arthritis.

Acute episodes of pain and swelling occur during the course of osteo-arthritis and may be due to an unnoticed minor injury, or episodes of crystal synovitis. Such episodes repond well to anti-inflammatory drugs and physiotherapy. Analgesic and anti-inflammatory drugs are often effective in relieving rest pain in osteoarthritis but are disappointing when pain is mainly on weight bearing. In this circumstance, active physiotherapy improves muscle control and may be more effective. Chronic post-traumatic synovitis and chronic synovitis due to osteoarthritis are managed along lines similar to any other synovial inflammation but the expectation of improvement is rather less.

When conservative measures fail, the choice of second-line medical treatments is more limited in non-rheumatoid synovitis.

Immunosuppressive drugs are effective both in psoriatic arthropathy and in the skin lesions of psoriasis, but the hazards of their use remain. Gold and some of the other slow-acting drugs may also be beneficial in psoriatic arthropathy. None of this group of drugs has been shown to be of benefit in ankylosing spondylitis or other types of inflammatory arthropathy.

14.4   Operations for inflammatory arthritis of the knee

Correct timing of orthopaedic surgical procedures in the management of patients afflicted by inflammatory arthritis depends not only on a knowledge of the natural history of the particular disease and its likely response to non-operative measures, but also on familiarity with appropriate surgical procedures and their hazards. In most instances this is best achieved by the orthopaedic surgeon and the rheumatologist seeing together those patients in whom operation may be indicated. A plan of management for each patient can be agreed at a single visit.

14.4.1   INDICATIONS FOR OPERATION

There are three major indications for operation in inflammatory joint disease:

(1) *Diagnosis*: synovial biopsy is discussed on page 326.

(2) *Prophylaxis or cure*: synovectomy will be discussed in the next section.

(3) *Reconstruction and salvage*: some patients with rheumatoid arthritis and other inflammatory arthropathies will experience a remission of their disease before permanent damage has occurred in their joints. In the remainder, who have continuing active inflammation, even the best conservative management at present available will not arrest or delay the progress of the disease in every case. If the joint has already been damaged, deterioration will continue in the absence of inflammation due to secondary osteoarthritis. This is particularly true of a complex weight-bearing joint such as the knee, and there will be a continuing need for many years for the development of improved techniques of arthroplasty.

14.4.2 SYNOVECTOMY

Volkmann first reported successful synovectomy in 1877 for tuberculous synovitis. Reports in nontuberculous synovitis followed in 1887 and 1894 (Speed, 1924). Swett (1924) described good results following synovectomy of the knee for rheumatoid arthritis, but stressed the importance of operating early in the course of the disease. In 1955 London reported good results after two years in two-thirds of a series of 32 patients; the poor results were related to the extent of damage to the joint at the time of operation and to continuing active rheumatoid disease. As interest in surgical treatment of inflammatory joint disease increased, there was a resurgence of enthusiasm for synovectomy (Aidem and Baker, 1964; Stevens and Whitefield, 1966; Barnes and Mason, 1967). In most series, however, the proportion of good results diminished as follow-up was extended beyond three years. Several authors also noted the regeneration of synovium which in many cases could not be distinguished from active rheumatoid synovium (Patzakis *et al.*, 1973).

Despite the large number of follow-up reports there is a dearth of controlled studies of synovectomy compared with non-operative treatment. In the UK multicentre synovectomy trial (Arthritis and Rheumatism Council, 1976) there was less pain and tenderness, smaller effusions and less radiological deterioration in the operated knees. Unfortunately, numbers were smal and the study was terminated at three years. The outcome of a multicentre trial from the USA was less encouraging (Arthritis Foundation, 1977) and only soft-tissue swelling was significantly less in the operated group at three years. This topic is reviewed by Taylor and Hill (1978).

There is no doubt that synovectomy of the knee, carried out before the development of marginal erosions or significant damage to cartilage, is effective in the short term in relieving pain and swelling. It is an attractive hypothesis that removal of aggressive inflamed synovium would protect the joint from further damage, but despite a number of anecdotal reports there is unfortunately no convincing evidence to support this. Synovectomy carried out within the first 12 months of the disease is probably not indicated because of the possibility of spontaneous remission. Yet when operation is delayed until after the first year significant damage will already have developed in a proportion of knee joints and the benefits of early synovectomy will have been lost. These difficulties, together perhaps with improvements in non-operative management, have made synovectomy less popular; and in our own unit the number of synovectomies carried out for inflammatory joint disease has fallen steadily during the past few years. We now only consider synovectomy of the knee when there is continuing pain and synovial thickening in one or both knees which has not responded to medical management for six months or more and in the absence of active generalized joint disease.

(a) Irradiation synovectomy

When radioactive particles of a suitable size are injected intra-articularly they are taken up by the synovium, thus administering ionizing radiation locally to the diseased tissue in rheumatoid arthritis. If successful, such radiation synovectomy (synoviorthesis) would not only avoid the morbidity of surgical synovectomy and the need for post-operative rehabilitation, but, by ablating the whole of the diseased synovium, would also be more complete than surgical synovectomy.

Ansell *et al.* (1963) reported a good response in 16 of 30 knees a year after intra-articular injection of gold-198, with some improvement in a further seven knees. Typical of many subsequent uncontrolled studies is that of Topp *et al.* (1975) who noted clinical improvement at six months in 81% of knees injected with gold-198, but with a decline to only 50% over five years. Benefit may not appear until three months and is probably maximal at one year. Some joints will need more than one injection. Most of the radioactive material remains localized in the injected joint but there is leakage to regional lymph nodes, and to the body generally, to an extent which varies from patient to patient and with the preparation injected. Gold-198 is both a beta and a gamma-ray emitter and because of the penetration of gamma rays carries a greater risk of extrasynovial irradiation. Its use has now been largely abandoned in the knee in favour of yttrium-90 which has a similar half-life and is a powerful pure beta emitter with average penetration in soft tissue of 3.6 mm. Extrasynovial leakage can be reduced by concomitant intra-articular administration of corticosteroid and by resting the injected limb (either by splinting or by bed rest after injection for up to 3 days). Recently Onetti *et al.* (1982) have used phosphorus-32 colloidal chromic phosphate in the hope that the larger particle size would mean greater retention in the joint.

The intra-articular injection of radioactive material is followed by an increase in the number of circulating lymphocytes showing damaged chromosomes (Stevenson *et al.*, 1973). To some extent the amount of damage is related to the degree of extrasynovial escape of radioactivity (Gumpel, 1978). Up to the present, there have been no reports of increased malignancy, but radiation damage to skin and local tissues may result from injudicious choice of isotope and from faulty injection technique.

Controlled trials of radiosynovectomy against placebo (Bridgman *et al.*, 1973) and against surgical synovectomy (Gumpel and Roles 1975; Nissila *et al.*, 1978) suggest that the overall efficacy of surgical and radiation synovectomy is similar. The preliminary reports of another study comparing yttrium-90 with inactive yttrium in chronic knee effusions showed no benefit in the treated knees at two years (Yates *et al.*, 1977).

Radiation synovectomy is usually reserved for patients over the age of 45 who might otherwise be considered for surgical synovectomy. Radiation may be marginally more successful than operation when there are longstanding changes in the knee. If radiation is unsuccessful then surgical synovectomy can be considered later. There is a useful editorial review by Lee (1982) and a review in greater detail by Gumpel (1978).

(b) Chemical synovectomy

Attempts have been made to ablate rheumatoid synovium by the intra-articular injection of chemicals other than radioactive colloids. Numerous substances have been tried but interest has been greatest in osmic acid and in alkylating agents such as Thiotepa. Reported success rates with osmic acid vary and there may be a risk of cartilage damage. Despite some early enthusiasm controlled studies do not show significant benefit from intra-articular Thiotepa (Currey, 1965; Ellison and Flatt, 1971).

14.4.3 HAZARDS ASSOCIATED WITH SURGERY

(a) Cervical instability

The cervical spine may be affected in many types of inflammatory arthritis and is frequently involved in the rheumatoid arthritis. This may occur within the first year of the illness (Winfield *et al.*, 1981) and is usual in late or severe rheumatoid disease. Cervical subluxation can be demonstrated in a quarter of hospital patients with rheumatoid arthritis (Mathews, 1969) and carries a risk of cord compression and tetraplegia (Marks and Sharp, 1981). This is a hazard which should be considered before any rheumatoid patient is given a general anaesthetic.

Anterior atlantoaxial subluxation usually reduces when the neck is extended by can be detected on a lateral radiograph taken with the neck fully flexed. A view in extension is not needed unless the flexion film is abnormal or the odontoid is fractured or severely eroded. Subaxial subluxation is less common that atlantoaxial subluxation but is more likely to result in cord compression. The presence or severity of subluxation is not by itself an indiction for cervical fusion. This operation is indicated if there are symptoms or signs of spinal cord compression, or if intractable pain cannot be relieved by a collar. When any degree of cervical instability is present in a patient undergoing operation, the anaesthetist and operating room staff should be warned, and it is out custom to send such patients to the anaesthetic room wearing a soft collar.

(b) Steroids and surgery

Patients who have been treated with systemic corticosteroids or with ACTH should be presumed to have an impaired response to stress of the hypo-thalamic–pituitary–adrenal axis. This response may remain impaired for some years after steroid therapy has stopped. Simple tests of adrenal function alone, such as the plasma cortisol response to an injection of tetracosactrin (Synacthen), are not sufficient to exclude a failure of normal response by the

340

hypothalamus or pituitary. Testing of hypothalamic and pituitary function is complex and even the most elaborate testing cannot ensure that there will be a normal response to the stresses of general anaesthesia and surgery.

In practical terms the safest course is to give supplementary steroid cover routinely during the operative period to:

(1) Any patient who has received systemic treatment with steroids or ACTH for more than two or three weeks within the preceding twelve months.

(2) Any patient who has received more prolonged treatment within the preceding two years.

Elaborate steroid regimes are not necessary. The pre-operative regime should be continued up to the time of operation and the same regime should be resumed as soon as is practicable afterwards. In addition, the patient should be given intramuscular hydrocortisone succinate to supplement endogenous cortisol secretion (usually 100 mg is given with the pre-medication, 100 mg with the post-operative analgesic and 50 mg or 100 mg every 8–12 hours for 24 to 48 hours depending on the magnitude of the procedure).

Some anaesthetists also infuse hydrocortisone during prolonged and major operations. If it is not possible to resume the pre-operative steroid regime within 24 hours of the operation then cover with intramuscular hydro-cortisone may need to be prolonged. Post-operative collapse, which might in any way be due to steroid depletion, should be treated immediately by intravenous injection of 100 mg hydrocortisone succinate.

There are theoretical grounds for supposing that systemic steroid treat-ment might lead to an increase in wound infection and poor healing: this problem is considered later. Patients taking corticosteroids are also at risk of developing pulmonary tuberculosis, hypertension and diabetes mellitus. Hypokalaemia may be a problem and the patient is doubly at hazard of potassium depletion if diuretics are being given concurrently to control oedema or hypertension.

(c) Slow-acting (remission inducing) drugs and operation

In general non-steroid anti-inflammatory drugs should be continued for symptomatic control over the period of surgery. Patients taking slow-acting drugs require careful supervision. Admission to an orthopaedic ward may disturb the usual pattern of routine monitoring which may itself be a hazard to the patient. Penicillamine and gold may induce renal damage shown by proteinuria. Many of the slow-acting drugs carry a risk of thrombocytopaenia or neutropenia which would present particular difficulties during the operative period. Infection is a theoretical problem with immunosuppressive drugs, though in practical terms this seems not to be important. Penicillamine may rarely cause a syndrome resembling myasthenia gravis. This could be a danger if muscle-relaxing drugs were used during the anaesthetic.

The beneficial effects of these second-line drugs develop slowly and there is seldom any deterioration when the treatment is withheld for a few days or even one or two weeks. It is usually wise to discontinue slow-acting drugs a few days before operation unless the physician is able to continue to supervise administration and monitoring for toxic effects during the operative period. If immunosuppressant drugs are being used to control rheumatoid vasculitis, the treatment may need to be continued and careful consideration should be given to this when surgery is planned.

(d) Anaemia in inflammatory joint disease

Patients suffering from inflammatory joint disease may be anaemic. Appropriate investigations may disclose a remediable cause for the anaemia. There will remain a number of patients, usually with a normochromic normocytic or perhaps microcytic anaemia for which no cause can be found other than the association with inflammatory joint disease, and in whom the anaemia responds poorly to haematinic therapy. The serum iron is usually low, but in contrast to the finding in iron deficiency anaemia the total serum iron binding capacity is also low. It is suggested that iron stores present in the body are for some reason not available for utilization in normal erythropoesis. In some rheumatoid patients there is also reduced red cell survival. If the anaemia is severe it may be necessary to transfuse such a patient before operation. The benefit is temporary and after transfusion the haemoglobin will slowly return to the pre-transfusion level. The decision to transfuse should be taken jointly by the physician and orthopaedic surgeon, and the transfusion should be given a few days before the operation to allow any disturbance of fluid balance to recover, but not so long before that the haemoglobin has fallen again.

(e) Wound healing

Patients suffering from longstanding generalized rheumatoid arthritis are frequently rather frail. Such patients are more than usually susceptible to infections including pneumonia, bronchitis and pyelonephritis. Rheumatoid joints are also unusually prone to septic arthritis resulting from a haematogenous spread of organisms. In longstanding rheumatoid arthritis there is a measurable generalized loss of skin collagen. This loss is accentuated in patients who have been treated with corticosteroids, resulting in friable, atrophic skin, particularly on the extensor surface of the hands, forearms and legs. Chronic leg ulcers may develop following minor trauma or they may indicate the presence of vasculitis. Felty's syndrome (leucopenia, splenomegaly and rheumatoid arthritis) is associated with a tendency to cutaneous infection and leg ulcers. However in a study of 100 rheumatoid patients compared with 100 non-rheumatoid patients undergoing various orthopaedic operations (Garner et al., 1973) there was no significant difference between the two groups in the time taken for wound healing, although failure to heal by first intention occurred more frequently in the rheumatoid patients.

Wound healing in this study was not affected by disease severity or duration, but corticosteroid therapy was important. Forty-nine of the rheumatoid patients had been treated with steroids in doses varying from 2.5 to 15mg of prednisolone daily, and in this group there was an increased incidence of wound infection. There was also a significant delay in wound healing (20.3 days ± 11 days compared to 16.6 ± 7.5 days) in patients who had received steroids continuously for more than three years, and this effect depended on duration of treatment rather than daily dose. In practice it is seldom necessary to delay mobilization or removal of sutures beyond the normal time for operations on patients with non-inflammatory joint lesions.

Penicillamine inhibits the conversion of soluble to insoluble collagen in skin thereby altering elasticity and delaying the maturation of newly formed collagen. On theoretical considerations this drug might therefore be expected to reduce tensile strength in recent scar tissue and this has been shown experimentally in rats (Youseff et al., 1966). There is a case report of wound breakdown after thoracotomy in a patient treated with penicillamine (Burry, 1974) though this patient also had rheumatoid vasculitis which may have played a part. Prospective studies in rheumatoid patients undergoing orthopaedic surgery have not shown this to be a problem. In one study, delay in wound healing was no greater than in those patients who had been treated for more than three years with corticosteroids (Schorn and Mowat, 1977) and, in another, in which patients were receiving up to 1 g of penicillamine daily, there was no evidence of delay (Ansell et al., 1977). There is no absolute need therefore to discontinue penicillamine in patients undergoing ortho-paedic surgery: nevertheless, because of the practical difficulties in admin-istering and monitoring penicillamine therapy during the operative period, it is reasonable to withdraw it temporarily.

Rheumatoid vasculitis may cause serious delay in wound healing and necrosis of skin flaps. Patients in whom active vasculitis has been recognized should not undergo elective surgery until this complication of their disease has been brought under control.

(f) Vasculitis and necrobiotic nodules

Arterial inflammation has been noted in muscle and rectal biopsies, and at post-mortem, in a variety of tissues in patients with rheumatoid arthritis. Histologically, the lesions may be indistinguishable from those of poly-arteritis nodosa. Rheumatoid factors, immunoglobulins and complement have been demonstrated in the vascular lesions and it has been suggested that immune-complex deposition is responsible for the arterial damage. When arteritis is widespread there may be a lowering of serum complement levels. Patients in whom there is widespread visceral vasculitis may be ill and toxic with evidence of systemic rheumatoid complications such as pericarditis, scleritis and peripheral neuropathy. Bowel perforation due to vasculitic infarction can occur. Less florid cutaneous vasculitis, which may present as ulceration of the leg or around the ankles, is more dangerous because it is more likely to be overlooked. There may be areas of dermal necrosis (often as small as 2–3 mm across) on the arms, legs or trunk due to local infarction. The development of unexpected areas of haemorrhagic necrosis over pressure points (such as in the toes, heels, malleoli, hips, sacrum or ischial tuberosities) in bed-fast patients should be regarded as pointers to the presence of vasculitis. Occasionally there may be small infarcts in the pulps of the fingers or around the nail folds. These digital infarcts may herald widespread cutaneous vasculitis but are usually associated with medial arterial thickening which is probably more benign.

The presence of active vasculitis can lead to serious wound breakdown and widespread necrosis of skin flaps. When vasculitis is suspected elective operations should be postponed.

Subcutaneous nodules occur in 20–30% of patients with definite rheumatoid arthritis. The basis of the rheumatoid nodule is an inflammatory granuloma with an ischaemic centre. These nodules may undergo spontaneous necrobiosis and liquefy. Sometimes a sinus forms and the nodule discharges creamy matter, frequently described as 'pus', although the nodule is sterile unless secondarily infected. Once the skin is broken the risk of this occurring is high and the early use of an appropriate antibiotic is essential to prevent haematogenous spread of organisms to joints and operation sites. Spontaneous necrobiosis of rheumatoid nodules or small infarcts in the skin over existing rheumatoid nodules, even at points of pressure such as the olecranon surface of the elbow, suggest the possibility of vasculitis.

14.5 Popliteal cysts and synovial rupture

The differentiation of deep venous thrombosis from synovial rupture or from sudden enlargement of a pre-existing calf cyst is important (Katz et al., 1977). Untreated venous thrombosis carries a risk of pulmonary embolism and of chronic swelling of the leg. Unnecessary anticoagulation is also hazardous, particularly in patients who may be taking steroids or non-steroid anti-inflammatory drugs, who may be anaemic and who are prone to peptic ulceration.

14.5.1 INTRA-ARTICULAR PRESSURE

At rest, the intra-articular pressure in a normal knee when the subject is lying down, with the knee relaxed and extended is similar to the venous pressure and is about equal to or slightly below atmospheric pressure (Jayson and Dixon, 1970a, Levick, 1979). A strong isometric quadriceps contraction may induce a negative pressure of as much as -100 mm Hg (Jayson and Dixon, 1970b). When an effusion is present, or if the knee joint is distended by the introduction of saline or plasma, there is a slight positive pressure at rest and strong quadriceps contraction may generate positive pressures greater than 300 mm Hg (Caughey and Bywaters, 1963). Flexion of the knee causes even higher pressure, up to 1000 mm Hg. Mean pressures are higher in rheumatoid patients than in healthy control subjects (Jayson and Dixon, 1970b). In physiological terms, these are very high pressures and rupture of the knee joint may occur both in cadaver experiments (Dixon and Grant, 1964) and in healthy and rheumatoid volunteers. The synovium usually ruptures posteriorly where the capsule is weakest between the medial head of gastrocnemius and the insertions of semimembranosus and semitendinosus, but occasionally a pre-existing popliteal cyst may rupture. Rupture of the suprapatellar pouch is uncommon but has been reported.

14.5.2 JOINT RUPTURE

Spontaneous rupture of the knee presents with usually sudden, but occasionally gradual, onset of pain and stiffness in the muscles of the calf followed by swelling and tenderness in the calf with pitting oedema around the ankle (Dixon, 1964; Good, 1964). There is sometimes an episode of sudden pain in the popliteal fossa or a sensation of something giving way at the onset, but this is not usual. Homan's sign is usually positive. By the time the patient presents there is seldom a tense effusion in the knee but there may be a history of preceding swelling which has subsequently reduced. Synovial rupture occurs in osteoarthritis, but is more common in inflammatory disease. It has also been reported in subjects whose knees were apparently normal prior to the episode (Kilcoyne et al., 1978; Macfarlane and Bacon, 1980). In rheumatoid arthritis, synovial rupture is more likely to occur early in the illness before fibrosis of the capsule has occurred, and patients may first present for medical advice with this problem. Rupture can occur, however, at any stage of the disease and may happen more than once in the same patient.

In rheumatoid arthritis, the synovial fluid contains polymorphonuclear leucocytes and is rich in enzymes and inflammatory mediators. The escape of such fluid produces oedema, pain and tenderness extending down the calf to the ankle. Bleeding at the time of rupture also contributes to inflammation in the calf. Synovial rupture in septic arthritis has even more serious consequences.

14.5.3 SYNOVIAL CYSTS

Synovial cysts in the popliteal fossa may be enlargements of bursae or may arise directly by herniation from the back of the knee joint.

Recurrent, or chronic, synovial leakage may result in the formation of a cyst in the calf. Occasionally, a cyst forms after a single episode. Such cysts lie deep to gastrocnemius and sometimes deep to the soleus muscle. They may extend along the fascial planes of the muscles in the calf and can become so large as to present as a swelling at the ankle. Rarely the cyst may extend upwards between the muscles of the thigh. The wall of such a cyst is formed of fibrous connective tissue lined by fibroblasts and chronic inflammatory cells. Occasionally, a lining resembling synovial cells may be seen. The cyst contains fluid similar to synovial fluid and frequently large masses of fibrin clot.

Arthrography usually shows that fluid under pressure passes from the knee joint into the cyst. When the intra-articular pressure is increased so is the synovial fluid pressure in the cyst. If the knee is aspirated, however, the cyst usually remains tense. It is rarely possible to show that contrast injected into the cyst will pass into the knee. Jayson and Dixon (1970c) postulate the presence of a valvular mechanism which allows fluid to be pumped from the knee into the cyst, but not to return. This may have a protective effect by acting as a safety valve and preventing the development of very high intra-articular pressure during use (Genovese et al., 1972).

14.5.4 INVESTIGATION OF SYNOVIAL RUPTURE AND CALF CYSTS

The diagnosis of acute synovial rupture can occasionally be established on the history and findings. Where there is doubt, an arthrogram is a simple procedure and will usually confirm synovial rupture or cyst. An acute rupture may heal which makes confirmation difficult if the arthrogram is delayed more than a few days. A water-soluble radio-opaque dye is injected into the joint. The contrast medium leaking from the back of the knee typically has an ill-defined feathery outline in acute rupture in distinction to the well-defined margins of a cyst in the calf. The leak may not be shown unless the intra-articular pressure is raised by exercise; it is important that the patient should either walk about after injection of the contrast medium or do static quadriceps exercises and gentle knee bending. Screening may be helpful but is not essential since plain films taken before and after exercise can give all the necessary information.

Ultrasonic scanning may show the presence of a cyst but not usually of acute rupture.

Positive findings in the arthrogram do not entirely exclude a coexisting venous thrombosis (Gordon et al., 1979; Simpson et al., 1980; Belch et al., 1981). If there is doubt a venogram will be needed and, if emergency venography is readily available, this investigation may be preferred to arthrography. In the absence of thrombosis, the venogram may show distortion of the peroneal and popliteal veins due to the mass in the calf. This reduces the velocity of venous blood flow, and false positive results may be reported if ultrasonic scanning of flow in the popliteal and femoral veins by the Doppler technique is relied on as evidence of thrombosis. Radioiodine-labelled fibrinogen studies may also give false positive results probably due to the presence of fibrin and clot in the cyst or in the calf muscles.

14.5.5 MANAGEMENT OF SYNOVIAL RUPTURE AND SYNOVIAL CYSTS

The aim of treatment is to reduce the volume and pressure of fluid in the knee joint. Conservative measures to reduce synovitis are usually all that is required to control acute, or even recurrent, synovial leakage.

Acute synovial rupture or an acutely painful cyst should be managed by resting the knee joint, on a splint if necessary, and by giving analgesics. If there is active synovitis in the knee, the effusion should be aspirated and an intra-articular injection of corticosteroid may be given. Steroid will pass from the knee into a cyst but not in the opposite direction. If a cyst is aspirated it will usually refill within a few hours or days if there is still an effusion in the knee.

Indications for operation

When conservative treatment fails then an anterior synovectomy may be necessary, but operation on the back of the knee or on the cyst is not needed. If the synovitis abates, or after synovectomy, most popliteal and calf cysts will become smaller and may disappear (Jayson *et al.*, 1972; Pinder, 1973). Excision of a cyst without treating the synovitis of the knee is unsatisfactory and leads to recurrence or even to failure to heal with fistula formation. On those rare occasions when it is necessary to excise a synovial cyst in the calf, anterior synovectomy of the knee should be done at the same time if the synovitis is still active.

References

Aidem H P, Baker L D. Synovectomy of the knee joint in rheumatoid arthritis. *J Am Med Assoc* 1964;187:4–6.

Ansell B M, Crook A, Mallard J R, Bywaters E G L. Evaluation of intra-articular colloidal gold Au-198 in the treatment of persistent knee effusions. *Ann Rheum Dis* 1963;22:435.

Ansell B M, Moran H, Arden G P. Penicillamine and wound healing in rheumatoid arthritis. *Proc R Soc Med* 1977;70: Suppl 3:75–6.

Arthritis Foundation Committee on Evaluation of Synovectomy. Multicentre evaluation of synovectomy in the treatment of rheumatoid arthritis. Report of results at end of three years. *Arthr Rheum* 1977;20:765–71.

Arthritis and Rheumatism Council and British Orthopaedic Association. Controlled trial of synovectomy of knee and metacarpophalangeal joints in rheumatoid arthritis. *Ann Rheum Dis* 1976;35:437–42.

Asher R. The dangers of going to bed. *Br Med J* 1947;ii:967–8.

Bacon P A, Collins A J, Ring F J, Cosh J A. Thermography in the assessment of inflammatory arthritis. *Clin Rheum Dis* 1976;2:51–65.

Ball J, Lawrence J S. The epidemiology of the sheep cell agglutination test. *Ann Rheum Dis* 1961;20:235–43.

Barnes C G, Mason R M. Synovectomy of the knee joint in rheumatoid arthritis. *Ann Phys Med* 1967;9:83–102.

Belch J J F, McMillan N C, Fogelman I, Capell H, Forbes C D. Combined phlebography and arthrography in patients with painful swollen calf. *Br. Med J* 1981;282:949.

Boardman P L, Hart F D. Clinical measurement of the anti-inflammatory effects of salicylates in rheumatoid arthritis. *Br Med J* 1967;4:264–8.

Boyd R V, Hoffbrand B I. Erythrocyte sedimentation rate in elderly hospital in-patients. *Br Med J* 1966;i:901–2.

Brewerton D A, Caffrey M, Hart F D, James D C O, Nicholls A, Sturrock R D. Ankylosing spondylitis and HL-A27. *Lancet* 1973;i:904–7.

Brewerton D A, Caffrey M F P, James D C O. The histocompatibility antigen (HL-A27) and its relation to disease. *J Rheum* 1974;1:249.

Bridgman J F, Bruckner F, Eisen V, Tucker A, Bleehen N M. Irradiation of the synovium in the treatment of rheumatoid arthritis. *Q J Med* 1973;42:357–67.

Burry H C. Penicillamine and wound healing – a potential hazard? *Postgrad Med J* 1974;50: August Suppl, 75–6.

Bywaters E G L, Ansell B M. Monoarticular arthritis in children. *Ann Rheum Dis* 1965;24: 116–22.

Calin A, Fries J F. The striking prevalence of ankylosing spondylitis in 'healthy' W27 positive males and females. A controlled study. *New Engl J Med* 1975;293:835–9.

Caughey D E, Bywaters E G L. Joint fluid pressure in chronic knee effusions. *Ann Rheum Dis* 1963;22:106–9.

Cruickshank B. Interpretation of multiple biopsies of synovial tissues in rheumatic disease. *Ann Rheum Dis* 1952;11:137–45.

Currey H L F. Intra-articular thiotepa in rheumatoid arthritis. *Ann Rheum Dis* 1965;24:382–8.

Dick W C. The use of radioisotopes in normal and diseased joints. *Semin Arthr Rheum* 1972;1:301–25.

Dick W C, Neufeld R R, Prentice A G, Woodburn A, Whaley K, Nuki G, Buchanan W W. Measurement of joint inflammation. A radioisotopic method. *Ann Rheum Dis* 1970; 29:135–7.

Dixon A St J. Acute rupture of the knee in rheumatoid arthritis. *Proc R Soc Med* 1964;57:1129–30.

Dixon A St J, Grant C. Acute synovial rupture in rheumatoid arthritis, Clinical and experimental observations. *Lancet* 1964;i:742–5.

Dresner E, Trombly P. The latex fixation reaction in non-rheumatic diseases. *New Engl J Med* 1959;261:981–8.

Duthie J J R, Brown P E, Truelove L H, Barager F D, Lawrie A J. Course and prognosis in rheumatoid arthritis patients. *Ann Rheum Dis* 1964;23:193–202.

Ellison M R, Flatt A E. Intra-articular thiotepa in rheumatoid disease. A clinical analysis of 123 injected M.P. and P.I.P. joints. *Arthr Rheum* 1971;14:212.

Fassbender H G. *Pathology of rheumatic diseases.* Berlin, Heidelberg, New York: Springer-Verlag, 1975.

Fletcher M R, Scott J T. Chronic monarticular synovitis. Diagnostic and prognostic features. *Ann Rheum Dis* 1975;34:171–6.

Gardner D L. *The pathology of rheumatoid arthritis.* London: Edward Arnold, 1972.

Garner R W, Mowat A G, Hazleman B L. Wound healing after operations on patients with rheumatoid arthritis. *J Bone Joint Surg [Br]* 1973;55–B:134–44.

Genovese G R, Jayson M I V, Dixon A St J. Protective value of synovial cysts in rheumatoid knees. *Ann Rheum Dis* 1972;31:179–82.

Goldie I F. Soft tissue operations. In: *Arthritis of the knee.* Freeman MAR. ed. Berlin, Heidelberg, New York: Springer-Verlag, 1980; 132–5.

Good A E. Rheumatoid arthritis, Baker's cyst and 'thrombophlebitis'. *Arthr Rheum* 1964;7:56–64.

Gordon G V, Edell S, Brogadir S P, Schumacher H R, Schimmer B M, Dalinka M. Baker's cysts and true thrombophlebitis. Report of two cases and review of the literature. *Arch Intern Med* 1979;139:40–2.

Gumpel J M. Radiosynoviorthesis. *Clin Rheum Dis* 1978;4:311–26.

Gumpel J M, Roles N C. A controlled trial of intra-articular radiocolloids versus surgical synovectomy in persistent synovitis. *Lancet* 1975;i:488–9.

Harris R, Copp E P. Immobilisation of the knee joint in rheumatoid arthritis. *Ann Rheum Dis* 1962;21:353–8.

Harris R, Millard J B, Banerjee S K. Radiosodium clearance from the knee joint in rheumatoid arthritis. *Ann Rheum Dis* 1958;17:189–95.

Hilton J. *The influence of mechanical and physiological rest.* London: Bell and Daldy, 1863.

Hollander J L. Intrasynovial corticosteroid therapy. In: *Arthritis and allied conditions. 8th ed.* Hollander J L, McCarty D J. eds. Philadelphia: Lea & Fibiger, 1972; 517–34.

Hollander J L, Jessar R A, McCarty D J. Synovialsis: an aid in arthritis diagnosis. *Bull Rheum Dis* 1961;12:263–4.

Jayson M I V, Dixon A St J. Intra-articular pressure in rheumatoid arthritis of the knee. 1 Pressure changes during passive joint distension. *Ann Rheum Dis* 1970a;29:261–5.

Jayson M I V, Dixon A St J. Intra-articular pressure in rheumatoid arthritis of the knee. III Pressure changes during joint use. *Ann Rheum dis* 1970b;29:401–8.

Jayson M I V, Dixon A St J. Valvular mechanisms in juxta-articular cysts. *Ann Rheum Dis* 1970c;29:415–20.

Jayson M I V, Dixon A St J, Kates A, Pinder I, Coomes E N. Popliteal and calf cysts in rheumatoid arthritis. Treatment by anterior synovectomy. *Ann Rheum Dis* 1972;31:9–15.

Katz R S, Zisic T M, Arnold M D. The pseudothrombophlebitis syndrome. *Medicine* 1977;56:151–64.

Kilcoyne R F, Imray T J, Stewart E T. Ruptured Baker's cyst simulating acute thrombophlebitis. *J Am Med Assoc* 1978;240:1517–18.

Kirk J A, Kersley G D. Heat and cold in the physical treatment of rheumatoid arthritis of the knee. *Ann Phys Med* 1968;9:270–4.

Lawrence J S, Behrend T, Bennett P H, Bremner J M, Burch T A, Gofton J, O'Brien W, Robinson H. Geographical studies on rheumatoid arthritis. *Ann Rheum Dis* 1966;25:425–31.

Lee P. The efficacy and safety of radiosynovectomy. *J Rheum* 1982;9:165–8.

Levick J R. An investigation into the validity of sub-atmospheric recordings from synovial fluid and their dependence on joint angle. *J Physiol* 1979;289:55–67.

London P S. Synovectomy of the knee in rheumatoid arthritis. *J Bone Joint Surg [Br]* 1955;37–B:392–9.

McCarty D J, Hogan J M. Inflammatory reaction after intrasynovial injection of microcrystalline adreno-corticosteroid esters. *Arthr Rheum* 1964;7:359–67.

McConkey B, Crockson R A, Crockson A P. The assessment of rheumatoid arthritis. A study based on measurements of the serum acute-phase reactants. *Q J Med* 1972;41:115–25.

Macfarlane D G, Bacon P A. Popliteal cyst rupture in normal knees. *Br Med J* 1980;281:1203–4.

Marks J A, Sharp J. Rheumatoid cervical myelopathy. *Q J Med* 1981;50:307–319.

Mathews J A. Atlanto-axial subluxation in rheumatoid arthritis. *Ann Rheum Dis* 1969;28: 260–6.

Nissila M, Antilla P, Hamalainen M. Comparison of chemical, radiation and surgical synovectomy for knee joint synovitis. *Scand J Rheum* 1978;7:225–8.

Onetti C M, Guttierrez E, Hliba E, Aguirre C R. Synoviorthesis with ^{32}P-colloidal chromic phosphate in rheumatoid arthritis. *J Rheum* 1982;9:229–38.

Partridge R E H, Duthie J J R. Controlled trial of the effect of complete immobilisation of the joints in rheumatoid arthritis. *Ann Rheum Dis* 1963;22:91–8.

Patzakis M J, Mills D M, Bartholomew B A, Clayton M L, Smyth C J. A visual, histological and enzymatic study of regenerating rheumatoid synovium in the synovectomized knee. *J Bone Joint Surg [Am]* 1973;55–A:287–300.

Pekin T J, Zvaifler N J. Hemolytic complement in synovial fluid. *J Clin Invest* 1964;43:1372–82.

Phelps P, Steele A D, McCarty D J. Compensated polarised light microscopy. Identification of crystals in synovial fluids from gout or pseudogout. *J Am Med Assoc* 1968;203:508–12.

Pinder I M. Treatment of the popliteal cyst in the rheumatoid knee. *J Bone Joint Surg [Br]*

349

1973;55–B:119–25.

Ragan C. The general management of rheumatoid arthritis. *J Am Med Assoc* 1949;**141**:124.

Revell P A, Mayston V. Histopathology of the synovial membrane of peripheral joints in ankylosing spondylitis. *Ann Rheum Dis* 1982;**41**:579–86.

Ropes M W, Bauer W. *Synovial fluid changes in joint disease.* Cambridge, Mass: Harvard University Press, 1953.

Ropes M W, Bennett G A, Cobb S, Jacox R, Jessar R A. Diagnostic criteria for rheumatoid arthritis. 1958. Revision. *Ann Rheum Dis* 1959;**18**:49–51.

St Onge R A, Dick W C, Bell G, Boyle J A. Radioactive xenon (^{133}Xe) disappearance rates from the synovial cavity of the human knee joint in normal and arthritic subjects. *Ann Rheum Dis* 1968;**27**:163–6.

Schlosstein L, Terasaki P I, Bluestone R, Pearson C M. High association of an HL–A antigen W 27, with ankylosing spondylitis. *New Engl J Med* 1973;**288**:704–6.

Schorn D, Mowat A G. Penicillamine in rheumatoid arthritis: wound healing, skin thickness and osteoporosis. *Rheum Rehab* 1977;**16**:223–30.

Schumacher H R, Kulka J P. Needle biopsy of the synovial membrane – experience with the Parker–Pearson technique. *New Engl J Med* 1972;**286**:416–9.

Seward C W, Osterland C K. The pattern of anti-immunoglobulin activities in serum, pleural and synovial fluids. *J Lab Clin Med* 1973;**81**:230–40.

Simpson F G, Robinson P J, Bark M, Losowsky M S. Prospective study of thrombophlebitis and 'pseudo-thrombophlebitis'. *Lancet* 1980;**i**:331–3.

Soren A. *Histodiagnosis and clinical correlation of rheumatoid and other synovitis.* Stuttgart: Georg Thieme. Philadelphia, Toronto: J B Lippincott, 1978.

Speed J S. Synovectomy of knee joint. *J Am Med Assoc* 1924;**83**:1814–20.

Stevens J, Whitefield G A. Synovectomy of the knee in rheumatoid arthritis. *Ann Rheum Dis* 1966;**25**:214–9.

Stevenson A C, Bedford J, Dolphin G W, Purrot R J, Lloyd D C, Hill A G S, Hill H F H, Gumpel J M, Williams D, Scott J T, Ramsey N W, Bruckner F E, Fearn C B D'A. Cytogenetic and scanning study of patients receiving intra-articular injections of gold-198 and yttrium-90. *Ann Rheum Dis* 1973;**32**:112–23.

Swett P P. Synovectomy in infectious arthritis. *J Bone Joint Surg* 1924;**6**:800.

Taylor A R, Hill A G S. Synovectomy. *Clin Rheum Dis* 1978;**4**:287–309.

Thompson M, Douglas G, Davison E P. Synovectomy of the metacarpophalangeal joints in rheumatoid arthritis. *Proc R Soc Med* 1973;**66**:197–9.

Topp J R, Cross E G, Fam A G. Treatment of persistent knee effusions with intra-articular gold. *Can Med Assoc J* 1975;**112**:1085–9.

Winfield J, Cooke D, Brooke A S, Corbett M. A prospective study of the radiological changes in the cervical spine in early rheumatoid disease. *Ann Rheum Dis* 1981;**40**:109–14.

Yates D B, Scott J T. Rheumatoid synovitis and joint disease. Relationship between arthroscopic and histological changes. *Ann Rheum Dis* 1975;**34**:1–6.

Yates D B, Scott J T, Ramsey N. Double-blind trial of yttrium-90 for chronic inflammatory synovitis of the knee. *Ann Rheum Dis* 1977;**36**:481.

Youseff S A, Geever E F, Levenson S M. Penicillamine effect on wound healing. *Surg Forum* 1966;**17**:89–90.

Zacharski L R. Erythrocyte sedimentation rate. *Br J Hosp Med* 1976;**16**:53–62.

Zvaifler N J. The immunopathology of joint inflammation in rheumatoid arthritis. *Adv Immunol* 1973;**16**:265–336.

CHAPTER 15	# Knee Replacement

William Waugh

There can be little doubt of the need for a satisfactory arthroplasty to replace the knee joints of those patients crippled by chronic arthritis. Much progress towards this end has been made over the past ten years and this chapter begins by reviewing the use of this type of operation at Harlow Wood Orthopaedic Hospital.

15.1 Experience at Harlow Wood Orthopaedic Hospital

Shiers (1965) published the early results of his hinge replacement, but in the late 1960s we felt that the Walldius prosthesis might be a better choice. One advantage was the relatively broad surfaces which covered a wide area of bone and which might, at least theoretically, reduce the incidence of loosening and 'sinking in' of the components. This complication was reported as occurring with the Shiers' prosthesis by Watson and Hill (1976). Considerable bone resection from the femur and tibia is necessary to insert any hinge, but this makes it possible to correct severe deformities without too much difficulty. Although the value of cement fixation was becoming accepted in the late 1960s, we continued to use the Walldius prosthesis without cement as its designer intended (Walldius, 1957) in the hope that this might make management easier if infection occurred.

At the same time, it was clear that there was a group of patients with rheumatoid arthritis who had very painful knees with such severe loss of articular cartilage that synovectomy was contraindicated, but who did not have so much deformity that a large implant was needed. One of us (WW) had visited Dr MacIntosh in Toronto and felt that the double hemiarthroplasty operation would have some advantages in this situation. Very little bone has to be resected from the tibia to insert the metal plateau prostheses and if a tight fit was obtained there was no need to use cement.

Two completely different operations were now available each with its own indications and limitations, and one of us (JPJ) concentrated his efforts on the Walldius replacement and the other (WW) on the MacIntosh hemiarthroplasty. This not only gave each of us greater experience of the operative technique of a single procedure, but enabled us to recognize more quickly the results which could be achieved. It also led to the study of the pathological anatomy of the knee to try to define the indications for each operation. Stress radiographs (both anteroposterior and lateral) were used to determine the amount of instability, and tomography made it possible to recognize the extent and depth of areas of bony collapse. These investigations were certainly instructive and we learnt about some aspects of the gross changes occurring in the rheumatoid knee which were not generally appreciated at the time.

However, experience of hip replacements had clearly demonstrated that a metal-on-bone articulation was not satisfactory and that metal-on-polyethylene gave considerable advantages over metal-on-metal. Our two operations which had seemed to be reasonably satisfactory (provided expectations were modest) had become old-fashioned, at least in principle.

The Freeman–Swanson replacement was first reported at a meeting of the British Orthopaedic Association at Oxford in September, 1971, (Freeman and Swanson, 1972). In 1972 we embarked on what turned out to be a long involvement with this operation and with the changes in technique which were introduced in subsequent years.

A major orthopaedic meeting devoted to the knee joint was held in Amsterdam in 1973. Various new arthroplasties were described and we decided to begin to use a prosthesis (other than a hinge) which had some inherent stability. A choice lay between the Attenborough (1974) 'stabilized gliding total knee replacement' and the prosthesis described by Sheehan (1974). The former appeared rather complicated and the Sheehan was chosen by us for intuitive rather than scientific reasons.

At this time it seemed likely that there might well be an indication for a 'smaller' implant to replace knees at an earlier stage of destruction and which could be regarded as a 'modern' version of the MacIntosh hemiarthroplasty.

The Manchester replacement seemed to fulfil this requirement (Shaw and Chatterjee, 1978).

Between 1975 and 1978 we were using three types of replacement (Freeman, Sheehan and Manchester) which made it possible to deal with most of the difficulties provided by the wide variety of pathological changes which occur in chronic destructive arthritis. We never chose a prosthesis without visiting the surgeon who had invented it. Not only should the operative techniques be learnt first-hand, but it is equally important to try to understand, by personal discussion, the principles which lie behind the design. It also seemed essential to build up experience with a limited number of methods, rather than be tempted to do a small number of each new arthroplasty.

During these years, a better understanding of the problems of knee replacement gradually developed. This came through an appreciation of the pathological anatomy of the rheumatoid and osteoarthritic knee which has been well summarized by Freeman (1980). The need for carrying out an appropriate soft-tissue release in order to achieve correct alignment represented an important step forward. Furthermore, instruments were designed which went some way to ensuring that the bone cuts were made accurately.

Finally, two additional arthroplasties have been introduced at Harlow Wood which have superseded the Walldius and Manchester prostheses. In spite of the theoretical objections and the reported complications following constrained hinges (Arden and Kamdar, 1975), there does seem a need for this type of operation in knees which are very severely damaged in old people and to replace smaller implants which have failed. The Stanmore hinge (Lettin et al., 1978) is a well-designed metal-on-plastic joint with a 7° valgus angle and it has been used at Harlow Wood since 1978.

Our results from the Manchester replacement were not satisfactory and the author was invited to take part in the trial of the Oxford Knee. This is an entirely original design, yet to be proved in clinical use, but it demands very little bone resection and so can be regarded as a conservative procedure.

We recognized in 1972 that it was essential to follow-up patients at regular intervals for an indefinite period. A Knee Assessment Clinic (with two rheumatologists) was set up and we also held two follow-up clinics each month. Initially records were kept in a form based on that used at the London Hospital (Freeman, 1980), but for the past three years a new method of assessment has been introduced. This is based on standardized questions and functional testing carried out by non-medical personnel; the information recorded by the surgeon is reduced to a minimum (Waugh, Tew and Johnson, 1981; Waugh, 1982). A statistician attached to the clinic is responsible for the collection of data and also for tracing patients who fail to attend. This has enabled us to maintain a constant review of our results which influences our policy of management.

353

Table 15.1 Primary knee replacements at Harlow Wood Orthopaedic Hospital

Name	Year introduced	Total (to 1981 inclusive)
Walldius	1968	82
MacIntosh	1971	54
Freeman	1972	215
Sheehan	1974	115
Manchester	1975	65
Stanmore	1978	19
Oxford	1980	33
		583

Table 15.2 Primary knee replacements at Harlow Wood Orthopaedic Hospital in 1980 and 1981

Freeman	27
Sheehan	5
Stanmore	13
Oxford	32
	77

Table 15.1 gives the number of primary knee replacements carried out at Harlow Wood Orthopaedic Hospital and the year in which each was first introduced. The present practice is shown in Table 15.2 which gives the type and number of replacements carried out in the years 1980 and 1981.

The remainder of this chapter will deal with various aspects of knee replacement and will be based on the author's experience which has been broadly described. Other prostheses will be discussed in relation to points of principle. It clearly is not possible to deal with all the different designs which have been produced, particularly since the number of new prostheses has increased greatly during the last few years.

15.2 Indications for knee replacement

Not all orthopaedic surgeons would agree with Insall's claim that the results of knee replacement can approach the excellence achieved by replacement of the hip joint (Insall et al., 1979). This reference was made in a paper describing the new total condylar prosthesis. In spite of its success this implant has already been modified and Insall et al. (1982) now use almost exclusively the posterior stabilized total condylar prosthesis.

The cautious surgeon, who has observed the progressive changes made in the design of a number of implants, will wish for information which will give some indication of the durability of the many new models which are often reported with a relatively short follow-up. Theoretical arguments may give grounds for optimism, but we really do need to know the results in patients observed for at least ten years. Until this is achieved, it is wise to restrict knee replacements to those patients whose knees are producing severe pain and disability and who cannot be treated by any other method.

Consideration needs to be given to the age of the patient, the degree of destruction in the individual's knee and the involvement of other joints by the disease process.

Tibial osteotomy must remain the operation of choice for medial compartment osteoarthritis in patients up to the age of 65 years. Middle-aged men who have unilateral osteoarthritis with advanced changes (bony collapse of more than 1 cm) are still best treated by arthrodesis. When both knees are affected, knee replacement may be justified at a rather earlier age; but tibial osteotomy must still be considered even when the radiological changes are beyond the limit at which the operation can be expected theoretically to give the best results (see Chapter 13).

Lateral compartment osteoarthritis is relatively less common and usually occurs in women (Waugh, 1981). There are mechanical reasons (Hagstedt, 1974) which explain why patients with this condition do not present until the changes in the joint are relatively advanced. This may also be related to the suggestion that patients with a valgus deformity are able to achieve some compensation during walking for the high lateral compartment loads which are assumed from static calculations (Johnson and Waugh, 1980). Many patients present with a deformity of greater than 30° of valgus and are often more than 60 years of age, so knee replacement may be the only possible treatment other than arthrodesis. When lateral compartment osteoarthritis follows lateral meniscectomy, the deformity is likely to be less and a supracondylar osteotomy will be indicated (these points are also considered in more detail in Chapter 13).

In rheumatoid arthritis the choice may be particularly difficult and a very wide variety of individual problems present themselves. For example, juvenile rheumatoid arthritis may produce a deformity by asymmetrical epiphyseal growth. There may also be an active synovitis, and if the knee becomes painful at the age of, say, twenty, then an intra-articular supra-condylar osteotomy or a double osteotomy (Benjamin, 1969) is likely to be the most satisfactory procedure. Synovectomy may be indicated where there is a persistent synovitis which is not controlled by medical treatment. It is generally accepted that the results will be best when there is little or no loss of articular cartilage. While this is probably true, a 'late' synovectomy must be considered in young and middle-aged women even when the indications are not ideal. The operation may well relieve pain for a number of years and this is valuable time gained.

355

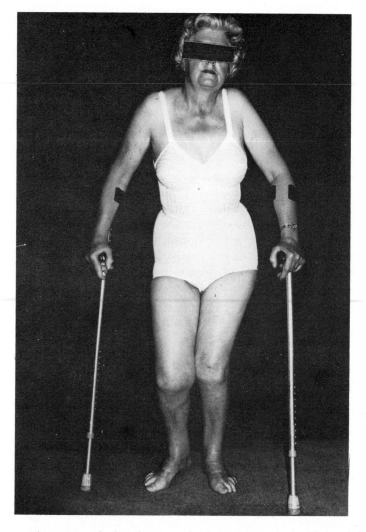

Fig. 15.1 This patient who has rheumatoid arthritis is severely disabled with flexion contractures of both knees. Her pain is such that knee replacement has to be considered even though she is relatively young.

A woman, say, 40 years old with two very painful knees, each with a flexion contracture of 30° or 40°, presents a particularly difficult problem (Fig. 15.1). The articular changes are likely to be advanced and there seems to be little alternative to bilateral knee replacement. The early result may well be spectacularly successful, but it remains difficult to predict the outcome. Loosening may well occur in five or ten years time, but even then it may be possible to insert another prosthesis. But what will be the situation at the age of 60 years? Furthermore, haematogenous infection can also be a risk at any time. Many of these patients are so miserable and so handicapped that they are prepared to accept the risks and indeed they may fail to appreciate the explanation which must be given to them. It is true that the progression of arthritis in other joints, or other medical diseases, may limit their activities before their knee joints fail. Most surgeons, rheumatologists and their patients find it difficult to accept the idea of a wheel-chair life in middle-age and probably it is right to proceed with knee replacement. It will, however, be best to use a prosthesis which needs the resection of the least possible amount of bone for its insertion (provided that deformity can be corrected and stability achieved).

Older patients with longstanding rheumatoid arthritis and secondary osteoarthritis present a less difficult problem. Their joints are so badly damaged that replacement may be the only way of restoring function. It is, however, wise not to be too ambitious with those who have given up the attempt to walk and who are bed-ridden. There may well be both physical and psychological reasons why these patients cannot be successfully re-habilitated even if they have technically satisfactory operations. If, however, the patient can stand and take a few steps (even with the aid of two people) the prospect will be very much better. It is sometimes the case that hip replacement is also necessary and our experience of patients who have had both hips and both knees replaced has been reported by Espley and Herbert (1981).

Table 15.3 summarizes what might be regarded as the best indications for the operations which have been discussed. Many factors have to be considered in the approach to each individual patient. The aims to be achieved must be realistic and the possible outcome needs to be fully explained to the patient.

Table 15.3 The indications for operations for chronic arthritis of the knee

	Age	Deformity	Disease*	Other joints involved
Synovectomy	Under 45	None	RA	Multiple
Tibial osteotomy	Under 65	Flexion <15° Varus <5°	OA	Unilateral or bilateral
Supracondylar osteotomy	Under 65	Flexion <15° Valgus <15°	OA	Unilateral or bilateral
Arthrodesis	Under 65	Any	OA	None
Knee replacement	Over 65†	Any	OA RA	Multiple

* RA, rheumatoid arthritis; OA, osteoarthritis.
† The age limit for knee replacement can be reduced when multiple joints are involved and in the presence of severe deformity of the knee.

15.3 Types of knee replacement

It is difficult to devise any comprehensive classification of knee prostheses, but there is some sense in grouping replacements according to size since this gives an indication of the amount of bone which has to be removed for them to be inserted. The following types can be recognized:

(1) Compartmental   (Manchester, Oxford)
(2) Condylar   (Freeman, Insall)
(3) Semiconstrained   (Sheehan, Attenborough)
(4) Constrained hinge   (Walldius, Stanmore)

Some replacements will not fall neatly into such groups; for example, Insall's total condylar prosthesis which was relatively unconstrained has been superseded by the posterior stabilized total condylar which is described as semiconstrained.

Various design features may influence the surgeon's choice of a particular prosthesis, but the pathological anatomy of the knee to be operated on needs to be taken into consideration. Although the patterns of involvement are different in rheumatoid arthritis and osteoarthritis, the changes in the knees where replacement is being considered can be described in three phases:

(1) There is loss of articular cartilage, but the bony configuration is normal (Fig. 15.2) and there is no, or only very slight, deformity present (flexion; valgus or varus). The ligaments are intact and so it should be possible to use a small compartmental prosthesis.

(2) When a deformity develops, bony collapse of the overloaded femoral and tibial condyles will occur in one side of the joint (medial in varus, lateral in valgus). The collateral ligaments on the concave side of the deformity may become shortened. A soft-tissue release is necessary to achieve the correct alignment (a coronal tibiofemoral angle of 7° of valgus). Bone has to be resected in order to achieve a flat surface on which to place a prosthesis and the gap created is best filled by a condylar type of prosthesis.

(3) At the final stage, lateral subluxation of the tibia may occur (Fig. 15.3). This associated with attrition of both cruciate ligaments and the collateral ligaments may be stretched. In this situation, stability can be most satisfactorily maintained with a semiconstrained or constrained prosthesis.

In general terms the aim should be to remove as little bone stock as possible compatible with the restoration of alignment and stability. The statements which have been made can all be debated and various points in relation to them will be considered later in the chapter in dealing with our experience of the various prostheses used at Harlow Wood Orthopaedic Hospital. First it may be helpful to make some general observations about operative technique and design.

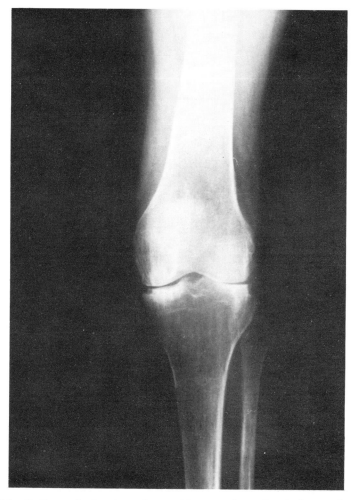

Fig. 15.2 Radiograph showing a knee with severe loss of articular cartilage, but there is no deformity and the bony outline is preserved.

5.4 Instrumentation and the bone cuts

5.4.1 THE TIBIAL CUT

It is essential that the tibial component is inserted so that it is at right angles to the tibial axis in both planes (Fig. 15.4). Since the tibia is often bowed, this axis is represented by a line drawn from the centre of the knee to the centre of the ankle, but it is difficult to know where the centre of a badly disorganized knee lies. A tibial intramedullary jig ought to be helpful, but will not necessarily lead to the centre of the ankle if there is a bend in the shaft. An

359

external jig applied to the subcutaneous surface is not always easy to direct to the centre of the ankle when the ankle and foot are wrapped in towels or plastic sheeting. Jigs, therefore, can only be an aid to accuracy and undoubtedly some surgeons are better than others in achieving a correct cut; perhaps the less skilful need to make a special effort to acquire the art. It is after all possible to practice with instruments on cadaveric knees or on skeletons.

It is not only necessary to make the cut at the correct angle, but also at the right level. This is determined to some extent by the type of implant being

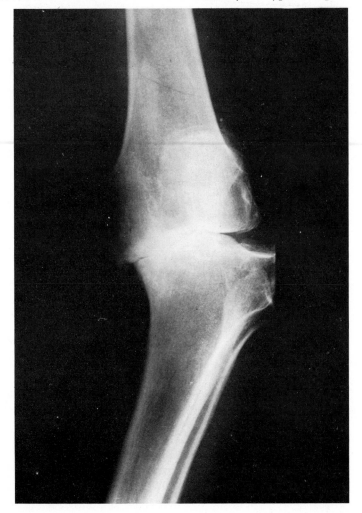

Fig. 15.3 Radiograph of a severely affected knee with a varus deformity and more than 1 cm of bony collapse in the medial tibial condyle and lateral subluxation of the tibia.

used, but there is room for variation. In the first place it is important to remove as little bone as possible so that the flat surface of the component can lie on the hard subchondral bone rather than the soft cancellous bone which is present only a few millimetres distally. It is also recognized that the strength of the bone diminishes with the depth below the surface (Kaufer *et al.*, 1978). But a deep area of collapse in one tibial condyle may mean that a flat surface cannot be achieved without resecting to a depth of 1 cm or more – and even then the lowest point of the hollow may not be reached. Compromise is necessary between having a flat surface and an area of unsupported cement which will be unavoidable when an intact cortical rim is not present. There is no certain way of knowing what area of defect in relation to the area of flat surface is acceptable. The component can be supported by screws inserted vertically into the tibia and the cement re-enforced by vitallium mesh (Hood *et al.*, 1981). If the area of collapse is both extensive and deep, an intramedullary stem may be needed for fixation.

The assumption in the foregoing discussion has been that the tibial cut is made straight across the top of the bone which implies removal of the intercondylar eminence. Where the design of the implant is such that the cruciate ligaments are retained, two separate cuts are necessary and it is rather more difficult to judge them separately.

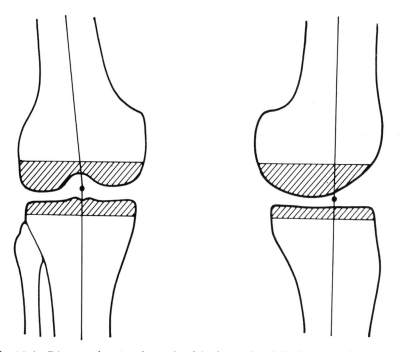

Fig. 15.4 Diagram showing the angle of the femoral and tibial cuts in relation to the axis of the shafts of the bones.

Furthermore, in these more limited operations it is not so easy to expose the whole circumference of the tibial articular surface and there is no doubt that full exposure does make it easier to achieve the correct cut. The other advantages of removing the posterior cruciate ligament are more important and relate to the path of movement of the replaced knee and the shape of the tibial component. This is a point on which Freeman and Insall are in complete agreement (Freeman *et al.*, 1977).

15.4.2 THE FEMORAL CUT

The angle at which the lower end of the femur is cut is critical because it determines the correct coronal tibiofemoral angulation (7° valgus). Unfortunately, an intramedullary jig (or a femoral component with an intramedullary stem) will not necessarily guarantee correct alignment. The medullary canal is often wide, and even if a very long jig is used, it may well be placed at a significant angle to the axis of the shaft (perhaps as much as 2° or 3° in either direction). The introduction of the tenser (Freeman *et al.*, 1978) is one method of attempting to overcome this difficulty. This instrument, which is inserted after the tibial cut has been made, has two flat blades each of which can be opened independently. This makes it possible to alter the angle between the femur and tibia. Alignment is assessed by a long rod which passes through the instrument; the proximal end should lie over the femoral head and the distal end over the centre of the ankle. If this cannot be achieved, the appropriate (medial or lateral) soft-tissue release is carried out. It is difficult to locate the centre of the femoral head which is often taken to be three finger-breadths medial to the anterior superior iliac spine. Apart from the crudeness of using finger-breadths as a form of measurement, the bony landmark is often lost beneath a layer of fat or beneath the towels used to isolate the operation site. Most surgeons (including the author) believe that it is important to be accurate within 2° or 3° in the coronal tibiofemoral alignment, but have to accept imprecise technical methods. Possibly the use of an image intensifier in the operating theatre might provide a solution, but there are practical difficulties which, although not insuperable, prevent its routine use at the present time.

As with making the tibial cut, the various instruments available provide a valuable guide, but the femoral cut is also often made correctly by a combination of technical and intuitive surgical skill.

15.5 The design of the tibial component

The shape of the tibial component in compartmental and condylar replacements is a compromise between the requirements of stability and fixation. O'Connor *et al.* (1982) have demonstrated that a completely flat tibial component will provide the least resistance to the shear forces which are likely to produce loosening and this is achieved in the Oxford replacement with the use of meniscal bearings. These articulate with a flat metal tibial plate, but their upper surface is concave to provide stability with the curved femoral component.

Walker *et al.* (1981a) have carried out mechanical tests on 12 different types of tibial component. Compressive load was applied with antero-posterior force, rotational force and valgus–varus moment. The relative deflections between component and bone were measured. Best results (the least deflections) were found with one-piece components which incorporated a metal tray. This finding has been confirmed by three-dimension finite element stress analysis (Lewis *et al.*, 1982).

If the shape of the tibial and femoral components is such that an element of constraint is introduced to avoid anterior subluxation and lateral translation then the fixation must be correspondingly improved. The total condylar prosthesis (Insall *et al.*, 1979) has quite a large intramedullary post on the tibial component (Fig. 15.5). This will be even more critical in the posterior stabilized total condylar which is described as 'semiconstrained' which Insall (1981) now uses exclusively. The benefits of constraint and fixation are thus finely balanced.

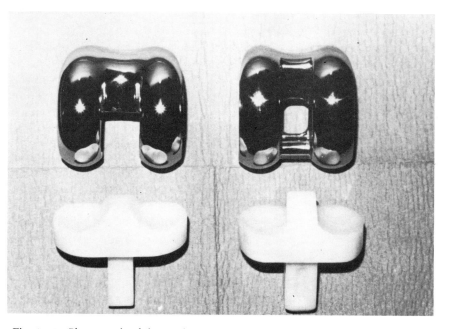

Fig. 15.5 Photograph of the total condylar prosthesis, models I and II. Insall now uses the posterior stabilized model (on the right) exclusively. (With acknowledgements to Dr J. N. Insall, Hospital for Special Surgery, New York.)

15.6 Wear and creep of polyethylene

Wear of the socket in a hip replacement is so slight (Charnley, 1979) that it scarcely constitutes a problem in clinical practice. In the knee, however, the situation is different and wear cannot be entirely ignored. Certainly a localized area of high loading which may occur when there is a residual varus or valgus deformity after operation will produce deep wear, so that complete penetration or fracture of the plastic can occur (Fig. 15.6). Alignment is to a large extent under the control of the surgeon and better technique should at least decrease the incidence of this type of wear. Nevertheless, removed prostheses frequently show evidence of pitting wear after a relatively short period (two or three years). This may be related to the inclusion of acrylic or bone debris between the articular surfaces which can occur in most designs of

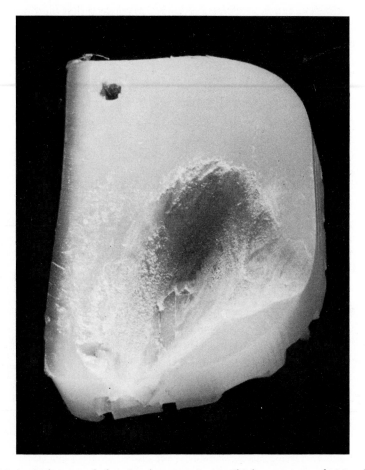

Fig. 15.6 A photograph showing deep wear in one tibial component of a Manchester replacement which was removed after four years.

replacement (Fig. 15.7). Walker *et al.* (1981b) have studied wear in what they regarded as 'a reasonable simulation of the situation in the condylar replacement type of knee prosthesis'. More conforming and thicker plastic tibial components were considered to be needed to diminish the penetration rate. But again it was recognized that a compromise has to be achieved between this and the fact that low conformity provides freedom of movement and prevents excessive forces and torques from being transmitted to the implant–bone interface.

Aside from the mechanical consequences of wear, the biological effect of polyethylene debris on the tissues is important. Charnley (1979) believes that the particles from unconstrained knee replacements are significantly larger than those he has seen with the small diameter femoral head prosthesis. The larger particles may provoke a macrophage response which could be a factor in producing loosening. Freeman *et al.* (1982a) confirm that there are always likely to be radiolucent lines at the bone–cement interface which may well be static and benign. Anything which stimulates macrophage activity will lead to progressive osteoclasis and widening lucent lines: products of cell death, bacteria and foreign particulate matter are suggested as possible stimuli.

Creep of polyethylene is also an important consideration and may be seen in knee replacements as the length of follow-up time increases. It remains to be seen whether attempts at containment with metal bands or trays is

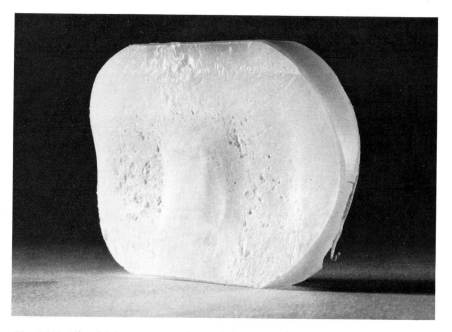

Fig. 15.7 The tibial component of an early Freeman after six years' active use. There is diffuse abrasive wear, partly from particles of acrylic cement.

effective. Black (1978), in an excellent review article, concludes that problems of excessive wear and creep encountered in total knee replacements are the direct result of failing to allow adequately in the design for the properties of the material.

New materials will undoubtedly become available to substitute for the polyethylene (and perhaps metal) components. Polyethylene impregnated with carbon fibre is now available in some replacements, but the results of clinical evaluation with this material have not yet been reported.

15.7   The need for intramedullary stems

There are perhaps two reasons for using components with medullary stems.

First, better fixation can be achieved and such stems are clearly essential for constrained hinges. The length needed is debatable, but the femoral and tibial stems of the Stanmore are 150 mm and 145 mm long. Semiconstrained prostheses theoretically are less liable to loosening and so their stems may be correspondingly shorter (for example, in the Attenborough and sphero-centric). The Sheehan replacement, with stems 135 mm and 114 mm long, probably represents a reasonable balance between fixation and constraint. The importance of good cement technique is now recognized: fragile cancellous bone and fatty marrow must be curetted out, followed by vigorous irrigation. Retrograde injection after blocking the medullary canal also seems desirable. Each component should be cemented in separately and the knee kept flexed in order to avoid sinkage or lateral movement which could occur as the knee is fully extended.

Second, it is sometimes suggested that intramedullary stems provide a reliable guide to alignment. This certainly is not always the case as has already been pointed out when discussing the way the femoral cut is made. A long thick stem may help, but variations in bone size would make it impractical to stock a series of prostheses with all possible combinations of length and thickness.

Many surgeons, however, have a strong determination to avoid invasion of the medullary canal and are rightly concerned about the extensive bony destruction which may be associated with loosening or infection. The initial Freeman–Swanson prosthesis was especially designed to avoid penetration of the bone and its lack of constraint was thought to demand relatively less fixation. The large number of designs now available illustrate the various degrees of compromise which are possible between the two extremes. Unfortunately, there is at present no certain answer, but the middle position seems to be held by the modern type of condylar replacements which already have been mentioned and which will be discussed later in this chapter.

Finally, in this section, it seems appropriate to introduce the question of femoral and tibial shaft fractures in patients with the knee replacements. The incidence seems to be low: two fractures only have occurred in our series of

583 operations. There are, nonetheless, theoretical reasons for anticipating a higher risk of fractures in prostheses which are constrained to a greater or lesser degree, and which have medullary stems. This is another factor to add to the balance in choosing the type of prosthesis to use.

15.8 Soft-tissue releases

15.8.1 MEDIAL AND LATERAL

Freeman *et al.* (1978) and Insall *et al.* (1979) drew attention to the need for a release procedure when it can be shown that correct coronal tibiofemoral angle cannot be achieved in extension because of tightness of the soft tissues on the concave side of the lateral deformity. This can be demonstrated by using a tenser (Freeman *et al.*, 1978).

The first step is to divide all the adhesions in the paracondylar gutters. In a varus deformity, the capsule, medial ligament and pes anserinus are then stripped from the upper end of the tibia as far distally as necessary. Alternatively, the medial ligament can be detached from the medial femoral condyle and if this is done it is particularly noticeable that when the posteromedial corner of the capsule is released, not only will the varus deformity be corrected, but, if there has been a flexion contracture, the knee can also be extended easily.

To correct a valgus deformity it may be necessary to divide the iliotibial band and this should be done through a separate incision proximal to the knee. The lateral intermuscular septum should also be cut. The lateral capsule and collateral ligament are then detached from the lateral femoral condyle. The principle, as on the medial side, is to slide the soft tissues from the bone and to maintain them in continuity.

Most orthopaedic surgeons accept that a medial or lateral soft tissue release is often needed to restore 'ligamentous balance'. Goodfellow (1981) disagrees and argues that the only structure which can be 'contracted' is the posterior capsule. He is able to demonstrate before operation that valgus or varus deformities can usually be corrected when the knee is held in 20–30° of flexion (Fig. 15.8(a) and (b)). Furthermore, when spacers of the height needed to give correct ligamentous tension are inserted at operation, alignment will be achieved, but a flexion contracture may be produced (or if one is already present it may be made worse). The residual flexion contracture should decrease gradually in the weeks (or months) after operation, but full extension is not always regained. Those surgeons who wish to obtain correction of varus or valgus deformity in full extension will find it difficult to accept this view and may prefer to carry out the releases which have been described, but this should not be done if the Oxford Knee is being used (Goodfellow, 1981).

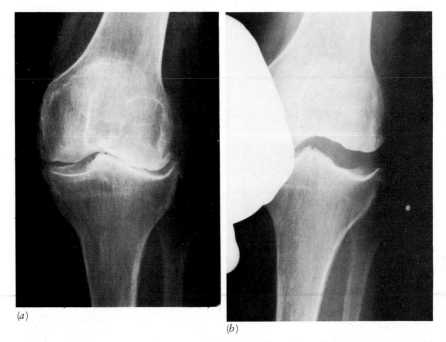

(a)

(b)

Fig. 15.8 (a) Shows the radiograph of a knee with a valgus deformity which could not be corrected when the knee was in maximal extension. (b) When the knee was flexed 30° and a correcting couple applied normal alignment could be achieved. (With acknowledgements to Mr J. Goodfellow.)

15.8.2 POSTERIOR

A flexion contracture is always associated with shortening of the posterior capsule and there may be adhesions between the capsule and the back of the femoral condyles. In addition to this, there may be a contracture of the anterior cruciate ligament (Somerville, 1960) or a bony block at the front of the condyles (Waugh *et al.*, 1980). Any degree of flexion deformity can, of course, be corrected by resection of bone, but this may lead to the removal of an excessive amount and also produce relative lengthening of the extensor mechanism. In most types of knee replacement the posterior part of the femoral condyles is removed and this allows access to the posterior capsule so that it can be stripped from the posterior surface of the femur. Full extension can then be achieved without further bone resection.

15.8.3 POPLITEUS

When there is a flexion contracture this tendon is often shortened and it should be divided to remove one of the forces which may produce lateral translation of the tibia on the femur. This is particularly important with the

Freeman replacement which has no constraint to this abnormal movement. The tendon can easily be found at its insertion to the lateral femoral condyle.

15.8.4 PATELLA

In a valgus knee, the patella may be dislocated laterally and it is essential that this is corrected by release of the lateral capsule. This should be done from within the joint and carried proximally as far as is necessary to allow the patella to remain in the midline during flexion and extension.

15.9 Patellar replacement

Many prostheses have a patellar replacement available, but there is still some disagreement about the need for this procedure, although it is being increasingly advocated.

Some implants (for example, all compartmental types and the Sheehan arthroplasty) do not present a metallic femoral surface to the patella, so the patient is left with the patellofemoral articulation as before operation (apart from the removal of osteophytes and correction of alignment). Other replacements (such as the Freeman and Stanmore) have a metal 'trochlear' surface. There are then certainly theoretical reasons for replacing the patella, although it remains to be proved that this will produce a substantial improvement in the overall results.

Whether or not the patella is replaced, it is essential to achieve central alignment and to demonstrate at the end of the operation that the patella stays in the midline when the knee is flexed and extended. The importance of a lateral release has already been emphasized. It is equally important to ensure that the external rotation deformity (which is frequently present in the flexed valgus knee) is corrected. These patients often also have a rigid valgus foot so that overcorrection of the external rotation has to be avoided.

The various difficulties with the patella after knee replacement have been described (Mochizuki and Schurman, 1979). It is undesirable to excise the patella subsequently and it should be possible to avoid secondary procedures (such as transposition of the tibial tuberosity).

Most patellar 'buttons' which are available have a convex surface (for example, for the Insall total condylar and for the Kinematic prosthesis). There has been some theoretical concern about the wear of polyethylene on convex surfaces and for this reason the Freeman patellar replacement is concave. The amount of wear in each type is not yet known.

The slippery and relatively shapeless posterior surface of the replaced patella may increase the incidence of subluxation after operation (Freeman et al., 1981). It is, therefore, essential to carry out the various steps which have been described to prevent this complication. Further, the femoral component should have a central groove to maintain the patella in position, at least while the medial capsular incision is healing. This is present on the Insall and the Kinematic replacement and also on the new Freeman–Samuelson prosthesis.

If lateral dislocation of the patella occurs the knee will become unstable, full active extension will be lost and a valgus–external rotation deformity may occur. The consequences are, therefore, disastrous and since minor procedures are unlikely to be satisfactory, it may be necessary to revise the replacement in order to be certain of correcting the alignment of the patella and the external rotation of the tibia which may well be present.

15.10 Comments on individual prostheses

The discussion in this chapter has so far been concerned with general principles and it now seems appropriate to consider briefly our experience with the prostheses which have been used at Harlow Wood Orthopaedic Hospital.

15.10.1 WALLDIUS

This is certainly a large prosthesis which demands considerable bone resection for its insertion. The articulation is a metal-on-metal bearing with the disadvantage of high friction and the production of metallic debris. Although Phillips and Taylor (1975) reported what appeared to be satisfactory results, this operation is properly regarded as obsolete in the 1980s. Nonetheless, our overall re-operation rate in 82 primary replacements of this type was 11.0% which is lower that that for some of the more 'modern' types of replacement in our series. This may be partly explained by the fact that most patients were old and were so very disabled before operation that they did not regain a high level of activity afterwards. The incidence of loosening, may, therefore, have been less and some degree of pain tolerated. Furthermore, although a small number of loose Walldius prostheses have been replaced by a Stanmore hinge, secondary operations have been avoided if possible. The incidence of deep infection has, however, been higher than with any other type of operation. Ten Walldius prostheses have been removed and arthrodesis attempted for this complication which, more often than not, occurred months or years after the operation. On the other hand, only three arthrodeses were performed for infection in 215 Freeman replacements, and two out of 117 Sheehan replacements. There have been no deep infections requiring removal of the prosthesis in 65 Manchesters.

15.10.2 MACINTOSH HEMIARTHROPLASTY

Our experience with this operation began in 1972 and the last was performed in 1975 (with a single exception in 1979). Although MacIntosh and Hunter (1972) reported good results, our re-operation rate in 1981 was 27.8% from

54 operations. An arthrodesis was carried out in two knees (one for infection), but the remaining 13 were converted to another type of replacement. These knees all showed sclerosis and then collapse of the bone in the femoral condyles. The process is, however, usually slow and the average time between the first operation and the subsequent revision was 58 months, which is longer than was the case with the re-operations which were needed for failed Manchester and Freeman replacements. In spite of this the quality of the results in the remaining hemiarthroplasties was never as good as that which would be expected from an arthroplasty in which both elements of the joint are replaced.

15.10.3 MANCHESTER

This small compartmental replacement represented a simplification of the original Gunston arthroplasty (Gunston, 1971). Deep slots had to be cut in the femoral condyles to receive the curved femoral components. The tibial components were slightly dished and were provided in different sizes. Although good results were reported by Shaw and Chatterjee (1978), our experience has been disappointing. We carried out 65 operations between 1975 and 1979. By the end of 1981, 18 (27%) had failed and needed a conversion operation at an average interval of 35 months between the first and second operations. No doubt some of our early failures were due to poor operative techniques. There were no jigs to help in making the tibial cuts and the components were sometimes put in tilted. Furthermore, at times we tried to correct a more severe deformity than is possible with any compartmental replacement. The knee may become unstable and anterior subluxation was not uncommon. Failure was associated with increasing pain and deformity. At re-operation there was usually evidence of loosening of some (or all) of the four components (Fig. 15.9). The slots cut in the femoral condyles were commonly enlarged to at least twice their original width and there might also be destruction of bone beneath a loose tibial component. The polyethylene was often worn and deeply grooved (Fig. 15.6) as if tracking had occurred; this would occur, for example, on the medial tibial component in association with a varus deformity. Finally, synovitis caused by polyethylene debris was sometimes present. These changes were variable and not easy to classify, but the degree of bone destruction has nearly always made it necessary to use a stemmed replacement (such as the Stanmore hinge) in order to secure fixation. Williams *et al.* (1978) reported a high incidence of failure when the prosthesis is used in osteoarthritic knees, but satisfactory results were obtained in rheumatoid arthritis although the follow-up was relatively short. We have not yet been able to demonstrate any causal relationships in our group of patients in whom the operation has failed. Our experience of the relatively early failures of the Manchester operation (and the difficulties of conversion) led us to stop using this prosthesis in 1979. We do, however, see some patients who after five or six years have an excellent clinical result with no radiological evidence of loosening.

15.10.4 OXFORD

The development of the operation and the biomechanical principles involved have been described by Goodfellow and O'Connor (1978) and Goodfellow *et al.* (1981). A more recent paper (O'Connor *et al.*, 1982) deals in particular with the fixation of the tibial components, but also describes the early clinical results in 98 arthroplasties carried out since 1976.

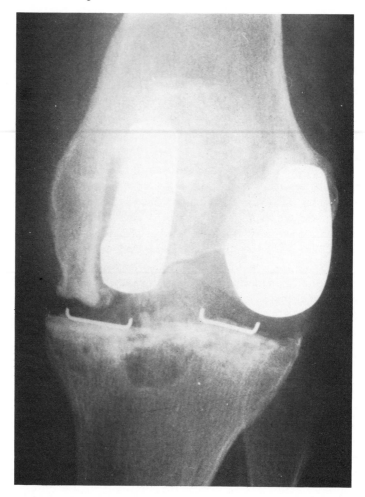

Fig. 15.9 Radiograph shows a clearly unsatisfactory Manchester replacement after two years' use. There is obvious widening of the tracks cut for the femoral components.

The replacement consists of two sets of three components to be inserted and Fig. 15.10 shows the assembly of one set. The curved femoral component has a single stud and the flat tibial component has a flange for fixation. Both components are cemented in position. The unique feature is the mobile meniscal polyethylene bearings which are inserted between the fixed metal components. These 'menisci' allow rotation and can conform to the path of movement which may be imposed by the remaining cruciate ligaments. There are eight different heights of bearing which, after testing with spacers, allows adjustment of ligamentous tension on each side of the joint so that correct coronal alignment will follow. This is in accordance with Goodfellow's view about the state of the ligaments and capsule in arthritic knees which has already been discussed in relation to soft-tissue release (page 367). We have certainly found that a flexion contracture is often present at the end of the operation and that the knee does not always achieve full extension over the subsequent months. Ten of our 33 Oxford replacements had a flexion of 15° or more after six months. It remains to be seen how much this will spoil the quality of the functional result. We have not been able to relate the flexion contracture after operation with the amount of flexion contracture before or with the degree of valgus or varus deformity which was present. This is not

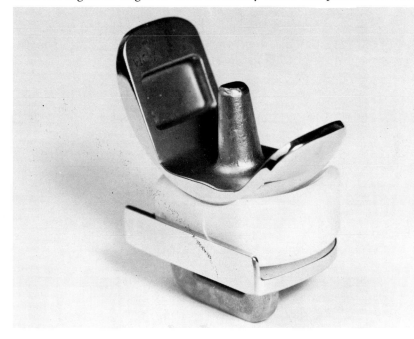

Fig. 15.10 Photograph showing the components inserted for an Oxford replacement. A similar set is placed in the opposite side of the joint. There is only one size for the femoral components, but the flat tibial component is in three sizes. The meniscal bearings are provided in eight different heights.

surprising in such a small group of patients, but it may be advisable, at least in the first instance, to confine the operation to those knees in the relatively early stages of arthritis and which have less than 0.5 mm of bony collapse. No doubt the quality of the results and the precise indications for the operation will become more clear as greater experience is gained.

A report from Oxford of 118 operations with a 1–5 years follow-up is awaiting publication (Goodfellow, personal communication). Whilst it is too early to make predictions it does seem that this completely original design will have advantages over the more conventional types of compartmental replacements.

15.10.5 UNICOMPARTMENTAL REPLACEMENTS

No such operations have been carried out at Harlow Wood, but it seems appropriate to mention the particular problem which is posed by the knee in which one tibiofemoral compartment only is affected while the other is relatively normal. In these circumstances, it is tempting to consider replacing the affected side of the joint. Results from the standard Marmor modular prosthesis used as a unicompartmental replacement seem to vary, but Insall and Aglietti (1980) report a marked deterioration in the results after 5–7 years. At Harlow Wood most of our patients have knees in which we either feel a tibial (or supracondylar) osteotomy would be satisfactory, or one so badly damaged that a total replacement seems justifiable.

15.10.6 FREEMAN

The early design of the Freeman–Swanson (ICLH) Knee has been modified in a series of stages over the past ten years with the aim of improving elements in the application of the original concept. Freeman (1980) summarized the timing of the various changes in both the design of the implant and the instruments used for its accurate insertion.

The tibial component was increased in area so that its edges overlap the cut surface of the bone. Fixation is now obtained by two 'osteointegration' pegs which produce an immediate interlock and eliminate the use of acrylic cement. Freeman et al. (1982b) have described their experience of this technique; there was no incidence of loosening in 56 knees which were followed up for an average of two years. A high anterior flange was added to the femoral component to improve articulation with the patella and a bicondylar shape introduced which allows removal of cement from the back of the joint. A technique for fixation of the femoral component without cement, using pegs similar to those in the tibial component, has been developed, but the results have not yet been published. A concave patellar button can be used with or without cement.

Instruments are available which make it more easily possible to achieve accurate bone cuts. The tenser is particularly helpful since it allows assessment of the need for a medial or lateral release and enables alignment to be obtained by 'steering' the femur so that the end of a long rod is brought to lie over the centre of the femoral head and the centre of the ankle (although the precise position of these points is not easy to estimate accurately).

Freeman has reported the improvement in the quality of the results which has been brought about by the various modifications (Freeman et al., 1978; 1982b; Freeman, 1980) and we have been able to demonstrate an improvement in alignment between one group of knees operated on in 1972 and 1973, and another in 1977, when the tenser and other new instruments were available (Waugh, 1983).

There is no doubt that the evolution of this type of replacement represents the outcome of much original thought and a willingness to make changes which appeared likely to lead to better results. Unfortunately, it has to be accepted that there is some confusion of nomenclature (for example, Freeman, Freeman–Swanson, ICLH and more recently Freeman–Samuelson) and it is difficult to record the overall results of our experience. The fact that we have carried out 215 'Freeman' replacements since 1972 and that our re-operation rate is now 16.7% (with an average interval of 46 months) is largely a reflection of the problems encountered with the early designs. In a statistical review (Tew and Waugh, 1982) we have divided the Freeman replacements into 'early' and 'late' models with the change occurring in 1977, but this is not an entirely satisfactory solution.

Finally, the new Freeman–Samuelson prosthesis (Fig. 15.11) has two major modifications. First, the femoral component has a central channel to help maintain the patella in the midline while healing of the medial capsule takes place. Second, a central eminence has been added to the tibial component to provide greater stability. All these changes will be welcomed, but it remains to be seen whether or not the quality of the results will be improved.

15.10.7 SHEEHAN

This prosthesis remained largely unchanged since its introduction, but in 1981 modifications were introduced to increase its strength and surface area (Fig. 15.12). Our 117 arthroplasties were mostly carried out between 1975 and 1979. A slight decrease in numbers in 1980 and 1981 was largely due to a desire to avoid the theoretical disadvantages of intramedullary cement. However, by the end of 1981 only eight (6.8%) had had a second operation (two of which were arthrodeses for late infection).

However, if we consider 'failure' to be not merely the need for a further operation, but to include those patients who have severe pain, then our overall 'failure rate' with the Sheehan prosthesis becomes much the same as with other types of replacement which have a higher re-operation rate (Tew

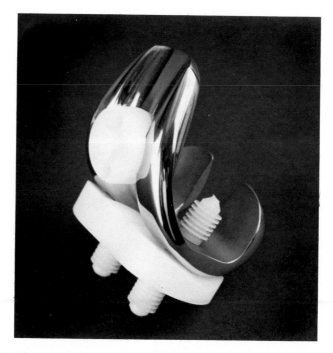

Fig. 15.11 Photograph showing the new Freeman–Samuelson prosthesis. There is a shallow groove on the femoral component to articulate with the patellar component and a central eminence on the tibial component to provide some lateral restraint. Osteointegration pegs in all three components allow fixation with cement. (With acknowledgements to Mr M. A. R. Freeman.)

and Waugh, 1982). It seems that there are a group of patients with Sheehan prostheses who complain of severe pain, but who do not have radiographic evidence of loosening or bone destruction. The reason for this is not clear, but minor degrees of 'sinkage' are difficult to detect and in some instances this may have occurred so that the remaining articular surfaces come into contact again (Fig. 15.13). We have only carried out a second operation where there were signs of loosening, deformity or breakage of the tibial stud.

The six knees which were revised all had a valgus deformity before their initial operation which had not been fully corrected to the desired 5–10° of coronal tibiofemoral valgus. Figure 15.14 relates the coronal tibiofemoral angle before and after operation in 92 knees and shows that with one exception (a patient who had previously had a tibial osteotomy and whose Sheehan arthroplasty developed a late infection) all varus deformities were adequately corrected. The same is not true for valgus deformities and it seems as though there may be a limit (say, 20° of valgus) above which we have not been able to be certain of achieving correction. The explanation might lie in the failure to carry out an adequate soft-tissue release or to loss of position if the knee is extended before the cement is set. These points also apply to varus knees, but the fixed external rotational deformity which is often associated with valgus may be an important factor. We have only seen wear of the polyethylene or breakage of the stud when there has been a residual deformity after operation (Fig. 15.15(a) and (b)).

Since this implant does not require removal of bone from the length of the tibia and femur (excavation rather than resection is carried out) it may be

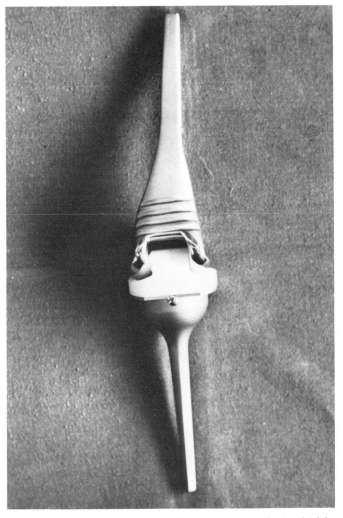

Fig. 15.12 Photograph showing a new Sheehan revision prosthesis which has a larger articulating surface on the femoral component with a corresponding increase in size of the tibial component, and a stronger tibial stud. (Acknowledgements to Deloro-Stellite Ltd.)

difficult to correct a flexion contracture. In a group of 60 unselected knees, 28% had a flexion contracture over 15° before operation and of these 76% did not obtain full extension afterwards.

These considerations lead to the tentative conclusion that this operation might be particularly suitable for severe varus deformities with lateral subluxation of the tibia and a flexion deformity of less than 15°. Undoubtedly

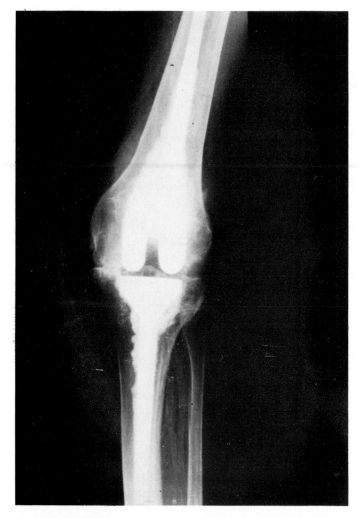

Fig. 15.13 Radiograph showing a Sheehan replacement where there may be sinkage and contact between the original articular surfaces on the medial side of the joint. Correct alignment has not been achieved and it can be seen that the intramedullary stems do not lie exactly in the axis of either the femoral or tibial shafts.

valgus deformities can be corrected satisfactorily, but in our hands this has been less predictable. Chen and Helal (1980) have also had failures when attempting to correct knees with very severe deformities.

15.10.8 STANMORE

This prosthesis (or variants of the present model) was first produced in the 1950s to replace bone resected for the treatment of tumours around the knee. The operations were usually carried out in relatively young people and according to Scales (1981) there has been no loosening in this group. The operation was subsequently carried out in patients with chronic arthritis and results were reported by Lettin *et al.* (1978).

This constrained hinge has to be set against the background which has already been discussed in this chapter. More recently a number of the American volume of the *Journal of Bone and Joint Surgery* contained three papers describing experiences with hinged replacements (Wilson *et al.*, 1980; Bargar *et al.*, 1980; Hui and Fitzgerald, 1980) and the editorial (Murray, 1980) concluded that the time had arrived for surgeons to become 'unhinged'. Reports are needed which give the incidence of loosening, sinkage and bone destruction with the Stanmore replacement over a 5–10 year period and it would be wrong to be too optimistic about our early experience. We

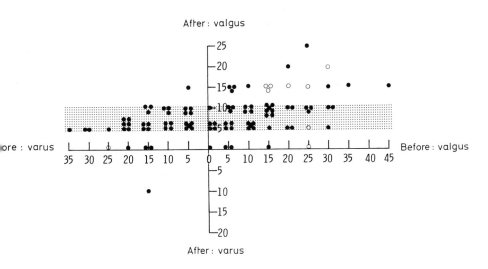

Fig. 15.14 Diagram showing the coronal tibiofemoral angle before and after 92 Sheehan replacements. This is a clinical measurement rounded to the nearest 5°. Some severe valgus deformities were not corrected to within the 5–10° valgus range. Knees which had a revision operation are indicated by the open circles. Correction of varus deformities was more successful and a second operation was only needed in one varus knee.

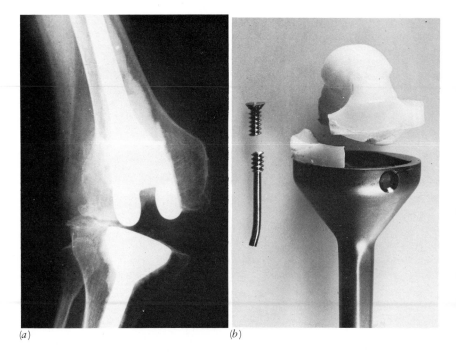

(a) (b)

Fig. 15.15 (a) The radiograph of a Sheehan replacement four years after operation in which the valgus deformity was not corrected. (b) A photograph shows wear and breakage of the tibial stud in this knee.

have used the prosthesis in 45 knees (19 primary operations and 26 conversions between 1978 and 1981) but most of the operations (35) have been carried out in the last two years. There has been one early infection which did not recur after vigorous initial treatment, and no late infections. The tibial component has become loose and been recemented in one patient two years after the first operation. At present we await with apprehension the complications (particularly late infection and loosening which seem likely to occur).

There are, nonetheless, a number of patients for whom this operation may well be indicated. In our group, primary replacements have been used to deal with severe valgus deformities in women aged over 75 years and occasionally in elderly patients with severe flexion contractures who could scarcely walk and in whom replacement of one or both hips (as well as both knees) was also being planned. These are patients in whom a simple operation is needed which will allow rapid rehabilitation. Their level of activity will also be low and it remains to be seen whether this can be regarded as compensation for the poor quality of their bones which may be responsible for poor fixation. Certainly cement technique is important: we now use intramedullary plugs of bone or polyethylene and retrograde filling with liquid cement. Each

380

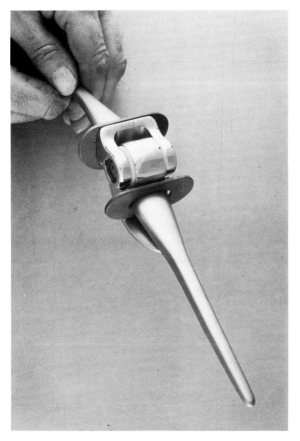

Fig. 15.16   This photograph shows the plateau plates in position in the femoral and tibial components of a Stanmore knee.

component is cemented separately with the knee in flexion. Scales (1981) has designed a set of plateau plates of varying sizes which cover the cut end of the femur and tibia (Fig. 15.16). This means that cement is retained when there is a bony defect and so pressurization is achieved. Further the surface contact between the prosthesis and bone is increased.

The prosthesis can be used for conversion from a smaller replacement which has failed and where there is extensive bony destruction. Whether or not there are better alternatives for this situation will be discussed in the next section.

15.11   The failed knee replacement

By the end of 1981, the 587 primary knee replacements at Harlow Wood had produced 69 revision or conversion operations and 22 arthrodeses. Ahlberg and Linden (1981) described a somewhat similar experience. Rand and Bryan (1982) reported that out of 5643 knee replacement operations at the Mayo Clinic, there were 626 revision operations. Their paper was based on an experience of 142 revision operations: of the knees concerned 95 had had one revision, 37 two and 10 three revision operations. The problem seems almost overwhelming, but surgeons now are having to deal with the failures of early knee replacements, many of which have already been abandoned. It certainly is to be hoped that the prostheses being used at present will not provide such an abundant harvest of revision operations.

Failure may be defined in a number of ways, but there are three major problems: first, infection; second, aseptic loosening and thirdly there is the group of patients whose knees are painful without any obvious cause. It has not been our policy to consider a second operation unless there is evidence of increasing deformity, abnormal anteroposterior or lateral mobility, or radiological signs of loosening and bone destruction. Those patients whose knees are painful, but which appear to be clinically and radiologically satisfactory are best advised to persevere, particularly as they are often better than they were before their operation, unless or until a cause is found to explain their symptoms.

15.11.1 INFECTION

Infection may often lead to the removal of the implant, but vigorous initial treatment of either early or late sepsis may be successful. An infected haematoma should be evacuated by reopening the wound without delay followed by closure and the insertion of three or four suction drains. The appropriate antibiotic must be given systemically in large doses. The same approach should be used for late haematogenous infections and antibiotics continued for many months.

Our experience with serious infections has fortunately not been great. A list of prostheses removed is given in Table 15.4 and in all these patients an

Table 15.4 List of prostheses removed

	Arthrodesis for infection	Total number of operations (primary and conversions)
Walldius	10	111
MacIntosh	1	54
Freeman	3	228
Sheehan	2	120
Manchester	0	65
Stanmore	0	45
Oxford	0	33

arthrodesis was carried out. We have not attempted secondary replacements in infected knees and an exchange operation may be a reasonable proposition provided it is carried out in the early stages (Elson, 1982).

It may be that some haematogenous infections can be prevented by the use of prophylactic antibiotics when these patients are especially at risk and Brause (1982) outlines a possible regime.

15.11.2 MECHANICAL FAILURE

Mechanical failure of the metallic components of modern prostheses does not seem to be a problem at the present and wear and breakage of the polyethylene has already been discussed (page 364). In our experience wear in itself has not yet been a primary cause of failure, but has been important only in relation to malalignment and loosening.

15.11.3 LOOSENING

Loosening can be regarded as a form of biological failure although mechanical factors are obviously involved. The presence of translucent lines of less than 1 mm is not important (Ritter *et al.*, 1981), but progressive widening and subsequent bone destruction is a serious complication which is associated with pain and instability. This has occurred and led to a further operation in 75 of our 587 primary replacements. The amount of bone which is removed at operation in a variety of replacements has been measured by Hankin *et al.* (1981). The major difficulty, however, is the amount of additional stock which is lost when there is progressive loosening and this may well prejudice the chances of achieving a successful arthrodesis or reconstruction. It is therefore important to recognize the early signs and to intervene before bone destruction has reduced the lower end of the femur and the upper end of the tibia to hollow cortical shells. No surgeon will want to operate before the patient has sufficient disability to warrant it (and this is not always the case in the early stages), but when serial radiographs clearly demonstrate progressive changes it is not sensible to delay (Fig. 15.17(a) and (b)).

15.11.4 SALVAGE OPERATIONS FOR MECHANICAL FAILURE

It has been possible to convert failed hemiarthroplasties to a standard Freeman replacement and on three occasions a Sheehan prosthesis has been removed and revised with a similar implant. There has, however, often been so much loss of bone associated with failure of the early Freeman and Manchester replacements that we resorted to what seemed to be the simplest solution and used a constrained hinge. Initially a Walldius prosthesis was chosen in the hope that if it became loose the absence of cement might be

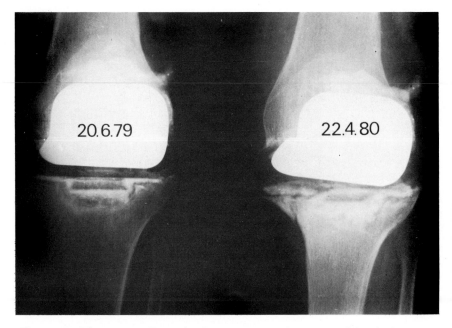

Fig. 15.17 These two radiographs show progressive loosening of the tibial component and bone destruction in an early model of a Freeman replacement.

associated with less destruction and that an arthrodesis might finally be possible. This was an illusion because metallic debris often caused an extensive granulomatous reaction. Since 1978 we have used the Stanmore hinge for most of our conversions, but it is difficult not to escape the thought of the possible consequences of late infection or loosening. The prostheses used as conversions are given in Table 15.5.

Table 15.5 Prostheses used for the salvage of non-infected failed knee replacements

Walldius	29	Sheehan	3
Freeman	11	Stanmore	26

There are now perhaps two better possible solutions to the problem of salvage operations. First, improved techniques of arthrodesis using internal and external fixation (Stulberg, 1982) should give a higher chance of success. Knutson and Lidgren (1982) describe success with a two-stage procedure in infected replacement. First, the implant is removed and a thorough excision of infected tissue is carried out. The cavity is packed with gentamycin beads. After four weeks in a plaster cast an arthrodesis is carried out using a massive cancellous bone graft and a long intramedullary nail for fixation.

Our policy now is to offer arthrodesis, particularly to patients under 60

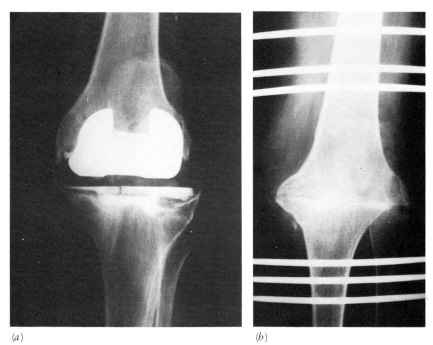

(a)   (b)

Fig. 15.18 (a) Loosening of the tibial component of an early Freeman replacement. (b) This was operated on before there was further bone destruction, so that it was possible to obtain satisfactory surfaces for arthrodesis without too much resection. This knee subsequently went to bony consolidation.

years of age, at a time when sufficient bone stock remains to make bony fusion possible without too much difficulty (Fig. 15.18). Unfortunately many patients reject this advice and ask to be given the chance of having another replacement. This leads to consideration of the second possible solution which is to use a less constrained prosthesis than a hinge which would theoretically be less likely to become loose. The Freeman–Samuelson revision replacement fulfills this requirement. The femoral component has a thick stem and there is a stemmed metal tibial component on which the polyethylene tibial component is fixed (Fig. 15.19). This produces better fixation and allows bony defects to make up with cement. Other semiconstrained prostheses are also available such as the stabilized condylar prosthesis in the Kinematic series (Fig. 15.20) which has a thick enough tibial component to make up considerable bone loss and restore tension in the ligaments. The Kinematic rotating hinge (Walker *et al.*, 1982) is another possibility.

Nevertheless, there will be some knees for which a constrained hinge will be needed and in a series of replacements at the Hospital for Special Surgery, a constrained total condylar III prosthesis had to be used in three revision operations (Hood *et al.*, 1981).

15.12 Where do we stand now?

Some orthopaedic surgeons are still proud to be able to say that they have
never done a knee replacement and certainly they have avoided the anguish of
having to deal with the failure of some of the models introduced in the early
1970s. The optimism of those who have designed their own prostheses

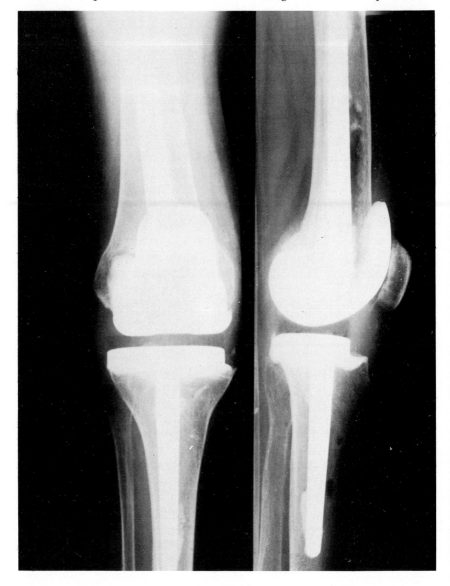

Fig. 15.19 The Freeman revision components are shown in this radiograph taken
shortly after operation.

remains undeterred since nearly all of them have made modifications which leads them to hope that they have at last found a satisfactory solution. Meanwhile another five or ten years have to go by before we really know the answer.

The attractions of a small replacement are evident to those who wish to conserve tissue and who would like an artificial knee to mimic nature's design. The Oxford prosthesis may go some way to realizing this philosophical aim and perhaps is the best replacement for those who wish to allow the posterior cruciate ligament to determine the path of movement. It is, however, important to define as precisely as possible the limits of its use in relation to the pathological changes in the knee which is being replaced. There must be many joints so badly damaged in which a small implant could not be expected to function reliably.

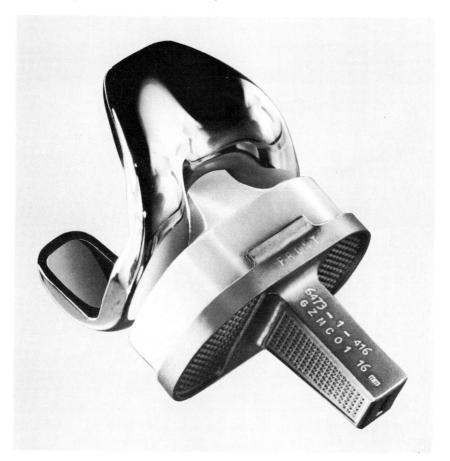

Fig. 15.20 A photograph of the Stabilizer Knee in the Kinematic series. (With acknowledgements to Howmedica.)

The present trends in the design of the condylar type of replacement which was initiated by Freeman and Swanson (1972) illustrate a broad approach in the balance between fixation and constraint. The Freeman–Samuelson knee now has an element of constraint and fixation with the possible advantage of eliminating cement. The Insall total condylar knee (Insall *et al.*, 1979) has now been superseded by the posterior stabilized total condylar (Scott and Schoscheim, 1982) which Insall uses almost exclusively (Insall, 1981). Fixation of the tibial component is by quite a large intramedullary peg and cement. The Kinematic series is based on Walker's biomechanical studies (Walker *et al.*, 1981a) particularly with regard to the tibial component: the polyethylene is housed in a metal tray and has a medullary peg for fixation with cement. The stabilized knee in this series looks somewhat similar in its basic design to the Insall–Burstein posterior stabilized total condylar prosthesis.

If the arguments for and against preservation of the posterior cruciate are left aside, we now seem to have reached a number of condylar replacements with varying degrees of constraint which may come as near as is possible to a 'universal' knee replacement with a very wide application. Differences, which may, or may not, be important, are likely to remain, but it is to be hoped that the designs will not continue to change.

There will probably always be some knees which will need a semi-constrained (or even wholly constrained) replacement with long intramedullary stems for fixation, but most surgeons will probably want to restrict their use of these large implants.

Judgements of choice remain difficult and will remain a matter for theoretical knowledge and intuition until more information becomes available. This will only be possible if surgeons combine their results so that large enough numbers of operations can be collected to allow useful statistical evaluation (see Chapter 16).

Ten years ago we were using prostheses which we have now abandoned and, although the future remains uncertain, some of the present generation of implants will probably still be in use at the end of another ten years. It is then that we shall really begin to know whether the results are as good as those achieved by hip replacement. Certainly, sufferers from chronic arthritis of the knee are very severely disabled and need help. Research may lead to the elimination of rheumatoid arthritis or at least to the reliable control of the inflammatory process by drug treatment, but osteoarthritis is likely to remain and affects the knee more commonly than the hip (Lawrence *et al.*., 1966). The need for a solution to the problems of knee replacement is therefore evident and the inventors of the current range of prostheses should be congratulated on the determination to provide relief for these very disabled patients.

References

Ahlberg A, Linden A. Secondary operations after knee joint replacement. *Clin Orthop Rel Res* 1981;156:170–4.

Arden G P, Kamdar B A. *Complications of arthroplasty of the knee. Total Knee Replacement.* London: Institute of Mechanical Engineers, 1975;118–22.

Attenborough C G. Stabilised gliding total knee replacement. *The Knee Joint.* Proceedings of the International Congress 1973. Amsterdam: Excerpta Medica, 1974.

Bargar L, Cracchiolo A, Amstutz H C. Results with the constrained total knee prosthesis in treating severely disabled patients with failed total knee replacements. *J Bone Joint Surg [Am]* 1980;62–A:405–511.

Benjamin A. Double osteotomy for the painful knee in rheumatoid arthritis and osteoarthritis. *J Bone Joint Surg [Br]* 1969;51–B:694–9.

Black J B. The future of polyethylene. *J Bone Joint Surg [Br]* 1978;60–B:303–6.

Brause B D. Infected total knee replacement. *Orthop Clin North Am* 1982;13:245–9.

Charnley J. Wear of hip sockets. In: *Low friction arthroplasty of the hip.* Berlin, Heidelberg, New York: Springer-Verlag, 1979;320–31.

Chen S C, Helal B. Preliminary results of the Sheehan total knee prosthesis. *Int Orthop* 1980;4:67–71.

Elson R A. Personal communication, 1982.

Espley A J, Herbert M. The replacement of both hip and knee joints in rheumatoid arthritis. *J R Coll Surg Edinburgh* 1981;26:214–7.

Freeman M A R. *Arthritis of the knee.* Berlin, Heidelberg, New York: Springer-Verlag, 1980.

Freeman M A R, Blaha J D, Insler H. Replacement of the knee in rheumatoid arthritis using the ICLH prosthesis. *Recon Surg Traum* 1981;18:147–74.

Freeman M A R, Blaha J D, Insler H. Cementless fixation of the ICLH tibial component. *Orthop Clin North Am* 1982b;13:141–54.

Freeman M A R, Bradley G W, Revell P A. Observations upon the interface between bone and polymethylmethacrylate cement. *J Bone Joint Surg [Br]* 1982a;64–B:489–93.

Freeman M A R, Insall J N, Besser W, Walker P S, Hallel T. Excision of the cruciate ligaments in total knee replacement. *Clin Orthop Rel Res* 1977;126:209–12.

Freeman M A R, Swanson S A V. Total prosthetic replacement of the knee. *J Bone Joint Surg [Br]* 1972;54:170.

Freeman M A T, Todd E C, Bamert O, Day W H. ICLH arthroplasty of the knee: 1968–1977. *J Bone Joint Surg [Br]* 1978;60–B:339–44.

Goodfellow J W. Personal communication, 1981.

Goodfellow J W, O'Connor J. The mechanics of the knee and prosthesis design. *J Bone Joint Surg [Br]* 1978;60–B:358–70.

Goodfellow J W, O'Connor J, Biden E. Designing the human knee. In: *Mechanical Factors and the Skeleton.* Stokes I A, ed. London: John Libbey, 1981;52–4.

Gunston F H. Polycentric knee arthroplasty: prosthetic simulation of normal knee movement. *J Bone Joint Surg [Br]* 1971;53–B:272–7.

Hagstedt B. High tibial osteotomy for gonarthrosis. Thesis (University of Lund) 1974.

Hankin F, Lowie K W, Matthews L S. The effect of total knee arthroplasty prostheses designs on the potential for salvage arthrodeses: measures of volumes, lengths and trabecular bone contact areas, *Clin Orthop Rel Res* 1981;155:52–8.

Hood R W, Vanni M, Insall J M. The correction of knee alignment in 225 consecutive knee replacements. *Clin Orthop Rel Res* 1981;160:94–108.

Hui F C, Fitzgerald R H. Hinged total knee arthroplasty. *J Bone Joint Surg [Am]* 1980;62–A:513–9.

Insall J N. Personal communication, 1981.

Insall J N, Aglietti P. A five to seven year follow-up of unicondylar arthroplasty. *J Bone Joint Surg [Am]* 1980;62–A:1329–37.

Insall J N, Lachiewicz P F, Burstein A H. The posterior stabilized condylar prosthesis: a modification of the total condylar design. *J Bone Joint Surg [Am]* 1982;**64–A**:1317–23.

Insall J N, Scott W M, Ranawat C S. The total condylar prosthesis. *J Bone Joint Surg [Am]* 1979;**61–A**:173–80.

Johnson F, Waugh W. Evidence for comensatory gait in patients with a valgus knee deformity. *Acta Orthop Belg* 1980;**46**:558–65.

Kaufer H B, Matthews L S, Sonsteeard D A. Total knee loosening. American Academy of Orthopedic Surgeons: *Symposium on reconstructive surgery of the knee.* St Louis: C V Mosby, 1978;308–25.

Knutson K, Lidgren L. Arthrodesis after infected knee arthroplasty using an intramedullary nail. *Arch Ortop Traum Surg* 1982;**100**:49–53.

Lawrence J S, Bremner J M, Bier F. Osteoarthrosis. Prevalence in the population and relationship between symptoms and X-ray changes. *Ann Rheum Dis* 1966;**25**:59–66.

Lettin A W F, Deliss L J, Blackburne J S, Scales J T. The Stanmore hinged knee arthroplasty. *J Bone Joint Surg [Br]* 1978;**60–B**:327–32.

Lewis J L, Ashew M J, Jaycox D B. A comparative evaluation of tibial component designs of total knee prosthesis. *J Bone Joint Surg [Am]* 1982;**64–A**:129–35.

MacIntosh D L, Hunter G A. The use of the hemiarthroplasty prosthesis for advanced osteoarthritis and rheumatoid arthritis of the knee. *J Bone Joint Surg [Br]* 1972;**54–B**:244–55.

Mochizuki R M, Schurmann D J. Patellar complications following total knee arthroplasty. *J Bone Joint Surg [Am]* 1979;**61–A**:879–86.

Murray D G. In defence of becoming unhinged. *J Bone Joint Surg [Am]* 1980;**62–A**:495–6.

O'Connor J, Goodfellow J W, Perry B. Fixation of the tibial components in the Oxford knee. *Orthop Clin North Am* 1982;**13**:65–87.

Phillips H, Taylor J G. The Walldius hinge arthroplasty. *J Bone Joint Surg [Br]* 1975;**57–B**:59–62.

Rand J A, Bryan R S. Revision after total knee arthroplasty. *Orthop Clin North Am* 1982;**13**:201–2.

Ritter M A, Gioe T J, Stringer E A. Radiolucency surrounding the posterior cruciate condylar total knee prosthetic components. *Clin Orthop Rel Res* 1981;**160**:149–52.

Scales J T. Personal communication, 1981.

Scott W N, Schosheim P. Posterior stabilised knee arthroplasty. *Orthop Clin North Am* 1982;**13**:131–9.

Shaw N W, Chatterjee R K. Manchester knee arthroplasty. *J Bone Joint Surg [Br]* 1978;**60–B**:310–13.

Sheehan J M. Arthroplasty of the knee. *The Knee Joint.* Proceedings of the International Congress 1973. Amsterdam: Excerpta Media, 1974.

Shiers L G P. Hinge arthroplasty of the knee. *J Bone Joint Surg [Br]* 1965;**47–B**:586.

Somerville E W. Flexion contracture of the knee. *J Bone Joint Surg [Br]* 1960;**42–B**:730–5.

Stulberg S D. Arthrodesis in total knee replacements. *Orthop Clin North Am* 1982;**13**:213–24.

Tew M, Waugh W. Estimating the survival time of knee replacements. *J Bone Joint Surg [Br]* 1982;**64–B**:579–82.

Walker P S, Ben-Dor M, Askew M J, Pugh J. The deformation and wear of plastic components in artificial knee joints. *Eng Med* 1981b;**10**:33–8.

Walker P S, Emerson R, Potter T, Scott R, Thomas W H, Turner R H. The kinematic rotating hinge: Biomechanics and clinical application. *Orthop Clin North Am* 1982;**13**:187–100.

Walker P S, Greene R D, Thatcher J, Ben-Dor M, Rutherford M S, Ewald F C. Fixation of tibial components of knee prostheses. *J Bone Joint Surg [Am]* 1981a;**63–A**:258–67.

Walldius B. Knee arthroplasty with prosthesis. *J Bone Joint Surg [Br]* 1957;**43–B**:187.

Watson J R, Hill R C J. The Shiers arthroplasty of the knee. *J Bone Joint Surg [Br]* 1976;**58–B**:300–4.

Waugh W. The clinical consequences of deformities about the knee joint. In: *Mechanical factors and the skeleton.* Stokes I F. ed. London: John Libbey. 1981;163–72.

Waugh W. Assessment of knee function. *Acta Orthop Belg* 1982;**48**:36–44.

Waugh W. Knee replacement. In: *Recent advances in orthopaedics.* McKibbin B. ed. London: Churchill Livingstone, 1983.

Waugh W, Newton G, Tew M. Articular changes associated with a flexion deformity in rheumatoid and osteoarthritic knees. *J Bone Joint Surg [Br]* 1980;**62–B**:180–3.

Waugh W, Tew M, Johnson F. Methods of evaluating results of operations for chronic arthritis of the knee. *J R Soc Med* 1981;**74**:343–7.

Williams E A, Hargadon E J, Davies D R A. Late failure of the Manchester prosthesis. *J Bone Joint Surg [Br]* 1978;**61–B**:451–4.

Wilson F C, Fajgenbaum D M, Venters G C. Results of knee replacement with the Walldius and geometric prosthesis. *J Bone Joint Surg [Am]* 1980;**62–A**:497–503.

CHAPTER 16

Evaluation
Marjorie Tew

16.1 The problems to be considered

The reasons for carrying out replacement operations are nearly always because the patient's arthritic knee causes him severe pain and impairs his mobility and sometimes because it feels insecure or is grossly deformed.

The objective of the replacement operation is to remedy all these defective conditions. The criterion of success is ideally the degree to which the artificial knee is a perfect substitute for a normal knee, but more realistically the degree to which the patient is satisfied in all respects with the results of the operation, in the long as well as in the short term.

In so far as the results are not completely satisfactory, orthopaedic surgeons are concerned to understand whether the cause of failure lies in the unsuitability of the prosthesis for its purpose, the quality of the surgery, some factor in the patient's general condition or the specific condition of his knee. Understanding is reached by evaluating evidence; in accumulating the necessary evidence the first problem is to select the condition about which information should be recorded. If general conclusions about the disordered knee and its treatment are to be drawn, the experience of individual patients has to be aggregated. Thus the second problem is to specify uniform criteria for measuring the conditions, so that homogeneous groups can be defined and comparisons made which have real meaning. Once the data have been collected, the third problem is to apply methods of analysis which are capable of leading to valid conclusions about related conditions and providing a reliable base for further advances in knee replacement surgery.

16.2   The records to be collected – review of data systems

Though the knee joint plays a unique and very important role in personal mobility, it is only one part of a complex mechanism and its satisfactory function is affected, directly or indirectly, by the fitness of the other parts, particularly the other joints of the lower limbs. It may possibly be affected also by the person's general health, psychological attitude and expectations. Satisfactory function of the knee depends on its anatomical and physiological characteristics, though no epidemiological study has established the limits within which these may vary without detriment, or measured the probability that certain conditions which pass as normal at one stage, including those following injuries, will be associated with ultimate abnormality.

Clearly the range of factors with a potential influence on knee function is very wide; it is not yet known how many of them have a causal relationship, or even a significant association, with an unsuccessful outcome of knee replacement. Therefore there is a case for recording information on every conceivably relevant variable in a form that would permit computer analysis and the correlation of variables.

Such systems have been designed for use in American clinics. One of these (Amstutz and Finerman, 1973) sets out to record up to 500 items of information about each patient and his knee, covering his general medical history and habits relating to health, the medical history relating to his knee including previous operations, the operative findings and his hospital course, as well as records before and after operation of his personal mobility and a wide range of anatomical and physiological measurements made by clinical examination and from radiographs. Since such a detailed account is too cumbersome for the routine assessment of the patient's post-operative progress, a compact knee rating schedule is also prepared, on which pain, walking ability, muscle power and range of movement, and independence of personal function are each graded on a 1–10 point scale, with points for residual flexion contracture and extension lag deductible from the total score.

In England, to evaluate the ICLH (Freeman–Swanson) prosthesis, a system on the same principle, adapted from that used in the Mayo Clinic (Coventry et al., 1973), was set up. 'We have deliberately included near exhaustive information on the Form so that this can in turn be transferred to the computer and used retrospectively for investigations which might not have been precisely defined at the outset of a particular study' (Freeman et al., 1977a). Here again the cumbersome detailed form has been supplemented for routine use by a short form covering only grades of pain and walking ability and the five clinical measurements assumed to be the most significant.

Besides the fact that comprehensive records become incomprehensible instruments for routine clinical management, there are other objections to such systems. Obviously it takes a great deal of medical time and skill to grade accurately every case under so many variables and a great deal of clerical time and skill to keep the records and prepare them for computer use. Not many hospitals have sufficient resources to devote to this task; and unless all the prescribed information is accurately recorded for every case in a series, the system defeats its own purpose, for the validity of the conclusions from any analysis of the data is reduced as the proportion of entries in the 'not recorded' sub-groups is increased.

In so far as the practical objections restrict the number of cases for which comprehensive information is available, the fundamental statistical objection becomes decisive. For even in the larger centres the number of cases in a single series is not great in statistical terms (see pages 404, 407, 408). Once they have been classified into all the specific sub-groups made possible by the detailed data, the numbers in each may well be too small to permit significant associations to be discerned between the variables cross-classified. This would be the more likely where, as in the case of deep infection, the incidence of the index condition is low and does not vary very greatly between the sub-groups of interest to compare.

To the cost of collecting the detailed data has to be added the cost of computer analysis and interpretation of results, which increases with the amount of material available. Perhaps it is the combined effect of all the objections which explains why so little use appears to have been made of all the data collected or at least prescribed. Freeman reported in 1977 (Freeman *et al.* 1977a) '. . . in the 5 years that the Form has been in use, we have used only a few pieces of the recorded information to evaluate our results'. These are the ones included in his shorter routine form. His later reports (Moreland *et al.*, 1979; Todd *et al.*, 1980) do not indicate wider analyses.

If all the detailed data so expensively gathered are not, or cannot be, used, resources would be more profitably directed at producing a narrower set of basic data, more likely when analysed to yield significant results. This would be within the capacity of more centres to collect and grading might be more reliable when effort was concentrated on a few items only. If several centres were to co-operate in gathering the same information, the limitations of small numbers would be reduced, but explicit and unambiguous criteria would have to be given for grading the variables and making the physical measurements to ensure that the resulting data were homogeneous and comparable.

Towards enabling the results after operation with different prostheses to be compared, the British Orthopaedic Association Research Subcommittee, after much deliberation and compromise, prepared a Knee Function Assessment Chart (Aichroth *et al.*, 1978). This purported to consist of 'only fundamental measurements recorded in a simple way' and so was to be suitable to be widely used. In addition to the patient's age, sex, diagnosis, duration of disease, state of other joints, his own assessment of his satisfaction with the operation and of how much his present disability was due to the affected knee, the variables to be graded before and after operation concern pain, five aspects of personal mobility and five physical measurements, graded on a 4, 5 or 6 point scale.

However, the grades as prescribed are not always mutually exclusive (allowing only one possible value for each knee) or exhaustive (together covering the possible values for all knees) and, as will be indicated below, it is doubtful that in practice, when applied to different series, the criteria for grading are sufficiently unambiguous to produce homogeneous, comparable groups. Given the inherent theoretical and practical difficulties this may be inevitable, for the 'fundamental measurements' to be recorded are of characteristics which are not simple and objective, but extremely complex and highly subjective to the patient, while the actual measurements depend on the personal judgement of the recorder.

16.3   Fundamental measurements and uniform criteria

16.3.1   PAIN

The first of these fundamental measurements must concern the severity of the patient's pain. To use the reduction of pain achieved as the test of success of knee replacement is to imply that pain can be measured and, if individual experience is to be aggregated, that it can be measured according to uniform criteria. But pain is essentially a subjective experience, which cannot be measured in an objective way. The patient's own grading, unqualified by the recorder's opinion, must be accepted, but as a result, subgroups of nominally the same grade may not in fact be homogenous or strictly comparable.

Pain is not simply a physical response to the stimulus of physical disorder. Common experience and scientific investigation confirm that, for any individual at any time, perception of pain and assessment of its severity are influenced by many other factors – emotional, psychological, circumstantial, social, cultural, and the use of drugs which blunt sensitivity. On any particular occasion, these factors may have a greater or lesser influence on the assessment of pain from a physical disorder. In turn, pain from a physical disorder may influence the assessment of other factors. For example, results of current research in Nottingham show that pain in the knee is very strongly associated with depressed mood, but there is no means of knowing how much, if at all, the former state is dependent on the latter. Also, pain-relieving drugs have been found to have very limited power to mask severe pain in the knee. Thus, though it cannot be claimed with certainty that an observed change in assessed pain between two occasions is due to a change in one single factor, the working assumption has to be that the dominant factor is a change in the physical condition of the knee, brought about by the replacement operation or by some later event or process. Since pain cannot be precisely measured, a 4 or 5 point verbal scale, ranging from very severe to no pain, is as likely to give a realistic classification of the facts as would the finer gradations of more sophisticated visual analogue or graphic rating scales.

The degree of distress which pain causes depends on its duration as well as its severity. Continuous pain of moderate intensity may well be rated as more distressing than intermittent severe pain. Thus assessment of severity may be usefully supplemented and qualified by an assessment of frequency. If pain is not present all the time, its occurrence and duration may best be graded by reference to the circumstances in which it is felt or the actions which provoke it – weight bearing in extension or in flexion, when the joint is moved or when it is still, when it has been used for too long or when it has been still for too long. This information may be more instructive and more reliably classified than information on the location of pain which many patients find difficult to describe precisely.

Only less disabling than severe pain is a sense of insecurity at the knee. It is often noted that this subjective instability occurs where laxity of the joint is not clinically observed and does not occur where it is (Freeman *et al.*, 1977a). It is, therefore, important to record the patient's evidence.

16.3.2 MOBILITY

The second area of fundamental measurement concerns the personal mobility of patients. Mobility, however, may be impaired by many conditions besides a disordered knee, hence it is necessarily a very unspecific indicator of knee function.

If we want to assess the effect of the knee replacement, we have to isolate the contribution that the affected knee makes to mobility before and after operation; and, so that proper comparisons of this contribution can be made, it is necessary to measure the performance of the same activity by each patient by the same standards on each occasion.

Such requirements cannot be fulfilled if information is gathered, as is customary in orthopaedic departments, by asking each patient how well he performs certain activities, such as walking or using stairs, in his own environment, which is always unique to him. Some people are more able than others to adapt their environment to accommodate their disability and to compensate for a disordered knee. Personal estimates of performance are usually very approximate and may relate to a maximum achievement or some kind of average. Groups obtained by aggregating records of nominally the same degree of mobility may in reality be far from homogeneous; and since the cases where the affected knee is, or is not, the limiting factor cannot be segregated, no legitimate conclusion about knee function could possibly be drawn from the resulting data.

These objections are obviated if knee function is measured directly in the clinic, by asking each patient at each assessment to perform certain standard tests which normally involve satisfactory knee function, then grading the difficulty with which he does so by specific criteria and assessing whether the difficulty is due to deficiency in the knee under review or to some other joint or condition.

Such a method currently being developed at Nottingham (Tew and Waugh, 1980) grades on a 1–5 point scale the competence of the knee to perform tests of standing, walking, negotiating steps and using a chair. The test of standing, which grades for how long (up to 12 seconds) the knee under review can bear the entire body weight, by itself and without pain, is considered to be a fair index of that knee's potential contribution to normal standing. Walking ability is graded by the time (seconds) patients take to walk a set distance of 23 m, a test considered to be a fair index of their relative ability to walk, measured by any objective test. To test their ability to negotiate stairs, patients step on to (with the affected leg leading) and down from (with the affected leg following) a set of four platforms, graded in height from 15–30 cm; they use no support except for balance and stop whenever the action becomes painful. As the patient sits down and rises from a firm armchair, 40 cm high, the observer and patient together assess how much the affected knee is contributing to the total activity. In all the tests only those cases where the knee is the limiting factor to the total activity can be included in an evaluation of knee function, and these are subdivided according to whether the limitation is due to pain, weakness or stiffness, or subjective instability in the joint.

These objective and standard tests, which require minimal equipment and can be carried out by non-medical staff, make possible a much more accurate assessment of the functional capacity of the knee before and after operation than do conventional records. But even so, they do not necessarily measure the potential capacity of the replaced knee, for the tests measure what the knee can do in its present state, not what it could do after continued exercise. Many patients, with one knee appreciably stronger, tend to spare a replaced knee, lest overuse should make it painful again. Though our tests show that certain patients regain virtually normal functional capacity of the knee in all or some of the respects tested, they cannot show whether others, equally relieved of pain, fail to do so because of an intrinsic deficiency in the prosthesis, or in its insertion, or in the physiology of the patient, or simply because of underuse. This last doubt could perhaps be resolved if all patients had rehabilitation therapy for a sufficient period after the replacement operation, to restore not only muscular strength and control, but also self-confidence.

16.3.3 ALIGNMENT

The third area of fundamental measurement concerns the alignment of the knee. The knee serves its purpose most efficiently when it is so aligned that it can extend and flex fully and when the mechanical axis joining the centre of the femoral head and the centre of the ankle passes through the centre of the tibiofemoral joint. Alignment can probably deviate to some extent from the ideal without causing appreciable loss of satisfactory function, but the safe limits of deviation have not yet been precisely determined. Therefore, the objective of the replacement operation is to leave the alignment of the knee as near the ideal condition as possible.

From measurements of the relevant angles much can be inferred directly about the condition of the underlying bone and soft tissue (Todd *et al.*, 1980), and perhaps indirectly about the relationship between the condition of these and the patient's pain and mobility. The angles produced under active control by the patient and under passive stress are not necessarily the same and the information each implies about the underlying structure may likewise be different. Each type of information may be useful to the orthopaedic surgeon in one or other aspect of his work, but each should be used appropriately and the records should not be confused.

Measuring angles might seem a straightforward exercise, capable of yielding a reliable body of objective data, divisible into homogeneous subgroups, but there are considerable practical difficulties. The size of a contained angle depends on the location of the extreme points to be joined and of the point of intersection. But identifying the correct marker points, particularly in patients who are obese or deformed, as many who require knee replacements are, has to be a matter of judgement and the judgement of even experienced clinicians is known to vary. Where the relationship between alignment of the knee and personal mobility is concerned, the material angles in both the sagittal and coronal planes are those attained when the patient bears weight, but the inconvenience for both the measurer and the patients who for any reason have difficulty in standing on the affected leg may make the measurements less reliable.

Accurate measurement of the angle of extension (or flexion contracture) is further complicated in the presence of a valgus or varus deformity and vice versa, as is the measurement of valgus/varus angles in the presence of rotation of the hip or tibia or a fixed deformity of the foot (see Chapter 2). Usually, valgus/varus measurements are relative to a neutral angle of 0° (or 180°), but sometimes they are expressed as angles of deformity and are relative instead to the angle of the normal knee, reckoned as 7° valgus (or 173°) – a diversity of practice possibly causing confusion. There are other causes of variation in measuring valgus angles under lateral stress and varus angles under medial stress. Stressing is painful to many patients; the force applied by the doctor will depend on his strength, his unwillingness to hurt the patient, his dexterity in handling the goniometer at the same time and whether he measures with the knee fixed in extension or flexed.

These inaccuracies would be minimized if standard techniques and scales of measurement were universally applied. Whether the remaining inevitable sources of error seriously distort conclusions derived from the measurements would be a matter for further investigation.

It might be thought that, in view of their shortcomings, the measurements of angles made by clinical examination should be replaced by objective measurements made from radiographs, but in fact these too have short-comings which cast doubt on their greater reliability. The desirability of full length radiographs, from femoral head to ankle, has been canvassed (Denham, 1980), but the practical objections to them have been found to be overriding (Hood *et al.*, 1981). Radiographs showing only part of the femur and tibia have perforce to be used, but it has been found that angles are measured just as accurately on these shorter 43 cm films, except in the relatively uncommon cases where the bone is bent (Lawrence, 1980).

However, a comparison of valgus and varus angles as measured on 43 cm radiographs with those for the same knee measured on the same day in the clinic in Nottingham has revealed a disappointing lack of concordance in an appreciable number of cases. Similarly, discrepancies have been noted between radiographs of the same knee on different occasions. These, however, can be seen to be due to the pictures having been taken with the knee in a different position: '. . . it is notoriously impossible to center the knee and X-ray beam in the exact position with each successive X-ray' (Ilstrup et al 1976) and few hospitals are at present equipped to use the sophisticated method developed in Sweden to standardize radiographic examination (Hagstedt *et al.*, 1980). Difference in positioning probably explains also the discrepancies between the radiographic and clinical measurements, but there is not as yet any means of knowing which of the conflicting measurements more accurately describes the condition of the knee. Nor is there any feasible method for the doctors or radiographers to overcome the problems of limb rotation in deformed patients.

Other information from radiographs, for example, on the quality of bone or the attitude of components, could with profit be linked systemically with the other data recorded. At revision operations loosening of a component in the failed prosthesis is often found. It is not known how often some degree of loosening is present in apparently successful implants, whether it is a necessary cause of failure or whether it only becomes a necessary cause of failure beyond certain limits or in association with some other condition. Nor is the significance yet known of certain radiographic signs, such as radiolucent lines, in forecasting loosening (Insall *et al.*, 1979a; Ritter *et al.*, 1981). It would be of great value if data could be gathered and analysed to provide such knowledge.

16.3.4 OTHER PHYSICAL CHARACTERISTICS

Measurements of extension lag and quadriceps function are sometimes recorded, but the results and their significance are rarely discussed. They seem only to be used as a minor component in some scores. This suggests that they are not thought to play so fundamental a role as other variables in the satisfactory function of the replaced knee. This may be true also of abduction, adduction and rotation, which are even more rarely mentioned in the literature and for which techniques of measurement do not seem to have been developed.

16.4 Analysing the data

Once it has been decided for which variables data should be collected and by which criteria each variable should be measured, the next stage is to consider how the accumulated data should be analysed in order that knee replacement operations may be properly evaluated.

16.4.1 MEASURING RESULTS IN A SINGLE SERIES

The first objective is usually to compare within a single series the outcome of operation with the pre-operative state of the patients. This may be done for each variable separately. For example, if, as in the British Knee Function Assessment Chart, the pain reported for all knees has been classified into four grades of severity before and after operation, the percentage of knees falling within each grade can quickly be calculated and the change presented in a simple table or histogram. Typically, reports of short-term evaluations show nearly all knees in the 'unacceptable' grades before operation and almost as many in the 'acceptable' grades afterwards. From this it is probably correct to assume that in nearly every individual case pain was greatly relieved and that the small minority with 'unacceptable' pain after operation were the same individuals who also had it before, so that they were not made worse by the operation. This assumption would be less tenable in variables where the distribution at each period was less uneven and the swing less complete. For even if the number in the favourable grades was greater after operation, this could have been made up of those favourable before operation plus others improved by the operation, but it could also have been made up entirely of those who had improved while those who had been favourable were made worse. Thus the simple statement of the percentage in grades might mislead as to the extent of improvement and the risk of deterioration in individual cases.

This pitfall is avoided if, for each variable, the values before and after operation for each individual are presented as graphs, from which it can be seen how many cases have improved and by how much, in how many cases an 'unacceptable' condition has been made 'acceptable' or 'excellent' and what risk there is, if any, of a deterioration (Freeman et al., 1978; Moreland et al., 1979).

To give a more rounded picture, knee rating scores have been compiled to combine in one statistic assessment of several variables reflecting the condition of the knee before and after operation. Individual scores can be aggregated and the averages at each period can be compared to show concisely the absolute or relative change. The scores after operation can be graded from excellent to failure to summarize the outcome.

But the method by which they are compiled means that scores can be misleading and obscure more than they illuminate. The choice of items to be included and the relative weight to be given to each are entirely arbitrary. The components of success depend on the judgement of the compiler, and the composition of reported scores reveals wide variety in judgement. No social survey has found out how the final arbiters – the patients – judge success; their judgement might be quite different. Percentage weights given to variables comprising the scores range from 30–50 for pain; 0–50 for personal mobility (or function); 5–30 for range of movement; −25 to +15 for deformity; −15 to +10 for extension lag; 0–10 for muscle function; and 0–30 for objective instability (or laxity). Subjective instability, of real importance to the patient, is never included. There is similar diversity in the items and their weights making up the separate subgroups in each scoring system (Convery and Beber, 1973; Evanski *et al.*, 1976; Freeman *et al.*, 1977b; Hungerford *et al.*, 1982; Insall *et al.*, 1976; Laskin, 1976; Marmor, 1976; Ranawat and Shine, 1973; Wilson, 1973; Yamamoto, 1979).

Some scores include only a few items, which are considered to subsume the rest (Freeman *et al.*, 1977b), but other scores include many items (Insall *et al.*, 1976). The more items, the more ways there are of making up the same score, so a comparison of scores at different assessments could obscure the extent of changes, and even contrary changes, in the subgroups included. Since after operation the knee is often not the limiting factor in personal mobility, particularly in cases of rheumatoid arthritis, scores which weight mobility heavily tend to understate the improvement following replacement in rheumatoid patients and lead to the mistaken inference that the rheumatoid *knees* benefit less than the osteoarthritic.

16.4.2 COMPARING RESULTS IN DIFFERENT SERIES

The danger of mistaken inferences is increased if scores are used in comparing the outcome with different prostheses: the 'excellence' of a set of results computed by one score may well not be the same as the 'excellence' of another set of results computed by a different score or of results relating to a population which includes a different proportion of rheumatoid and osteoarthritic knees.

Certain prosthetic designs are considered by some surgeons to be more appropriate for use with certain degrees of damage or with certain kinds of patient, while others are considered suitable whatever the condition of the knee or the patient. In practice, however, it is unlikely that prostheses are allocated to patients or pathological states in random fashion. For this reason, or because the same unambiguous criteria for grading are not universally applied, some series may be recorded as including a larger proportion of the worst cases than others. The disparity was certainly found to be highly significant in every variable (except age of patient) when the BOA Assessment Chart was used to grade knees in five separate series (Tew and Waugh, 1979). The relative improvement is likely to be greatest in series initially with the largest proportions of the worst knees, but that does not mean that the prosthesis involved is necessarily the best. To show whether or not different prostheses are equally capable of improving the worst cases, they would have to be used equally in the worst cases.

This reasoning, however, rests on the assumption that the post-operative state depends on the pre-operative state. This assumption may well not be valid in the case of all variables, and in particular for pain. A foreign body in an eye can cause mild to severe pain; removing the foreign body nearly always removes the pain completely, whatever the original severity. From reported results, which show unanimously that the prostheses concerned nearly always relieve pain greatly, one might infer that the knee replacement operation is a parallel case.

If this inference is correct, it would be proper, as in the example shown in Table 16.1 to compare the proportion of cases in each grade of pain after operation with different prostheses and use the chi-squared test to determine the statistical significance of observed disparities, without having regard to the pre-operative distribution by grade of pain in each series. The illustrative data relate to a random sample of 120 replacement operations using Freeman-ICLH and Sheehan prostheses, carried out over the same period at Harlow Wood Orthopaedic Hospital. The prostheses were used equally for the worst knees, 96% of which had 'unacceptable' pain (grades 1 and 2) before operation. Assessed about one year after operation, 94% had no or 'acceptable' pain; in no case had the pain been made worse. The difference in grades achieved by each prothesis might very easily have happened by chance ($p > 0.20$).

However, the inference may not be correct, for when the 120 individual pairs of assessments of pain before and after operation were correlated, the correlation was found to be low but just statistically significant ($p < 0.05$): to a very small extent the variance in the grades of pain after operation was explained by the variance in grades of pain before operation. A statistically

Table 16.1 Post-operative pain

Prothesis	Grade of pain				Total
	1	2	3	4	
Freeman-ICLH	1	1	12	46	60
Sheehan	1	4	5	50	60
All knees	2	5	17	96	120

significant result is not necessarily a practically important result and in view of the difficulties already mentioned in assessing pain and comparing assessments on different occasions, too great weight should not be placed on this marginal finding. But in so far as the level of post-operative pain does depend on the level of pre-operative pain, then the improvement produced by different prostheses would have to be measured separately for each grade of pre-operative pain, so that like could be compared with like. The average improvement of individual cases with the same grade of pre-operative pain, achieved by different prostheses, would have to be compared and the significance of observed disparities tested by an analysis of variance, as in the example below dealing with flexion contracture (Table 16.2).

How far personal mobility after operation is determined by the state before operation clearly depends on the degree of involvement of other conditions and the patient's motivation. Comparing mobility at both periods is irrelevant in evaluating the replacement operation unless cases where the knee continues to be the limiting factor can be segregated and the comparison relates to this subgroup only. Standardizing for motivation is well-nigh impossible.

How much the alignment of the knee after operation is determined by its alignment before operation depends on the ability of the operation to reduce (and avoid increasing) deformity. In all reported results the proportion of knees in normal grades of knee angles is considerably increased by operation. But the ability of different prostheses to correct the deformities concerned cannot be measured by a crude comparison of the proportion of knees in normal and deformed grades before and after operation.

The less a particular deformity has been corrected by a replacement, the greater will be the correlation between the 'before' and 'after' measurements of it. To calculate the degree of correlation, both these values have to be known for each individual knee. When, for example, the correlation between

Table 16.2 Reduction of flexion contracture in Freeman-ICLH and Sheehan replacements

Flexion contracture before operation	No. of knees (%)				Average reduction	
	Freeman-ICLH		Sheehan		Freeman-ICLH	Sheehan
0–9°	13	(22)	32	(53)	2.3°	0.4°*
10–19°	14	(23)	20	(33)	10.0°	8.8°*
20° and over	33	(55)	8	(13)	29.4°	15.6°†
All knees	60	(100)	60	(100)	19.0°	5.3°

Significance of difference * $p > 0.05$; † $p < 0.01$

the 'before' and 'after' measurements of flexion contracture was calculated for the random sample of Freeman–ICLH and Sheehan replacements referred to above, it was found to be strong in the Sheehan group (where variance in the 'before' measurements explained half the variance in the 'after' measurements), but virtually absent in the Freeman group. On this evidence both types of replacement had considerable ability to correct, but the Freeman had very much the greater.

The data permit the average amounts of correction achieved to be calculated, 19.0° by the Freeman, 5.3° by the Sheehan (Table 16.2), but this simple comparison would be liable to overstate the superiority of the Freeman operation since it was used in a greater proportion of initial deformities over 20° where the potential improvement was obviously greater. Comparisons of like with like become possible if the change is measured in subgroups of initial flexion contracture as in Table 16.2. In each subgroup the average reductions conceal some variance in reductions in individual knees. Using the statistical technique of analysis of variance (Moroney, 1978), it can be established that in the subgroups with less than 20° of initial deformity, the difference between the average reduction effected by each prosthesis was not significantly greater than the difference in reduction between individual knees whatever the prosthesis. But where the initial deformity was 20° or more, the reverse was true. This means that the Sheehan operation was not significantly less successful in reducing (or not increasing) initial flexion contractures up to 19°, but confirms the superiority of the Freeman operation beyond this range.

The ability of different types of implant to correct other deformities could be measured by the same method. This illustrates that informative, constructive and reliable findings can be derived only after appropriate statistical analysis. If the ability to reverse pathological changes possessed by different prostheses implanted in different centres is to be compared, there would have to be agreement to publish results in sufficient detail for the appropriate analyses to be carried out or to pool data for combined analysis before publication. In any case, data would very often have to be pooled to provide sufficient numbers to increase confidence that the events measured did not happen by chance and that conclusions reached can be generally applied.

The numbers of cases in published comparisons are typically too small to show up significant differences in the results. This was so when the results of 178 replacements using four different prostheses were compared (Insall et al., 1976), though when 220 total condylar prostheses were later included in the comparison the proportion of excellent results with these was significantly greatest (Insall et al., 1979a).

The problem of insufficient numbers is compounded by the fact that the design or methods of insertion of prostheses are frequently changed, so that the use of one particular type may have been discontinued before data from a large enough number of implants have been accumulated for valid analysis and even if this had been possible, the conclusions may have been rendered irrelevant.

For in practice few, if any, modifications or innovations have been prompted by scientific analysis of past experience. Information on the various aspects of pain, its severity, its location, its frequency and what provokes it has been recorded in the near exhaustive systems of data collection. Cross-classifying such information with clinical or radiographic observations might well reveal associations material to identifying the underlying physical causes of pain, particularly when this persists or recurs after replacement. If such analyses have been done, the results have not been made widely known. Yet such knowledge would seem valuable, even essential, when prostheses and methods of insertion are being designed or modified to overcome the deficiencies experienced with existing models. At least the results of such analyses might suggest further plausible hypotheses and the variables it would be worth measuring in order to investigate them, or they might justify the exclusion of certain records from the concise systems of data collection, feasible in smaller centres.

In practice the method of advance, necessarily pragmatic, has been to identify conditions present in the cases of early failure, total or partial, to assume that they caused the failure and to invent techniques to prevent them. Steps are not taken to measure how often these conditions are found in cases of apparent success and, indeed, it would often be difficult or impossible to do this. Freeman, for example, recognized that sinkage of the tibial component and some patellar pain were occurring after replacement with the early model of his ICLH prosthesis and modified the design to forestall future failures, apparently without analysing all his post-operative records to confirm that these conditions were in fact strongly associated with failure, plausible as this hypothesis might be (Freeman et al., 1978).

That a co-existing condition was in fact the cause of failure can probably be inferred if the condition does not occur with the appropriately modified prosthesis, though the inference would become increasingly dubious if more than one modification were incorporated at the same time. Few, if any, surgeons, once persuaded on theoretical grounds that a new or modified prosthesis is better, are sufficiently rigorous to carry out a controlled trial, inserting the unmodified and modified prostheses respectively in matched groups of patients and comparing the outcome. But in any case it is doubtful that satisfactorily matched groups could be obtained from populations necessarily limited in size, given the range of characteristics potentially influencing outcome.

In one sense it would be ideal if prostheses became available for general use only after exhaustive, scientifically valid, testing, but the price of this policy would be to deprive the majority of patients substantial relief, even if that relief were limited to a few years. For there is as yet insufficient experience on which to base reliable assessments of the long-term success of knee replacement with the types of prosthesis currently favoured.

405

16.4.3 COMPARING SHORT- AND LONG-TERM RESULTS

There are reasons to expect that the success rate will be lower in the long term than in the short. In addition to further degenerative or traumatic changes in the knee, adverse changes in the prosthesis, notably mechanical loosening of the components and wear of polyethylene, are likely to develop sooner or later. It is of fundamental relevance that the timing and extent of such deterioration associated with different prostheses should be measured.

Results usually reported relate to only one assessment with an average interval since operation of less, often much less, than four years. Insall, however, reviewing his first 50 total condylar prostheses, found no deterioration in the first five years, but contrasted that to the progressive deterioration in the other types of prosthesis he had studied (Insall *et al.*, 1979b). For example, good and excellent results following the Guépar replacement fell from 79% after one year to 58% after three (Jones, 1979). The deterioration was quantified also in a group of 159 polycentric prostheses, of which 13% were assessed as failures at five years and 28% failures at seven years (Bryan and Peterson, 1979); only 7% of 479 of the original series with this prosthesis had failed (been revised or caused severe pain) at two years after operation (Skolnick *et al.*, 1976).

The trend of such results might be extrapolated to estimate roughly how many years would pass before half, or indeed all, of the original implants have failed and the durability of different prostheses could be assessed by comparing the proportions of failures at given intervals. This could not be done by comparing only the average times from implant to revision – a statistic attractive because it is simply calculated from the most readily available data – for since these averages depend on the length of time the prostheses have been in use as well as on the time to revision, they are necessarily short in new series even when revisions are few. Moreover, not all results which must be accepted as failures are actually revised.

Much more can be learned about trends in failure rates if the method used to construct survivorship tables (Armitage, 1971) is adapted to analyse the survival time of knee prostheses. This method has the great advantage of making possible the maximum use of data, for it takes account of prostheses implanted at different dates and so having different follow-up periods and implants in patients who have died or been lost to follow-up. It enables the number of failures, however defined, in any year to be related to the average number at risk throughout the year; the annual survival rates – the inverse of the annual failure rates – can then be used to calculate the diminishing percentage of implants surviving satisfactorily after each year of service.

When the method was applied to the post-operative records of 365 knee replacement operations carried out from 1972 to 1980 at Harlow Wood Orthopaedic Hospital and followed up to September 1981, the average annual failure (revision) rate over the first two years (1.5%) was found to be very significantly (p <0.005) lower than that over the next two years (6.4%) (Tew and Waugh, 1982). Thereafter the annual failure rate rose further, but after the sixth year the number at risk became too small for generalizations to be made with a significant level of confidence about the rate of further increase and, hence, about the proportion thereafter surviving. Extrapolating the possible trends indicates that only about one-half to one-third of the prostheses would remain *in situ* after ten years; on a wider definition of failure the proportions surviving satisfactorily would be smaller.

The same pattern was observed in each of the four types of prosthesis making up the total, with the annual failure rate most often highest for the Manchester and lowest for the Sheehan. But when the incidence of annual failure is so low and the numbers at risk so small, it is hardly possible to identify significant differences between prostheses. Over the whole period, however, the actual number of Manchesters which failed was significantly greater (p <0.01) than the number expected, if each year their failure rate had been the same as the average of the four groups; the actual number of Sheehan failures was fewer than expected, but not significantly so.

The other two prostheses studied were the early and the later, modified, Freeman–ICLH. Between these there was, surprisingly, no difference in failure rates calculated either annually or over the whole period. Measuring simply the proportion of failures at five and seven years, Bryan found with the same surprise that 'the early polycentric models performed about as well as the more sophisticated models' inserted by more experienced surgeons (Bryan and Peterson, 1979). These findings point to the need for properly evaluating new or modified prostheses, for designs are changed to remedy conditions existing in cases of failure but not necessarily its cause.

More penetrating analysis of results might well direct design effort more profitably, for superficial analysis can certainly mislead. In the Harlow Wood study the annual failure rate was not affected by the patients' age, diagnosis or pre-operative deformity. By far the most important factor determining it was the length of time the prosthesis had been implanted – the shorter the time, the lower the rate. In so far as this finding is generally valid, it follows that the larger the proportion of recent implants in a series, the lower will the failure rate appear to be if, as is conventional, failure rates are expressed as the percentage of failures in the total number of implants. Thus newly introduced prostheses will necessarily appear to give better results than those of earlier vintage, without the appearance being substantiated. The pre-ponderance of recent implants in the later modified Freeman group studied completely explained why its conventional failure (revision) rate of 5% was significantly lower than the rate of 22% for the early model, which has not been used for over four years.

The annual failure rate may also be affected by the type of prosthesis and all may not show the same pattern. But where rates are low or margins small, significant differences can only be discerned in large samples – many times larger than are likely to be available in individual series. Thus once again the need is emphasized for many centres to collaborate in following up replacements regularly for many years and analysing their records by a method capable of leading to conclusive results.

16.5 Conclusions

This survey has shown that the problems of evaluating knee replacement operations are many, complex, interrelated and indeed circular. The solutions, if possible at all, imply far-reaching changes in the collection and analysis of the data of experience. The questions to be answered are:

(1) How far does knee replacement succeed in remedying the deficiencies of the disordered, arthritic knee in both the short and long term?

(2) Is one type of replacement operation more successful than another in all or particular objectives and at all or particular stages of the progressive destruction which occurs in chronic arthritis?

(3) Can the conditions which cause success or failure be identified?

It has to be decided what evidence – what data and how analysed – would give conclusive answers to these questions.

Data have to be collected before they can be analysed, but it is futile to collect data unless they are of the kind and in the form necessary for the application of valid statistical methods of analysis. Unless sound methods of analysis are used, efforts towards improving outcome are in danger of being misdirected to changing conditions which are not in fact the root cause of failure. So a plan for analysis should precede the selection of data to be collected. But the expectation from the soundest methods of analysis is frustrated if the data to be analysed do not describe sufficiently accurately those conditions material to evaluation, whose identification in turn may be proposed by plausible hypotheses but has eventually to be confirmed by sound analysis. If comparisons are to be made, and comparisons are the essential instrument of evaluation, uniform criteria of measurement must be agreed and applied to produce homogeneous, comparable groups, but the difficulties inherent in obtaining specific, accurate and repeatable measurements are not simple to overcome.

To ensure that conclusions are not based on evidence from unrepresentative samples of experience and that differences observed by comparisons are statistically significant, sufficiently large numbers of cases are required. Where differences to be detected are small, the numbers available from single series are unlikely to be sufficiently large. Thus data from different collaborating centres will have to be aggregated, which reinforces the need for using uniform criteria of measurement.

So far remarkably little attempt seems to have been made to use the data gathered to cross-classify the presence or absence of pain and subjective instability after operation with the other variables as measured by patients' testimony, or by clinical examination or by radiographs. Yet such association of data, sufficient in quantity and reliability, might well be more successful in identifying the real causes of failure, even than the inspired surmises of percipient surgeons, and so provide a surer basis for further improvements in this operation which has already brought so much relief.

References

Aichroth P, Freeman M A R, Smillie I S, Souter W A. A knee function assessment chart. *J Bone Joint Surg [Br]* 1978;60–B:308–9.

Amstutz H C, Finerman G A M. Knee joint replacement – development and evaluation. *Clin Orthop Rel Res* 1973;94:24–41.

Armitage P. *Statistical methods in medical research.* Oxford: Blackwell, 1971;408–14.

Bryan R S, Peterson L F A. Polycentric total knee arthroplasty: a prognostic assessment. *Clin Orthop Rel Res* 1979;145:23–8.

Convery F R, Beber C A. Total knee arthroplasty. *Clin Orthop Rel Res* 1973;94:42–9.

Coventry M B, Upshaw J E, Riley L H, Finerman G A M, Turner R H. Geometric total knee arthroplasty. II. Patient data and complications. *Clin Orthop Rel Res* 1973;94:177–84.

Denham R A. Radiological examination of the knee joint and other special investigations. In: *Arthritis of the knee.* Freeman M A R ed. Berlin: Springer-Verlag, 1980;77–109.

Evanski P M, Waugh T R, Orofino C F, Anzel S H. UCI knee replacement. *Clin Orthop Rel Res* 1976;120:33–8.

Freeman M A R, Todd R C, Barnett P, Day W H. ICLH arthroplasty of the knee. *J Bone Joint Surg [Br]* 1978;60–b:339–44.

Freeman M A R, Todd R C, Cundy A D. A technique for recording the results of knee surgery. *Clin Orthop Rel Res* 1977a;128:216–24.

Freeman M A R, Todd R C, Cundy A D. The presentation of the results of knee surgery. *Clin Orthop Rel Res* 1977b;128:222–7.

Hagstedt B, Norman O, Ollsen T H. Technical accuracy in high tibial osteotomy for gonarthrosis. *Acta Orthop Scand* 1980;51:963–70.

Hood R W, Vanni M, Insall J N. The correction of knee alignment in 255 consecutive total condylar knee replacements. *Clin Orthop Rel Res* 1981;160:94–105.

Hungerford D S, Kenna R V, Krackow K A. The porous-coated anatomic total knee. *Orthop Clin North Am* 1982;13:103–22.

Ilstrup D M, Coventry M B, Skolnick M D. A statistical evaluation of geometric total knee arthroplasties. *Clin Orthop Rel Res* 1976;120:27–32.

Insall J N, Ranawat C S, Aglietti P, Shine J. A comparison of four models of total knee replacement prostheses. *J Bone Joint Surg [Am]* 1976;58–A:754–65.

Insall J N, Scott W N, Ranawat C S. The total condylar knee prosthesis: a report of 220 cases. *J Bone Joint Surg [Am]* 1979a;61–A:174–80.

Insall J N, Tria A J, Scott W N. The total condylar knee prosthesis: the first 5 years. *Clin Orthop Rel Res* 1979b;145:68–77.

Jones E C, Insall J N, Inglis A E, Ranawat C S. Guépar knee arthroplasty results and late complications. *Clin Orthop Rel Res* 1979;140:145–52.

Laskin R S. Modular total knee replacement arthroplasty. *J Bone Joint Surg [Am]* 1976;58–A:766–72.

Lawrence M. The role of goniometry and radiography in the assessment of the tibiofemoral alignment and knee joint stability. B Med Sci Thesis (University of Nottingham) 1980.

Marmor L. The modular (Marmor) knee. *Clin Orthop Rel Res* 1976;120:86–94.

Moreland J R, Thomas R J, Freeman M A R. ICLH replacement of the knee: 1977 and 1978. *Clin Orthop Rel Res* 1979;**145**:47–59.

Moroney M J. *Facts from figures*. Harmondsworth, Middlesex, England: Penguin Books, 1978;371–457.

Ranawat C S, Shine J J. Duocondylar total knee arthroplasty. *Clin Orthop Rel Res* 1973;**94**: 185–95.

Ritter M A, Gioe T J, Stringer E A. Radiolucency surrounding the posterior cruciate condylar total knee prosthetic components. *Clin Orthop Rel Res* 1981;**160**:149–52.

Skolnick M D, Bryan R S, Peterson L F A, Combs J J, Ilstrup D M. Polycentric total knee arthroplasty: a two-year follow-study. *J Bone Joint Surg [Am]* 1976;**58–A**:743–8.

Tew M, Waugh W. Total replacement of the knee. *J Bone Joint Surg [Br]* 1979;**61–B**:225–8.

Tew M, Waugh W. Guide to recording information about knee replacements. Internal publication (University of Nottingham) 1980.

Tew M, Waugh W. Estimation of the survival time of knee replacements. *J Bone Joint Surg [Br]* 1982;**64–B**:572–8.

Todd R C, Freeman M A R, Gschwend N. Clinical Assessment. In: *Arthritis of the knee*. Freeman M A R, ed. Berlin: Springer-Verlag, 1980;57–76.

Wilson F C. Total replacement of the knee in rheumatoid arthritis. *Clin Orthop Rel Res* 1973;**94**:58–64.

Yamamoto S. Total knee replacement with the Kodama–Yamamoto knee prosthesis. *Clin Orthop Rel Res* 1979;**145**:60–7.

410

PART FOUR

Tumours

CHAPTER 17

The Diagnosis and Treatment of Benign and Malignant Tumours around the Knee

J.N. Wilson

Tumours arising in any long bone can often give difficulties both in diagnosis and treatment and those around the knee are no exception. They may present either as a swelling, which may or may not be painful; or as a vague feeling of discomfort or insecurity, with no visible evidence of tumour; or as a sudden catastrophic event, resulting from a pathological fracture.

The knee is one of the more common sites in which primary bone tumours may occur and in the records of the Bone Tumour Registry at the Institute of Orthopaedics 20% of all recorded tumours arose in the knee, and if secondary tumours were excluded from the totals this figure rose to almost 24%. The active growing epiphyses for the leg are around the knee and since the knee is particularly liable to injury, we have two factors which may be complementary, and could possibly have some bearing on the high incidence of tumours around the knee.

17.1 Classification

There are many different classifications for bone tumours. For the purposes of this chapter the temptation to choose the easy way and simply to divide the

413

lesions into benign and malignant, followed by a long list of the different varieties, has been resisted. Instead, the more common tumours around the knee have been classified according to their tissue of origin, or where this is in doubt, as for example in giant cell tumour, aneurysmal bone cyst or Ewing's tumour, they are classified by their special peculiarities. To clarify the differential diagnosis, conditions simulating bone tumours are illustrated at the end of the chapter. The classification chosen is illustrated in Table 17.1.

Table 17.1 Classification of bone tumours arising around the knee

Bone-forming tumours	Exostosis (osteocartilaginous exostosis)
	Osteoid osteoma
	Parosteal osteosarcoma
	Osteosarcoma
Cartilage-forming tumours	Chondroma (including enchondromatosis)
	Chondromyxoid fibroma
	Benign chondroblastoma
	Chondrosarcoma
Fibrous tissue tumours	Non-osteogenic fibroma
	Fibrous dysplasia
	Malignant fibrous histiocytoma
	Fibrosarcoma
Lymphosarcoma	
Metastatic tumours	
Tumours of unknown origin	Simple bone cyst
	Giant cell tumour
	Aneurysmal bone cyst
	Malignant round cell tumour (including Ewing's tumour)

17.2 Diagnosis

Although most bone tumours arising around the knee will be confined to the one area the clinician must always remain aware of the possibility that the local lesion is just one part of a more generalized condition; metastatic disease, fibrous dysplasia and hyperparathyroidism being good examples of such cases. A general physical examination is therefore mandatory in all suspected tumours of bone, looking for other possible abnormalities which may indicate the presence of systemic disease of which the lesion at the knee is merely the first presenting symptom.

17.3 History and clinical examination

Tumours in any part of the skeleton system may present in three ways: with

414

pain, with swelling, or with a pathological fracture, or sometimes all three. The most common presenting symptom, however, is pain. At first this may be transient and only reported when it becomes more constant. Early pain may be associated with a minor strain, possibly causing a stress crack in the weakened cancellous bone, or even a small haemorrhage within the tumour. Constant, unremitting pain is usually an indication of a rapidly growing lesion, probably of a malignant nature, which is producing an expanding lesion under tension.

When considering the cause of any pain around the knee joint it is important to remember that this may be referred from the hip and can be the first indication of bone or joint disease at a proximal level.

Pathological fractures, common in the lower end of the femur and often involving the articular surface, may be the final catastrophic event which follows a period of pain; or, in very benign lesions, as a sudden presenting incident without prior symptoms. As a broad generalization, a pathological fracture without prodromal signs indicates a benign, slowly growing lesion; whereas in frankly malignant tumours, such as osteosarcoma, or locally

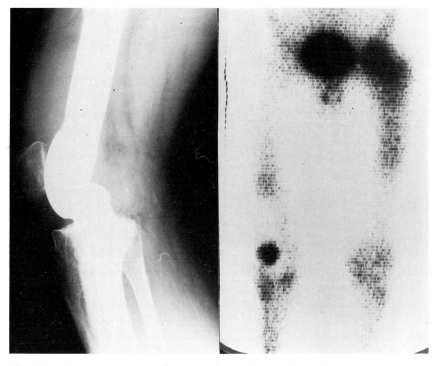

Fig. 17.1 Recurrence in the soft tissues after radical excision of bone tumours can be difficult to detect. This scan shows a recurrence in the region of the lower end of the femur which has been excised and replaced by an endoprosthesis. Careful local examination is mandatory at every follow-up visit.

415

malignant lesions such as giant cell tumours, pathological fracture is nearly always preceded by pain.

Localization of the pain is important, particularly if accompanied by tenderness; for it is very unlikely that in these circumstances the pain can be referred from elsewhere. Local tenderness may be an early warning sign of an impending pathological fracture.

The swelling is sometimes very obvious, but in the fat patient a small, diffuse prominence can be easily overlooked; and when there is a slow expansion of bone, such as occurs in giant cell tumour and chondrosarcoma, this may not become apparent until it has reached alarming proportions. The history that a swelling is increasing in size should never be neglected.

Sites of local tenderness should be carefully examined for irregularities, and the contours of the limb always compared with the normal side. Where there are obvious radiological signs that a tumour arises from bone a meticulous clinical examination must be carried out to exclude soft-tissue extension. This is particularly important when there has been a pathological fracture or when there is a history of previous operative interference. In these circumstances recurrence in the soft tissues after radical excision can be especially difficult to detect and the clinician must be constantly on the look out for it (Fig. 17.1).

Swelling due to an effusion or a haemarthrosis (in the absence of a pathological fracture) is unusual unless the synovium is involved. A marked effusion is more likely to be caused by arthritic disease, injury or infection; and chronic infection, such as tuberculosis, can be difficult to distinguish from tumour particularly when there is underlying bone disease (Fig. 17.2). However, the synovial thickening, the oedematous feel of the subcutaneous tissue and the increased warmth of the joint should alert the clinician to the alternative diagnosis.

17.4   Investigations

The characteristics of some bone tumours such as solitary osteocartilaginous exostoses, or certain fibrous lesions of bone, are so well known that very little investigation is required. Not infrequently, however, the diagnosis is uncertain, and particularly so if there is the possibility that the lesion is merely part of a generalized disease of the skeleton. In these circumstances a full skeletal survey and investigation of other systems are indicated.

17.4.1   THE WHOLE BODY ISOTOPE SCAN

This has largely replaced the X-ray skeletal survey which was used in the past, and radiographs of other bones are confined to any areas where there has been an increased uptake on the scan. The two main isotopes at present in use in whole body scanning are technetium 99m phosphonate and gallium 67

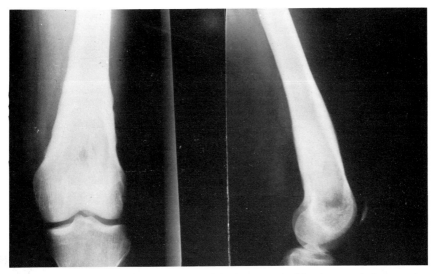

Fig. 17.2 Tuberculosis osteomyelitis of the lower end of the femur misdiagnosed as tumour. The clinical findings of oedema, generalized warmth of the joint and the Indian origin of the patient should have alerted the clinician to the correct diagnosis.

citrate. Technetium has a relatively short half-life of only a few hours which makes it convenient for completing the whole investigation as an out-patient, whereas the half-life of gallium is much longer, thereby delaying the final scan for 48–72 hours. Both have a high safety record and there is no radiation hazard. Technetium has the advantage of giving a very clear picture of the overall skeleton and is therefore probably the more useful; but gallium is said to be more selective and to have the ability to distinguish the activity of the lesion by the density of the scan (Simon and Kirchner, 1980). Technetium 99m, when linked with phosphate becomes specifically a bone-seeking isotope which gallium is not, but both are taken up selectively by any part of the skeleton where the bone turnover is increased (Fig. 17.3(b)). It must be made clear, however, that this does not necessarily mean that a bone tumour is present at every site of increased uptake, and Figure 17.3(c) illustrates how a 'second deposit' in the opposite knee was found to be merely due to the increased vascularity associated with osteoarthritis.

17.4.2 COMPUTERIZED TOMOGRAPHY (CT)

This technique has introduced a new dimension into the investigation of bone tumours, and is particularly useful in displaying the local extension of the disease into the soft tissues – giving valuable additional information if local resection is being considered. It is, however, still an expensive investigation and should be used with discretion. It is by no means essential in every case.

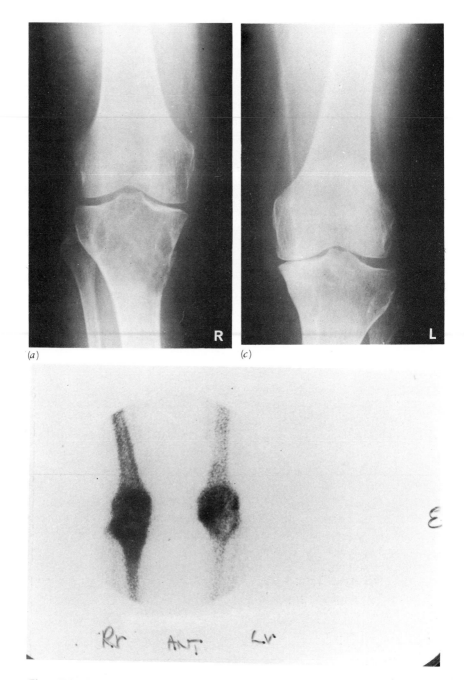

Fig. 17.3 Deceptive positive isotope scan. (a) Shows the radiograph of a giant tumour of the right tibia. Below is the technetium isotope scan (b) which shows a hot spot in both knees. (c) Shows the reason for the increased uptake in the opposite knee, which is due to arthritic changes in the joint. Isotopes merely demonstrate increased bone turnover.

17.4.3 RADIOLOGICAL EXAMINATION

Despite new innovations, X-ray studies continue to remain the most important investigation for any bone disease, and in the proper investigation of bone tumours *good quality* radiographs are essential. In addition to routine anteroposterior and lateral views, oblique projections and soft-tissue films may sometimes reveal important features. Tomography in two planes can be invaluable in locating deeply situated lesions, such as osteoid osteomata (Fig. 17.15); but arteriography, so popular in the past, is often of academic interest only and is rarely used except when it is essential to know the exact location of the main vessels. If major prosthetic replacement of the tumour bearing bone is contemplated careful radiological examination of the whole of the diseased bone is essential to avoid leaving behind skip lesions. For prosthetic replacement of tumours special measurement anteroposterior and lateral radiographs of the whole length of the femur and tibia must be taken at known anode-to-bone and bone-to-plate distances; or with a radio-opaque measurement marker alongside the bone. Routine chest films must also be taken in any tumour suspected of malignancy. Finally, it must never be forgotten that symptoms in the knee may, in the absence of local pathology, be referred from the hip.

17.4.4 BLOOD AND URINE EXAMINATION

It is rare for these investigations to add anything to the diagnosis, but nevertheless a basic set of tests should be done in every case where the diagnosis is uncertain (Table 17.2). Of these investigations the erythrocyte

Table 17.2 Routine investigations in suspected bone tumour

Blood	Erythrocyte sedimentation rate (ESR)
	Full blood count (with differential)
	Haemoglobin %
	Wasserman reaction
	Alkaline and acid phosphatase
	Serum proteins
	Serum calcium and phosphorus
	Blood urea
Urine	Proteins (Bence–Jones proteinuria)
	Blood
	Casts
Radiology	Chest
	Standard anteroposterior and lateral views
	Possibly special views and tomographs
Scans	Technetium whole body scan
	(Gallium scan is sometimes needed)
	CT scan in special cases

sedimentation rate is probably the most valuable. A significant rise may indicate the presence of infection or metastatic disease, and when combined with an alteration in the serum albumen–globulin ratio (and Bence-Jones protein in the urine), it is almost diagnostic of myelomatosis. Similarly, in Paget's disease a high erythrocyte sedimentation rate with a raised alkaline phosphatase should suggest the possible diagnosis of a sarcoma.

17.4.5 BIOPSY

However typical the clinical and radiological appearance, the diagnosis of any tumour will finally depend upon the examination of biopsy material. In most cases this is best obtained by open operation. Needle biopsies should be confined to sites not easily accessible to surgery, because the small amount of material obtained through a needle or trephine may be unrepresentative of the whole lesion and can therefore give rise to equivocal, or sometimes wholly incorrect reports. Open biopsy has the added advantage that the *macroscopic* appearance can be described: for example, its vascularity, whether it is cystic or solid, the presence of soft-tissue extension, the degree of encapsulation, and so on. All this can be valuable additional information, which should be recorded by the surgeon and passed to the pathologist. Such detailed description may also prove to be of considerable help later when planning definitive treatment.

Biopsy incisions should be planned with future surgical procedures in mind. This is particularly important where major prosthetic replacement for low grade malignant tumour is being considered because excision of the biopsy scar is desirable in such cases. Also, it should never be forgotten that a biopsy of a long bone may cause further structural weakness and can precipitate a pathological fracture. In these circumstances the limb should always be protected either by external splints or sometimes by internal fixation. Lastly, where it is essential to know the exact extent of the tumour (for example, when planning a prosthetic replacement), it may be necessary to carry out a second biopsy nearer to the proposed site of bone section.

17.4.6 THE PLACE OF A BONE TUMOUR ADVISORY PANEL

Although there are many bone tumours arising around the knee which are easy to diagnose and treat, it is clear from what has already been said that there are others where a consensus of opinion from experts of different disciplines can be valuable. The most convenient way to obtain this is by the formation of a panel of experts who can meet at short notice and *together* give an opinion on the diagnosis and advise on the best form of treatment. Of course, this can also be done by taking the case from department to department, but this is laborious and time consuming: one thing is certain – no one member should give his opinion in isolation without the benefit of the views of his other colleagues, for that is the sure way towards indecision, both in diagnosis and in treatment.

17.5   Treatment

There are basically three methods of treating any tumour of bone. These are:

(1) Surgical removal
(2) Radiotherapy
(3) Chemotherapy
or sometimes a combination or two or more.

17.5.1   SURGICAL REMOVAL

This can take several forms, varying from simple excision with bone graft to amputation of the whole limb. In the treatment of tumours of the knee four main methods need to be considered: local excision or curettage, with or without bone graft; massive graft replacement of tumour bearing bone with fusion of the knee; prosthetic replacement; and amputation.

(a) Local excision or curettage

This is the treatment of choice for all osteocartilaginous exostoses and most cystic or osteolytic lesions which have been proven benign or of a very low malignancy. Usually defects in one or other of the condyles of the femur or tibia demand that a filler is introduced to strengthen the articular surface, and this usually takes the form of an autogenous cancellous graft, often supplemented with homogenous bone from a bone bank, or from a heterogenous commercial source. If, on occasions, the defect is felt to be too large for grafting, or sufficient bone is not readily available, acrylic cement can be used as an infiller (Fig. 17.4) and some excellent long-term results have been reported (Woutters, 1974).

If curettage is to be carried out it must be meticulous and every small fragment of tumour removed until healthy bone is seen throughout the cavity. Copious irrigation with sterile distilled water is helpful after the curettage, not only to clear the bony crevasses, but also to destroy any residual tumour cells by osmosis. The cleaning of these cavities can be tedious and time-consuming, but it is essential if there is to be any hope of cure. Marcove et al. (1973) have reported considerable improvement in their results with curettage by using liquid nitrogen to cauterize the wall of the tumour cavity.

If an autogenous bone graft is to be used it can be obtained most easily from one or both iliac crests, and when needed further supplies of cancellous bone can be obtained from the greater trochanters. In the average-sized giant cell tumour involving the femoral or tibial condyles it is desirable to strengthen the articular surface with a strut of corticocancellous graft, either cut from the

421

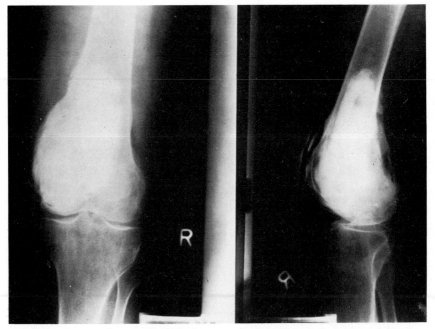

Fig. 17.4 Giant cell tumour of the lower end of the femur three years following currettage and cement infilling. (Reproduced by the kind permission of Mr K. H. Stone.)

ilium (Fig. 17.5(a)), or obtained as an intact rib from the bone bank (Fig. 17.5(b)). Following operation the weakened bone must be protected for the first month in a plaster or a Thomas splint, and then for many months in a weight-relieving caliper or a cast brace.

(b) Vascularized patella grafting

The author is indebted to Professor Merle D'Aubigne for the drawings shown in Fig. 17.6 which illustrate a technique of using the patella as a vascularized graft to fill defects either in the femur or the tibia following excision of one condyle for tumour. When used for repairing femoral defects the superficial anterior surface of the patella is used as the new articulation within the knee (as shown in Fig. 17.6). For tibial lesions the articular surface of the patella is directed proximally to form the new tibial plateau within the joint. The extensor mechanism is repaired by use of a capsular flap (Fig. 17.6(b)).

(c) Massive graft replacement of tumour bearing bone

Where curettage and cavity grafting have failed, or where the defect in the femur or tibia is so extensive that a simple infilling could not be expected to

422

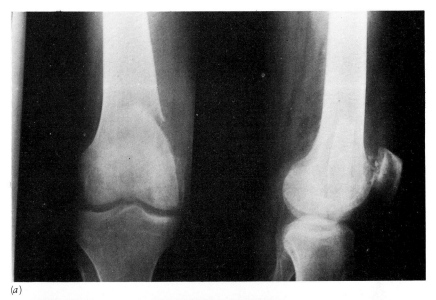

(a)

(b)

Fig. 17.5 (a) Corticocancellous graft used to strengthen the cavity grafting of a giant cell tumour. (b) Bone bank rib graft used to strengthen the cavity grafting of a non-osteogenic fibroma of bone.

succeed, the whole of the diseased bone can be removed by section at a distance from the tumour and the space filled with a massive graft cut from the femur or the tibia (according to which bone is being replaced) (Merle D'Aubigne and Dejouany, 1958). This procedure was first described by

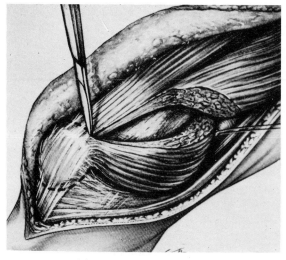
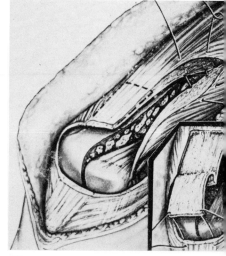

(a)   (b)

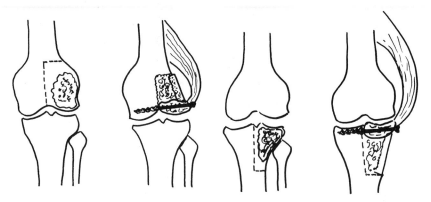

(c)

Fig. 17.6 Patellar vascular graft to fill defects in femur or tibia. (a) Shows the patella with its vascular pedicle of extensor muscle being mobilised, while (b) shows the method of restoring the extensor mechanism using a tendinous flap. (c) Shows the method of utilizing the patellar vascular graft to fill the defect in either the femur or tibia.

Juvara in 1929 and the principle of the operation (as illustrated in Fig. 17.7) remains unchanged. The tumour is approached through a long anterior incision extending from the anterolateral aspect of the mid-third of the thigh, across the knee and down the anterior crest of the tibia to its lower third. Whenever possible a tourniquet is used. The knee is widely opened and the tumour of the femur or tibial condyles fully exposed. The shaft of the affected bone is divided at least 5 cm beyond the limits of the tumour and the diseased

424

portion removed, complete with its articular surface. This is most easily accomplished by retrograde, extraperiosteal dissection, starting from the site of section through normal bone. Details of the technique of removing the tumour are described more fully in the section on prosthetic replacement. Once the tumour has been removed a 5 cm step is cut in the exposed end of the remaining shaft and the donor bone is divided longitudinally into half by a saw-cut in the coronal plane, the saw-cut being of sufficient length to produce a graft consisting of the anterior half of the shaft which will fill the defect created by the excision of the tumour. A Kuntscher nail long enough to extend the whole length of the femur and tibia and of the largest diameter possible is then inserted (Tormeno et al., 1978) by the retrograde method, making sure that in its final position it has engaged the tibia as far as its lower end. The split tibial or femoral half diameter graft is then turned upside down and screwed into the step in the resected bone and onto the remaining part of the donor bone at the knee. It has been pointed out (Merle D'Aubigne, 1982; Tormeno et al., 1978) that these large autogenous grafts are incorporated more rapidly if they are slid up or down rather than reversed. This allows cancellous to cortical bone contact which gives quicker union than an all cortical junction. The operation is completed by inserting tibial or femoral homografts (split longitudinally) over the defects above and below the knee and screwing the patella (with its muscular attachments intact but its articular surface removed) onto the autogenous graft to act as a source of blood supply.

Although this method can undoubtedly eradicate locally malignant tumours of the tibia or femur, the final result is marred by a stiff knee and sometimes fracture of the graft, or even of the nail. There is also a fairly high non-union rate. If facilities are available major prosthetic replacement is to be preferred. The use of massive allografts has been advised (Volkov, 1970; Parrish, 1973), but the complication and failure rate is too high for the method to be recommended in favour of prosthetic replacement.

(d) Prosthetic replacement of tumour bearing bone

With the introduction of the hinged knee prosthesis it has been a natural development to extend it in length to allow replacement of carefully selected bone tumours around the knee (Wilson et al., 1974; Sim and Chao 1979). Special radiographs for measurement must be taken for each patient to allow the design and manufacture of individual prostheses. The tumour bearing bone is totally removed as in the Juvara operation, but a mobile knee is preserved. Also, there is the added advantage that there are no problems of failure of bone healing at the site of resection. There are, of course, risks associated with mechanical failure of the endoprosthesis, or of its fixation to bone, both of which are inherent to any major joint replacement. However, already there are many replacements of one or other of the bony components of the knee which have remained successful over a large number of years – the longest known successful case being *in situ* for over 20 years (Wilson *et al.*, 1974).

Only tumours which are slow growing and of low malignancy are suitable for this treatment; the results are better when the tumour is still confined to bone, although a well circumscribed soft-tissue extension does not necessarily rule out the procedure. Highly malignant tumours, such as osteosarcoma or fibrosarcoma are unsuitable. They carry a high risk of local recurrence which, if it occurs, can be difficult or impossible to control, even by late amputation. Such an ill-judged conservative resection may even be responsible for a more rapid general dissemination of the disease. Major prosthetic replacement lends itself more easily to those bones which are

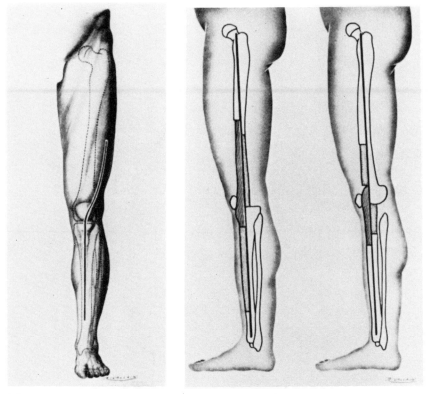

(a)

Fig. 17.7 Illustrative drawing of the 'turn-up/turn-down' bone graft of Juvara for repair after complete excision of lower end of femur or upper end of tibia. (a) Shows the incision used and diagrammatic representation of the method. The illustrations in (b) are drawings of the operative technique applied to a tumour of the upper end of the tibia. (Reproduced by the kind permission of Professor R. Merle D'Aubigne and the Editor of the *Journal of Bone and Joint Surgery* (see Merle D'Aubigne, 1958).)

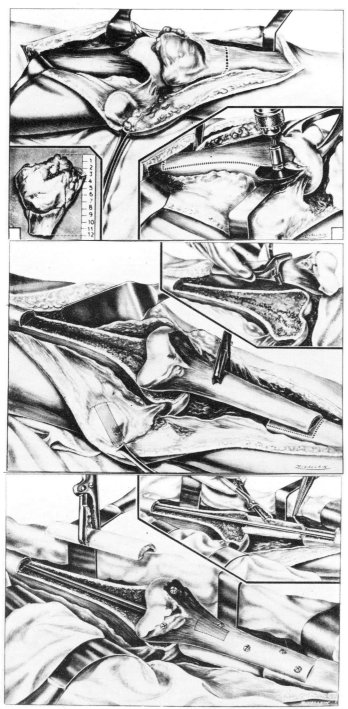

(b)

surrounded by muscle. The upper end of the tibia being superficial carries an increased risk of failure and has the added technical problem of reattaching the extensor mechanism of the knee.

(e) Operative technique

The operation is carried out through an anterolateral incision, extending to the mid-third of the thigh for resection of the lower third of the femur, and to the anterior mid-third of the shin if the upper tibia is to be resected. In either case the incision must be of sufficient extent to give wide access to the knee joint itself. A tourniquet can only be used easily for tibial resections and there is much to be said for temporary occlusion of the common femoral artery instead of using a tourniquet. It is wise to locate the external popliteal nerve early and isolate it with tape. The affected bone is exposed by extraperiosteal dissection – the femur through a posterolateral intermuscular approach between the vastus lateralis and the short head of biceps, the tibia by an anterolateral approach reflecting the muscles of the anterior compartment to the lateral side. Resection of the upper quarter of the fibula facilitates tibial removal. The previously decided level of resection should be defined early and the shaft of the bone divided at this level. Before this division is carried out the anterior surface of the healthy bone fragment is marked with a drill hole which can be lined up later with a corresponding mark on the prosthesis. The diseased portion of bone can then be most easily removed by retrograde dissection towards the knee, remembering that the main vascular supply to the femoral component is from the genicular vessels (particularly the short middle genicula artery) and that these must be carefully exposed and ligated during the last part of the dissection behind the knee. When removing the upper part of the tibia care must be taken to avoid damage to the division of the popliteal vessels into their anterior and posterior tibial branches, and much care is needed when separating the upper part of the anterior tibial muscles from the bone. It is at this stage that excision of the upper end of the fibula (usually removing it with the specimen) makes the dissection much easier.

Once the tumour has been removed and haemostasis achieved, the bone ends are reamed to receive the intramedullary fixation. All prosthetic replacements for bone tumours are 'custom made' from working drawings and the endosteal cavity must be reamed to just beyond the diameter of the intramedullary stem chosen for the particular patient, the size and curve of the stem being previously calculated from full length measurement radiographs of the involved bones. Motorized intramedullary reamers, with detachable heads increasing in size by 0.5 mm, are essential for this part of the operation. In the case of femoral replacements only a minimal amount of bone and cartilage, sufficient to allow room for the base of the tibial component of the hinged joint, is removed from the articular surface of the

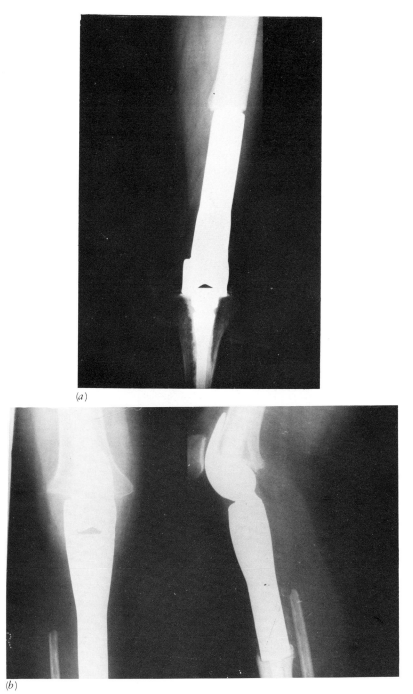

(a)

(b)

Fig. 17.8 (a) Lower femoral replacement showing the amount of bone removed in order to excise the tumour and to accommodate the knee hinge. (b) Upper tibial replacement showing the amount of bone removed.

tibia (Fig. 17.8(a) and (b)); whereas in upper tibial replacements enough bone must be removed from the femoral condyles to accommodate the whole of the hinge mechanism at the normal knee joint level (Fig. 17.9). A trial fit of the endoprosthesis must always be carried out before finally inserting the cement and a careful estimate made of tension in the extensor mechanism. If

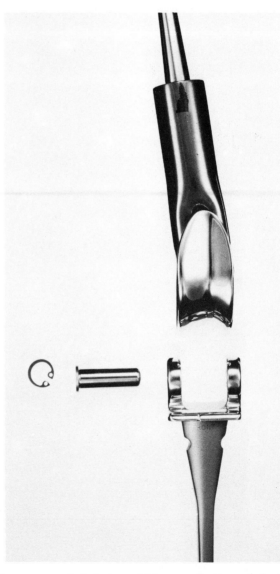

Fig. 17.9 Shows an exploded view of hinge mechanism of the Stanmore knee replacement.

430

in doubt it is better for this to be on the slack side rather than too tight. The cement for intramedullary fixation must be introduced with a cement gun (preferably of the pneumatic type), using a liquid rather than a paste mix, and whenever possible radio-opaque cement is preferred because it allows a more accurate assessment of the fixation during subsequent follow-up. Using the anterior marker drill hole in the bone the main component can be lined up to its own anterior mark, giving the correct rotation of the leg. After cementing in the other side of the prosthesis the metal axle used in the hinge is inserted as a push fit into the bearings of polyethylene already fixed in the femoral and tibial parts of the joint. The axle can be introduced from either side and secured in position by a circlip. Where the upper tibia has been resected the patellar tendon is sutured to a terylene sleeve previously secured to a slot in the lower part of the prosthetic replacement. The wound is closed in layers and two deep suction drains are left *in situ* for three days. The limb is rested in a suspended Thomas splint for three weeks, during which time the physiotherapist encourages the patient in gentle exercises. At three weeks the patient may begin to walk with crutches, using a back splint for protection. This can be discarded when 90° of controlled flexion has been regained and there is only minimal extension lag, or six weeks have elapsed since operation. The backslab will be required for longer in resections of the upper tibia in order to allow firm repair of the extensor mechanism of the knee and it is sometimes wise to fit the patient with a temporary caliper for use in the first few months.

In the author's personal series of 21 prosthetic replacements for tumours around the knee only two patients have failed to regain 90° of flexion and there have been no immediate post-operative infections. One patient has developed a low grade infection after five years, having previously had an excellent result. This infection was almost certainly from minor sepsis elsewhere (a chronic paronychia) and emphasizes the need to warn such patients of the risk of blood-borne infection and the need to use prophylactic antibiotics.

17.5.2 RADIOTHERAPY

In discussing the treatment of bone tumours in particular there are certain factors which must be taken into account when considering the use of radiotherapy. Firstly, very large malignant tumours, particularly if relatively radioresistant, are unlikely to be controlled by radiotherapy (Fig. 17.10); and in such cases it is probably wiser to advise immediate amputation. Secondly, cartilage and fibrous tissue tumours are very radioresistant and radiotherapy should never be used as a primary treatment merely to avoid the unpleasant alternative of amputation. Thirdly, serious necrosis of bone can occur as a result of heavy dose radiation, and even though the tumour tissue may have been completely eradicated the result may be marred by a pathological

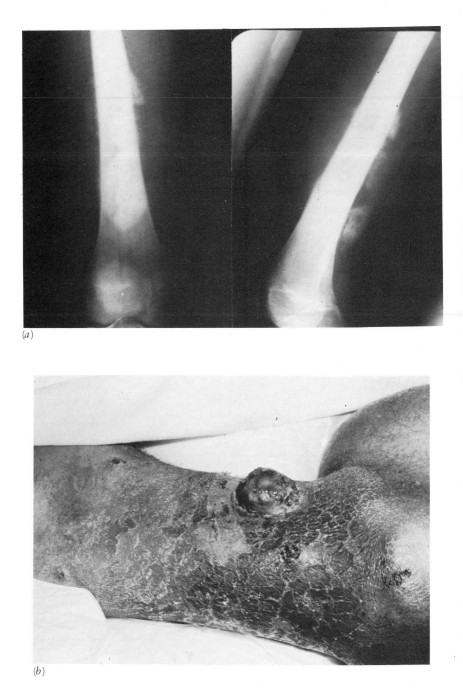

(a)

(b)

Fig. 17.10 This extensive osteosarcoma of the femur (a) was treated with radiotherapy. There was massive local recurrence (b).

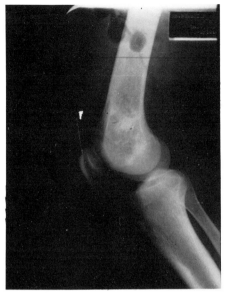

(a)

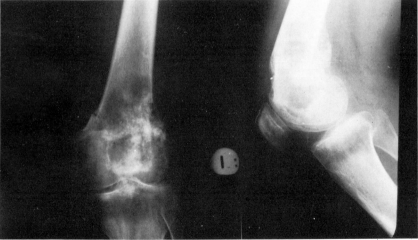

(b)

Fig. 17.11 This localized osteosarcoma (a) was successfully controlled by radiotherapy but a pathological fracture occurred six months after treatment (b). Amputation was carried out but no visible cells were found at the tumour site.

fracture (Fig. 17.11). Lastly, radiation used to control relatively benign tumours can be responsible after an interval of several years for the induction of a frankly malignant lesion.

In the treatment of bone tumours around the knee only malignant or locally malignant tumours are likely to be recommended for radiotherapy, with the possible exception of aneurysmal bone cyst which is highly radiosensitive and may be considered for treatment if surgery has failed or is impracticable. Among the primary malignant tumours only the variants of malignant round cell tumour (Ewing's sarcoma, reticulum cell sarcoma, lymphosarcoma) and Hodgkin's disease of bone are sufficiently radiosensitive to expect a dramatic control of the tumour growth; and even in these lesions there is no certainty that all the malignant cells will be destroyed by the radiation. In one comparative survey of malignant round cell tumours treated by radiation or by amputation there was a disturbingly high local recurrence rate in the cases treated by radiation alone and the early mortality was higher than in the amputation cases (Pritchard et al., 1975), and other workers studying the effect of adjuvant chemotherapy on the same tumour reached a similar conclusion (Bacci et al., 1978).

Chondrosarcoma is extremely radioresistant, and primary treatment by radiotherapy is not only a waste of time, but can be detrimental by masking the progress of the tumour within the soft-tissue reaction produced by the radiation. Fibrosarcoma, both of bone and soft tissue, is also very resistant to radiotherapy. For both these tumours treatment should be surgical. Osteosarcoma, although sometimes dramatically reduced in size by high doses of radiation, is generally radioresistant and it is only because of the very poor prognosis with any form of treatment that a conservative regime of local radiotherapy is sometimes advised. Moreover, with the advent of cytotoxic chemotherapy many clinicians feel that it is important to remove the main source of malignant cells at the primary site, and therefore amputation (or sometimes in carefully selected cases, prosthetic replacement) is considered to offer the best chance of survival.

It is tempting to advise the use of radiotherapy in the treatment of giant cell tumour and of one of its possible variants – aneurysmal bone cyst. Undoubtedly both tumours are very radiosensitive and can usually be controlled by therapy, although sometimes this ultimate effect is preceded by an alarming increase in size of the lesion. It must be emphasized, however, that radiotherapy for these tumours carries with it a definite risk of malignant transformation to a much more aggressive tumour, and that this transformation may occur several years after the apparent cure of the primary lesion.

Finally, it must be remembered that at the knee the high doses of radiotherapy required to control a tumour such as osteosarcoma will inevitably have serious effects upon the cartilage of the articular surfaces (and in a child the epiphysis), and can result in considerable stiffness, or even ankylosis.

17.5.3 ADJUVANT CHEMOTHERAPY

Although the first reports of the use of chemotherapeutic agents in the treatment of cancer date as far back as 1865, when potassium arsenite was used by Lissauer in the treatment of leukaemia (Shimkin, 1970), the modern era of treatment only started in the mid-1940s with the therapeutic introduction of nitrogen mustard. It had been observed during the trench warfare of 1914–18 that exposure to mustard gas (sulphur mustard) sometimes produced a dramatic fall in the white cell count, but it was not until after the Second World War that the possible therapeutic effect upon leukaemia was fully appreciated. This led to the introduction of nitrogen mustard (a slightly less irritant compound) and other alkylating agents, such as cyclophosphamide, into the treatment of leukaemia, lymphoid tumours and myelomatosis. These alkylating drugs are essentially antimitotic. They are thought to act by forming cross-linkages between DNA strands and by inhibition of protein synthesis. Whereas other cancer drugs, known as antimetabolites, compete with the metabolic processes of the cell.

There are now four main groups of chemotherapeutic agents in use for the treatment of malignancy. They are:

(1) *Alkylating agents* – Nitrogen mustards Cyclophosphamide
(Endoxan)
Phenylalanine mustard
(Melphalan)

(2) *Antimetabolites* – Methotrexate, which is a folic acid antagonist, is the best known example. Folic acid is an essential vitamin for cell growth and appears in its biologically active form as folinic acid which is required for the synthesis of purines and pyrimidines. The toxic effects of methotrexate on the marrow and other tissues can be reduced by following up the therapeutic dose with injections of folinic acid.

(3) *Steroid hormones* (with oestrogenic or androgenic activity) – These can be used in the treatment of hormone dependent tumours, such as those in the breast and the prostate.

(4) *Certain fungal and plant derivatives* (vincristine, adriamycin, etc.) – The vinca alkaloids (vincristine and vinblastine) are thought to interfere with the synthesis of DNA and RNA, while the antimitotic antibiotics (actino-mycin D, mithramycin and Adriamycin (doxorubicin) act as they do against bacteria, i.e. by inhibiting cell division.

Some chemotherapeutic agents are more effective on certain diseases, e.g. melphalan (phenylalamine mustard) for myelomatosis, mithramycin for the management of hypercalcaemia in myelomatosis. All are highly toxic, mainly to the bone marrow, but also to the myocardium. Regular monitoring of the red cells, white cells and platelets, as well as repeated ECG assessment of the myocardial function is essential. The use of these drugs is now so complicated that their control by an oncologist is to be recommended whenever possible. The protocol used in a trial of adjuvant chemotherapy in the treatment of osteosarcoma is shown below (Table 17.3) and gives some indication of the importance of strict control over the administration.

Table 17.3 Chemotherapy for osteosarcoma (1975 MRC trial of low dosage methotrexate)

Chemotherapy schedule for protocol A
3-*Drug group*
(a) Vincristine, methotrexate and citrovorum factor rescue
(b) Doxorubicin (adriamycin)
(a) and (b) are given alternatively every three weeks for a total of 9 cycles, i.e. *approximately 54 weeks.*

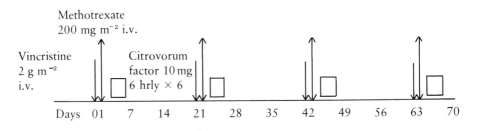

2-*Drug group*
Vincristine, methotrexate and citroborum factor rescue every three weeks for 18 cycles, i.e. *approximately 54 weeks.*

17.6 Specific tumours

In the following pages there are brief descriptions of bone tumours and tumour-like conditions which may appear around the knee. Space does not permit, nor would it be appropriate to describe these lesions in great detail and when seeking guidance on the management of one particular lesion the reader is referred back to the general points already made on treatment.

17.6.1 BONE-FORMING TUMOURS

These are: Osteocartilaginous exostoses
Osteoid osteoma
Parosteal osteosarcoma
Osteosarcoma

(a) Osteocartilaginous exostosis (Figs 17.12 and 17.13)

This benign tumour is frequently situated around the knee. It is usually a single lesion, but on occasions may be part of a diaphyseal aclasis. The tumour usually expands superficially from a narrow stalk and is always directed away from the main growing epiphysis. More rarely it arises from a broad base (Fig. 17.13). The lesion is almost certainly present at birth and gradually enlarges with growth. Increase in size after epiphyseal closure is rare and when it occurs should lead the clinician to suspect possible malignant change, although this is very uncommon and is usually associated with diaphyseal aclasis. Exostoses, however, are subject to local trauma and can sometimes fracture through their stem. Those in vulnerable positions and of appreciable size should be excised. However, it should be remembered that broad based exostoses arising from the back of the tibia (Fig. 17.13) can produce a challenging surgical exercise and are most easily approached by a posteromedial incision reflecting the medial head of gastrocnemius towards the midline.

(b) Osteoid osteoma (Fig. 17.14)

This is a rare lesion to occur around the knee (six in 254 cases, four of which were in upper shaft of tibia). It usually presents as an unexplained deep pain, often with a widespread radiation, worse at night and relieved by taking aspirin. Sometimes, when the tumour is located close to the bony cortex, the radiological diagnosis is easy – the classical appearance being one of marked sclerosis of bone surrounding an osteolytic area which contains a small bony nidus. In these cases the subperiosteal bone overlying the tumour will be irregular and thickened – a finding which is helpful when trying to locate the lesion at time of operation. There can be considerable difficulty, however, in locating these tumours when they are buried deeply in cancellous bone, for in these circumstances there will be no tell-tale sclerotic reaction in the cortex, and in such cases tomography (Fig. 17.15), isotope and possibly CT scanning may be valuable. Treatment is surgical, by local excision under radiological control. It is always wise to take a radiograph in theatre of the segment of bone removed to confirm that the tumour has been removed.

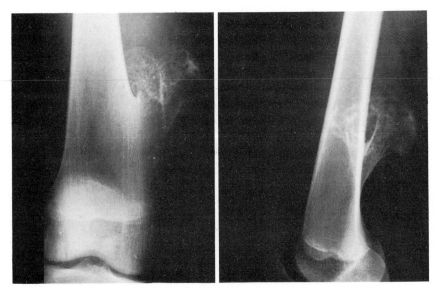

Fig. 17.12 Radiological appearance of a simple osteocartilaginous exostosis.

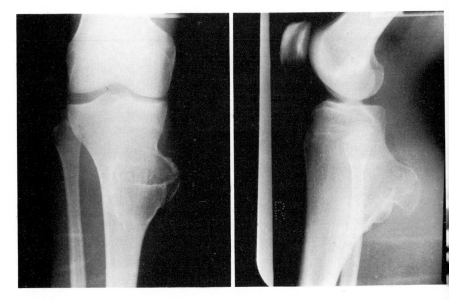

Fig. 17.13 Broad-based exostosis arising from the back of the tibia.

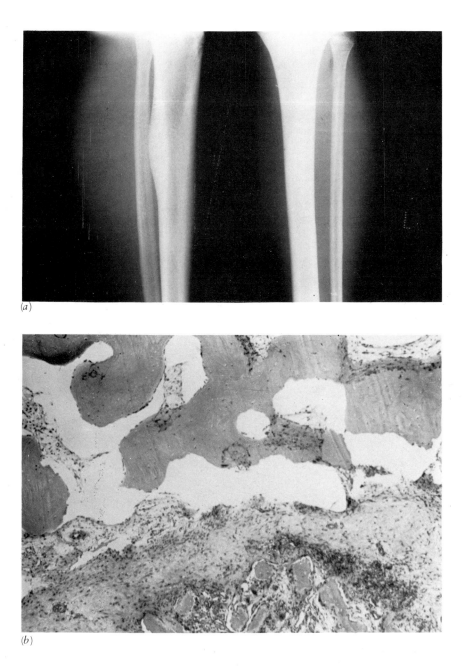

(a)

(b)

Fig. 17.14 Osteoid osteoma of the upper shaft of tibia may present as pain in the knee. It is usually eccentrically placed and has a characteristic thickening of the adjacent cortex (a). (b) Shows the classical microscopic appearance of dense bone surrounding a nidus of vascular matrix.

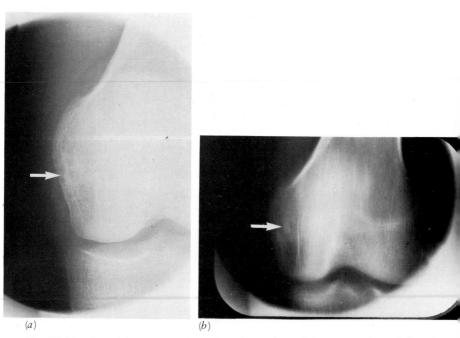

(a)   (b)

Fig. 17.15 Osteoid osteoma arising in a femoral condyle. Lesions buried deep in cancellous bone rarely have periosteal new bone to locate their position (a). Tomograms are essential (b).

(c) Parosteal osteosarcoma (Fig. 17.16)

This is a slow growing tumour of low malignancy most commonly seen around the knee joint, or in the upper part of the humerus. Although sometimes presenting with pain, more often it is swelling which brings the patient to the doctor. This tumour is always well demarcated from the soft tissues and seems to arise (as its name implies) from the periosteum, although in many cases there is also endosteal involvement. The diagnosis is usually made from the radiological appearance and the clinical history, for histologically it may be very difficult to demonstrate maglignant cells – the tumour consisting mainly of dense well-formed bone, interspersed with small nodules of fibrous matrix. The choice of treatment lies between prosthetic replacement of the whole of the tumour-bearing bone, or amputation. Limited resection of tumour alone has no place in the definitive management. The lesion is particularly suitable for prosthetic replacement, although, sadly, previous ill-advised local surgery makes this hazardous, or even impossible.

(d) Osteosarcoma (osteogenic sarcoma) (Fig. 17.10)

It is interesting to speculate why this most malignant of bone tumours should be so commonly sited around the knee, either in the lower femur or in the

440

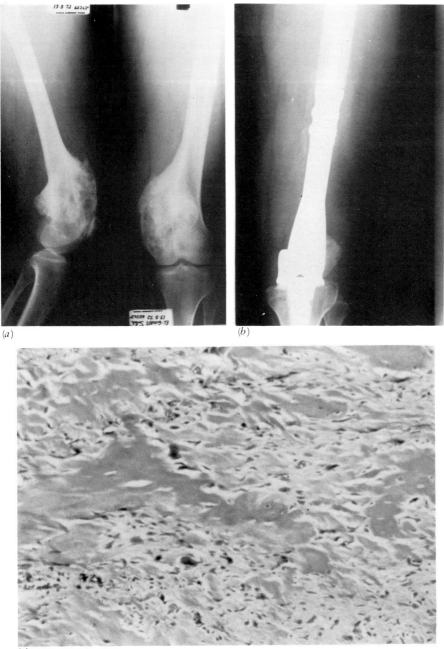

(a)

(b)

(c)

Fig. 17.16 A typical parosteal osteosarcoma of the lower femur (a) successfully replaced 12 years ago with a prosthetic lower half of femur and hinged knee (b). (c) Shows the classical microscopic appearance.

upper tibia; and to be reminded that it usually occurs in young people with active growth plates, and in a joint which is particularly susceptible to childhood injury. It is tempting to correlate a minor injury with a possible growth spurt, thereby initiating a state of uncontrolled repair. Could this infrequent and unfortunate timing of incidents be responsible for the very low and unexpected incidence of the tumour? Whatever the cause, it is a highly malignant lesion and quite different in its behaviour and prognosis from parosteal osteosarcoma. It usually presents with pain and swelling and only very rarely with a pathological fracture. Characteristically the radiological appearance is that of an endosteal bone-forming lesion, but quite often there are large areas of osteolysis where the soft-tissue tumour cells are expanding rapidly. The bone lesion soon breaks out from its periosteal confines and extends into the surrounding soft tissues – the reactive bone formation at the margins of the breakout being known as Codman's triangle (Fig. 17.17). Transverse strands of bone may radiate out into this soft-tissue mass as the so-called 'sun ray' spicules.

Histologically, the tumour is recognized by its pattern of pleomorphic and rapidly dividing cells forming a matrix which is interspersed with tumour bone (characterized by the absence of a lamellar pattern). Treatment must be radical if there is to be any hope of survival and should be by complete removal of tumour-bearing bone. This usually means an amputation. The radiosensitivity of the tumour is low and treatment by radiation should only be used when radical surgery is refused. Prosthetic replacement has little place in management and should only be considered in very small and very well defined tumours confined to bone. The use of cytotoxic drugs (combined with amputation) has changed a very gloomy prognosis to one with a limited ray of hope; and certainly there is no doubt that with this treatment the appearance of metastases has been delayed. Furthermore, whereas in the past to avoid stump recurrence, disarticulation of the hip was nearly always the treatment of choice for lower femoral lesions (Sweetnam 1973); it is now felt by many surgeons that in selected cases a through thigh amputation can be safely advised provided adjuvant chemotherapy is also to be used.

17.6.2 CARTILAGE-FORMING TUMOURS

These are: Chondroma
    Chondromyxoid fibroma
    Benign chondroblastoma
    Chondrosarcoma

(a) Chondroma

With the exception of deposits of enchondromatosis benign chondromata around the knee are infrequent. The lesions which eventually come to light do so because of pain and are usually patients in an age group where

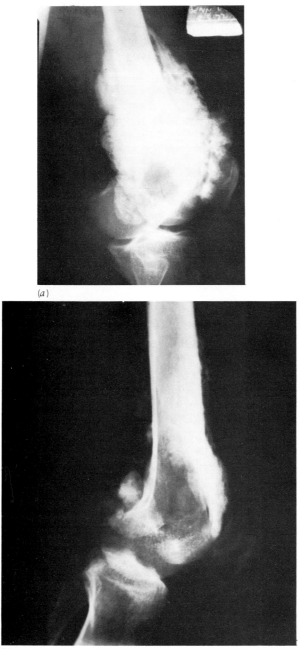

(a)

(b)

Fig. 17.17 Lateral radiographs of the lower end of a femur showing a limited resection ((a) and (b)). The inevitable recurrence has invaded the soft tissues making prosthetic replacement impracticable (b).

chondrosarcomatous change is likely to be occurring. Symptomless chondromatous deposits found accidentally in routine radiology surveys should be left strictly alone, unless they are increasing in size or producing other symptoms. Once discovered, however, it is mandatory to keep the lesion under a close radiographic surveillance. Smillie (1980) has described an osteochondroma which developed on the anterior surface of the lower femur. It had the appearance of a calcified subperiosteal chondroma and was responsible for painful limitation of patellar movement. Disabling new bone formation following simple excision was only prevented at a later operation by putting a sheet of Teflon over the raw bone surface.

(b) Chondromyxoid fibroma (Fig. 17.18(a))

This is a relatively uncommon destructive lesion, usually discovered before adult life and when it occurs around the knee nearly always affects the upper end of the tibia. It is difficult to distinguish radiologically from giant cell tumour (Fig. 17.18(b)) and non-osteogenic fibroma (Fig. 17.18(c)) and other factors, such as pain, rapidity of growth and age (all higher in giant cell tumour), must be taken into consideration in making the diagnosis. This lesion is non-malignant and can be successfully eradicated by meticulous curettage, followed by cavity grafting with bone bank and autogenous cancellous graft. Recurrence is rare and is easily treated by a second excision and graft.

(c) Benign chondroblastoma

This primary bone tumour was described many years ago as a 'chondromatous giant cell tumour' (Codman 1931) and at one time was thought to be exclusive to the upper end of the humerus. Jaffe and Lichtenstein (1942), however, who labelled the tumour a benign chondroblastoma, found the most frequent site to be around the knee. Radiologically it presents as an osteolytic lesion with some patchy endosteal calcification, situated in an epiphyseal segment of bone (Fig. 17.19(a)). Histologically, the tumour is a broad mixture of fibrous tissue, cartilage and bone, with a generous scattering of giant cells in the fibrous stroma (Fig. 17.19(b)). It is non-malignant, but if it is giving symptoms it should be treated by curettage and cancellous grafting.

(d) Chondrosarcoma

Although by far the most common site for a chondrosarcoma is in the upper third of the femur, it can arise around the knee, usually in the lower femur, but occasionally the upper end of the tibia is affected. It should always be considered in the differential diagnosis of a lesion presenting in the second

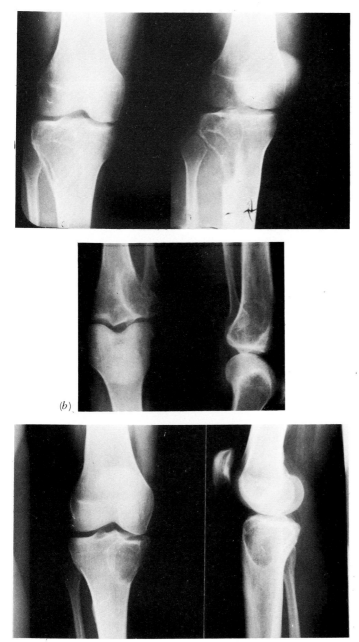

(a)

(b)

(c)

Fig. 17.18 Chondromyxoid fibroma of the upper end of tibia (a). Compare this with the appearance of an early giant cell tumour (b) and a non-osteogenic fibroma (c). In the early stages it is almost impossible to distinguish between these three conditions on radiological grounds.

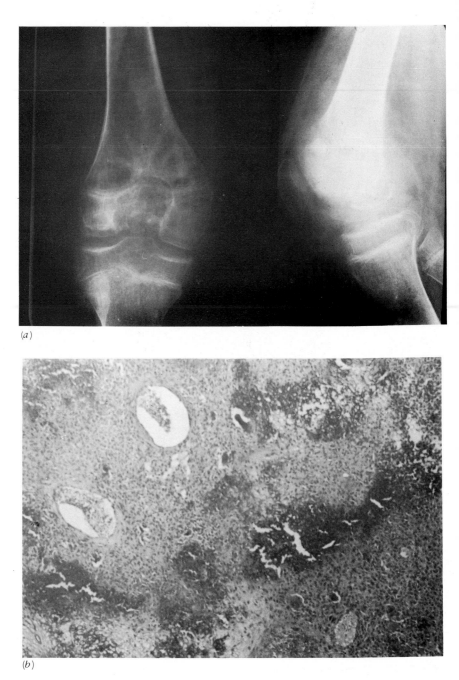

(a)

(b)

Fig. 17.19 A benign chondroblastoma of the lower end of the femur is shown in (a). The histology shows a mixture of fibrous tissue, cartilage and giant cells with intermingling patches of calcification (b).

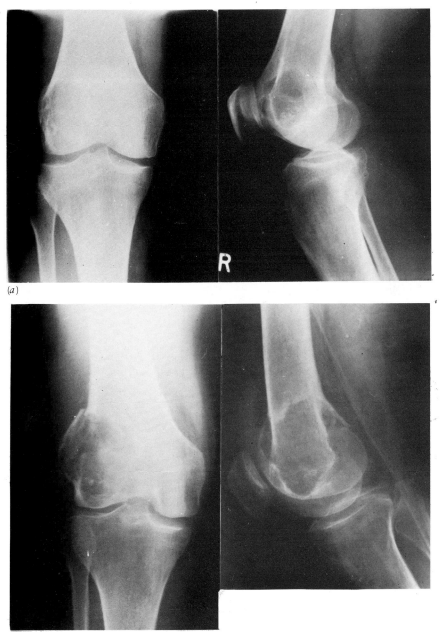

(a)

(b)

Fig. 17.20 An anteroposterior and lateral radiograph of a chondrosarcoma of the lower end of the femur is shown in (a). The patient refused further treatment at that time and was relatively free of pain until a pathological fracture occurred three years later (b).

half of life. A chondrosarcoma can be a very slow growing tumour and it may be several years before pain, swelling, or even a pathological fracture forces the patient to seek medical advice (Fig. 17.20). These lesions demand complete resection of the tumour-bearing bone, either by amputation, by massive bone graft, or by prosthetic replacement. Local curettage with or without cavity grafting is doomed to failure.

17.6.3 FIBROUS TISSUE TUMOURS

These are: Non-osteogenic fibroma
Fibrous dysplasia
Malignant fibrous histiocytoma
Fibrosarcoma

(a) Non-osteogenic fibroma

This may occur in the bones on either side of the knee and radiologically it is indistinguishable from giant cell tumour and other benign lesions (Fig. 17.18(c)). The content, however, is always solid and is not particularly vascular (as in giant cell tumour and aneurysmal bone cyst). Macroscopically and microscopically the tumour material is characteristic (Fig. 17.21) and the lesion usually presents at a much earlier age group than giant cell tumour. Histologically, the cellular structure is well-formed fibrous tissue interspersed with a few giant cells which may lead the unwary to diagnose a giant cell tumour. Treatment is by curettage and cancellous graft.

(b) Fibrous dysplasia

Although not strictly speaking a tumour, this condition, when monostotic, may present as an apparent cyst of any one of the bones around the knee. However, with the passage of time and the very considerable extension of the 'tumour' the real diagnosis becomes easier to make radiologically, and histologically the appearance is characteristic (Fig. 17.22(a), (b) and (c)). Treatment by local resection and bone graft is almost invariably followed by recurrence. Resection of the whole of the involved bone is required, followed by reconstruction with massive grafts or with a prosthetic replacement.

(c) Malignant fibrous histiocytoma and fibrosarcoma

These two malignant tumours are considered together because of their cellular and radiological similarity, and because the former is probably merely a less malignant variety of the latter. Both, however, can be very malignant and must receive radical treatment. Radiologically, the appearances only differ in the degree of demarcation (Fig. 17.23(a) and (b)); and histologically distinguishable features of the two conditions are by no means

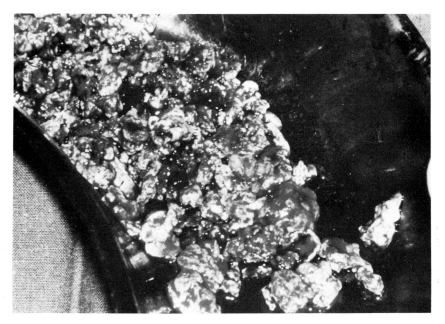

Fig. 17.21 Non-osteogenic fibroma of bone. The macroscopic appearance is quite different from giant cell tumour and has characteristic flakes of yellow tissue throughout the specimen.

clear cut, and their diagnosis is not uncommonly a source of disagreement between pathologists. However, in malignant fibrous histiocytoma there is a 'storiform' (mat-like) pattern to the fibrous stroma which, along with a relatively low cellular activity, is said to be a characteristic feature distinguishing it from the more aggressive stroma of a true fibrosarcoma. Provided the lesion is well contained, a malignant fibrous histiocytoma can be treated by complete resection and reconstruction with a massive graft or a prosthesis. But this method of treatment is not advisable in a rapidly growing fibrosarcoma where amputation is the treatment of choice. Radiotherapy has no place in the management of either lesion.

17.6.4 LYMPHOSARCOMA

This tumour can appear at any age group, but is more commonly seen in the latter half of life, and may sometimes be associated with Paget's disease. The tumour has no special distinguishing features and is only rarely found in the bones of the knee.

17.6.5 METASTATIC TUMOURS

Metastatic deposits must be considered in the differential diagnosis of any bone defect at all ages, and although clearly their diagnostic importance rises steeply in the second half of life a previous history of a primary malignant tumour elsewhere in the body should alert the clinician to consider metastases, even at a very early age. They are, however, rare around the knee (less than 1% in the Royal National Orthopaedic Hospital Bone Tumour Registry), usually favouring the shaft or upper end of the femur or humerus when they affect long bones. Being commonly osteolytic, metastases frequently present as pathological fractures.

17.6.6 TUMOURS OF UNKNOWN ORIGIN

These are: Simple bone cyst
Giant cell tumour and aneurysmal bone cyst
Malignant round cell tumour

(a) Simple bone cyst

This is an infrequent lesion around the knee, the usual site in the lower limb being in the upper end of the femur. Small subarticular cysts, or possibly

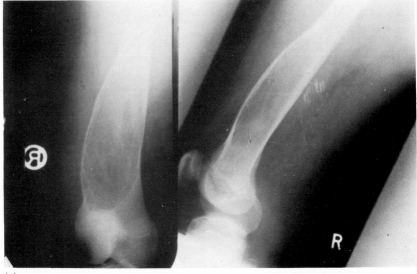

(a)

Fig. 17.22 Fibrous dysplasia of bone. (a) and (b) show radiographs of a case of fibrous dysplasia which was first diagnosed as a bone cyst (a). The considerable increase in size over a ten year period (b) suggests the correct diagnosis. The histological appearance is shown in (c) with the characteristic benign fibrous tissue interspersed with spicules of cancellous bone.

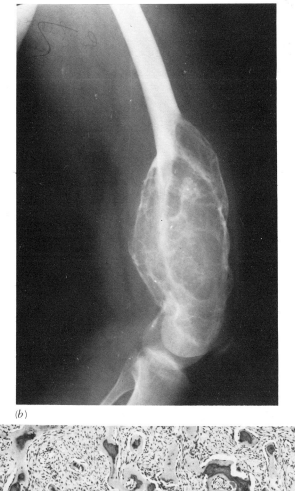

(b)

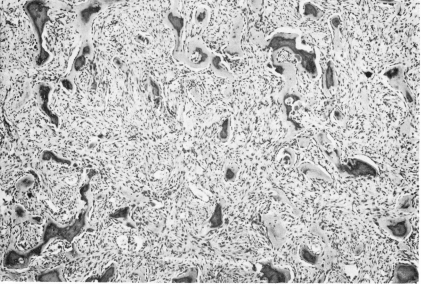

(c)

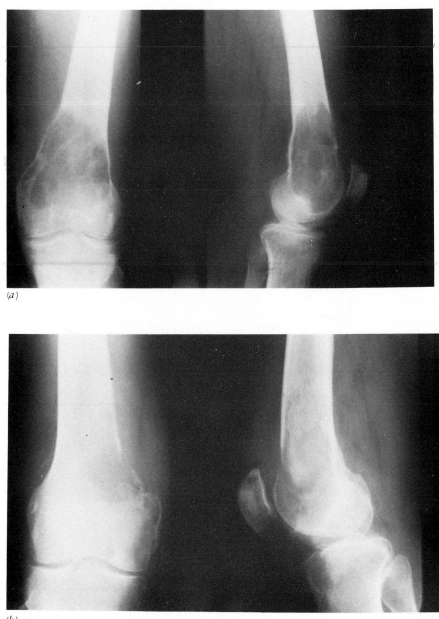

(a)

(b)

Fig. 17.23 Malignant fibrous histiocytoma and fibrosarcoma. A malignant fibrous histiocytoma (a) is usually better demarcated than its more malignant cousin fibrosarcoma (b).

ganglia arising from joint surfaces are occasionally seen (Fig. 17.24). If they give symptoms curettage and cancellous bone graft is the treatment of choice.

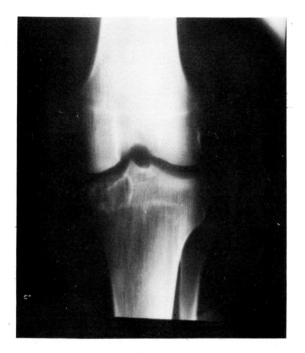

Fig. 17.24   A subarticular cyst of the tibia is seen in this anteroposterior tomogram.

(b) Giant cell tumour and aneurysmal bone cyst

These two conditions are considered together because they are so often misdiagnosed both radiologically and histologically, and not uncommonly the correct diagnosis depends largely upon the surgeon's description of the macroscopic appearance of the tumour at the time of the biopsy. Fig. 17.25(a) and (b) shows two identical lesions in the lower end of the femur, one of which is a giant cell tumour and the other an aneurysmal bone cyst. However, a clear distinction between the two conditions should be possible (Fig. 17.26(a) and (b)) and the differing features are summarized in Table 17.4. Although both giant cell tumour and aneurysmal bone cyst are very radiosensitive, treatment is usually surgical and radiotherapy reserved for those tumours in sites where adequate excision is impracticable. The occurrence of radiation-induced sarcoma in giant cell tumours some years after treatment by radiation is too well documented to go unheeded.

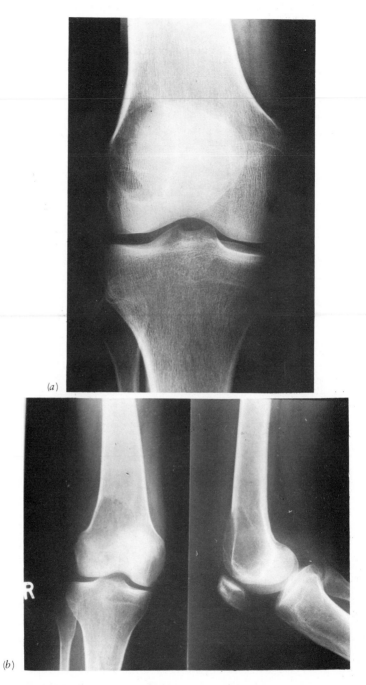

(a)

(b)

Fig. 17.25 The radiograph (a) is of an aneurysmal bone cyst and (b) is of a giant cell tumour, both arising in the lower femur in young adult women. Giant cell tumour and aneurysmal bone cyst can be indistinguishable radiologically.

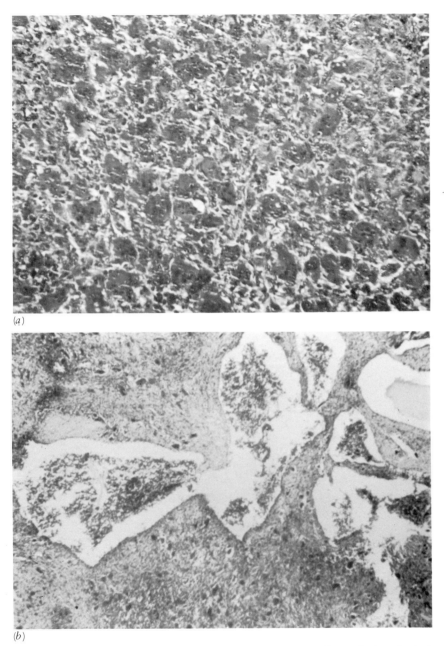

(a)

(b)

Fig. 17.26 Giant cell tumour and aneurysmal bone cyst. (a) Shows the histological appearance of a well-differentiated giant cell tumour. It is a solid lesion composed of fibrous tissue with a generous scattering of giant cells. Compare this with the large cystic spaces of an aneurysmal bone cyst (b), where the only solid tissue resembling a giant cell tumour is seen in the thickened cyst wall.

Table 17.4 Differences between giant cell tumour and aneurysmal bone cyst

	Giant cell tumour	Aneurysmal bone cyst
Age group	Adult lift up to early middle age	Adolescents and young adults
Site	Always in epiphysis and usually subarticular	Eccentric and may often involve shaft of bone
Radiological appearance	Osteolytic, extending into the corner of epiphysis	Osteolytic with aneurysmal bulging of cortex. Bony loculation usually present
Macroscopic appearance	Solid, containing vascular 'red currant jelly'	Cystic, filled with blood. Thick, 'velvety' lining with loculations of bone lined with similar tissue
Microscopic appearance (see Fig. 7.26)	Solid, but sometimes with small cystic spaces. The stroma is basically fibrous and vascular, containing many well formed giant cells	Mainly cystic with evidence of haemorrhage into these spaces. The cellular content of the lining of the cyst and septa resemble giant cell tumour

The usual initial treatment is by curettage and cavity bone grafting. Major resection of tumour bearing bone is reserved for cases of recurrence.

(c) Malignant round cell tumours

This rarely occurs in the vicinity of the knee except in the form of reticulum cell sarcoma, in which the basic round cell pattern is generously interspersed by a liberal amount of reticulum. The other variety of this tumour is Ewing's tumour which is essentially confined to the shaft of long bones and for all practical purposes never affects the knee.

17.6.7 LESIONS SIMULATING BONE TUMOURS

There are a number of conditions affecting bone which are not classified as tumour but which can be mistaken for them. These are illustrated in the composite Fig. 17.27. It is hoped that reference to these cases may be helpful in unravelling some of the diagnostic problems associated with bone tumours of the knee joint.

Fig. 17.27 (Pages 457 – 463) Lesions around the knee simulating bone tumours: (a) hydatid disease of lower femur; (b) Brodie's abscess (tuberculous osteomyelitis); (c) and (d) chronic osteomyelitis of upper tibia; (e) and (f) Paget's disease lower end of femur; (g) and (h) disappearing bone disease; (i) pigmented villonodular synovitis; (j) Gaucher's disease.

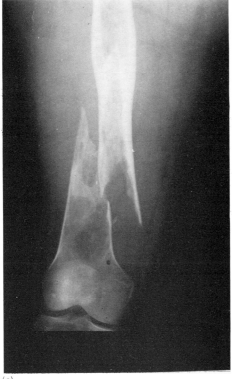

(a)

Fig. 17.27 (a) Hydatid disease of the femur with pathological fracture. The marked loculation, lack of fracture callus and Middle East origin of the patient should alert the clinician to the correct diagnosis.

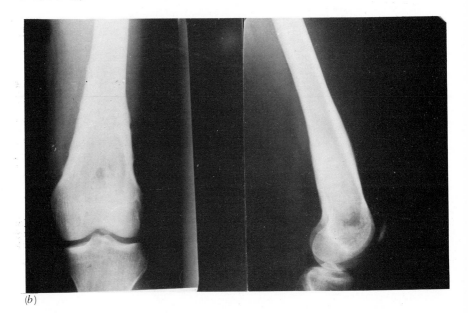

(b)

Fig 17.27 (b) Brodie's abscess (from tuberculous osteomyelitis). Note the irregular periosteal reaction around the lesion which is characteristic of chronic bone infection (also see legend of Fig. 17.2).

458

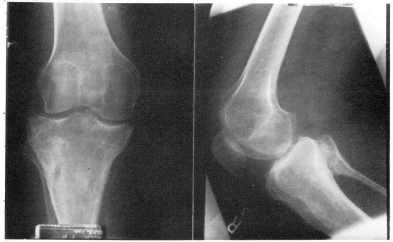

(c)

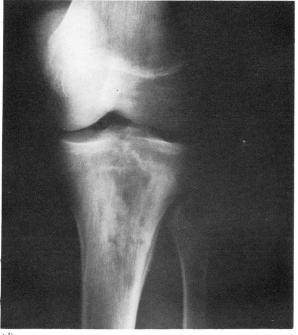

(d)

Fig. 17.27 (c) and (d) Chronic osteomyelitis of the upper tibia. This can be a particularly difficult diagnosis to make on radiographic findings alone and both malignant round cell tumour and osteosarcoma can present with the same appearance. ((d) Shows a similar case which later proved to be osteosarcoma.) Ancillary tests for infection may clarify the problem.

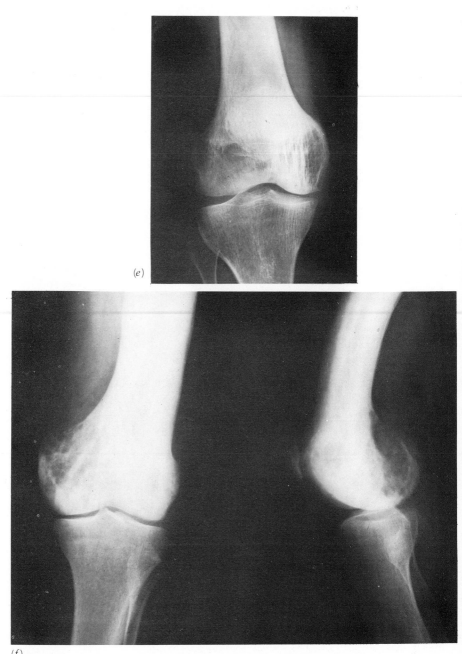

(e)

(f)

Fig. 17.27 (e) and (f) Paget's disease of lower end of femur. The coarse trabeculation of the medial femoral condyle combined with the typical, subarticular location of the lesion, makes the diagnosis. It must be remembered that such a lesion can undergo sarcomatous change, usually indicated by rapidly increasing destructive change (f).

460

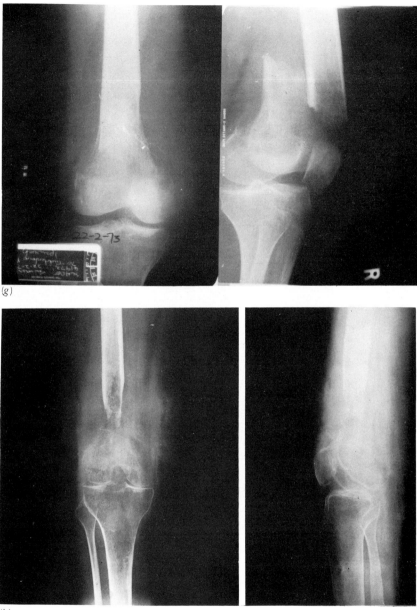

(g)

(h)

Fig. 17.27 (g) and (h) Disappearing bone disease (Gorham's disease). This rare condition of angiomatous osteolysis always presents as a pathological fracture through very osteoporotic, vascular bone (g). It is sometimes associated with large, subcutaneous angiomata. If left untreated fractures remain ununited and bone is gradually destroyed (h). Prosthetic replacement of the diseased bone is the treatment of choice.

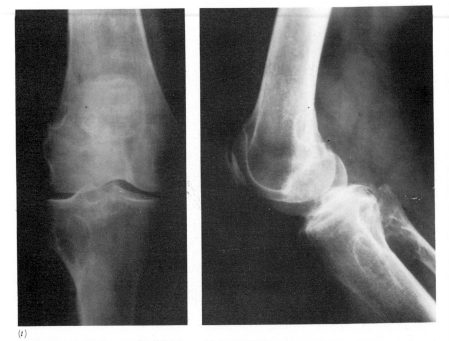

(1)

Fig. 17.27 (*i*) Pigmented villonodular synovitis (PVNS). Although sometimes referred to as a synovial tumour, the cause of this condition is unknown. It presents as a chronic swelling which is mildly painful. The synovial shadow is more dense than in rheumatoid disease due to haemosiderin deposits. The joint space is usually retained and there is no subchondral osteoporosis. Para-articular erosions are less common in loosely packed joints such as the knee where large synovial masses are often found.

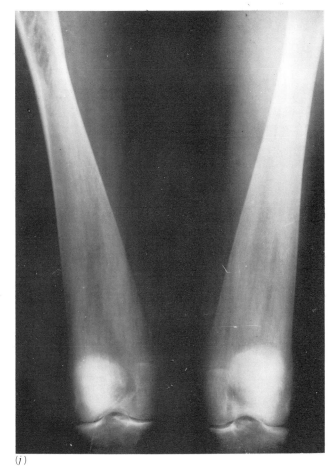

(j)

Fig. 17.27 (j) Gaucher's disease (lipid storage disease). A condition almost exclusively confined to patients of Jewish origin. When the condition affects the major long bones tubulation or modelling deformities occur, which in the lower end of the femur resemble an Erlenmeyer flask. Endosteal new bone may form, producing 'a bone within a bone' appearance. The finding of anaemia with splenomegaly should confirm the diagnosis. (Figs 17.27 (f), (i) and (j) are reproduced by the kind permission of Dr R. O. Murray and Dr H. G. Jacobson (1977) and Churchill-Livingstone.)

References

Bacci G, Campanacci M, Pagani P A. Adjuvant chemotherapy in the treatment of clinically localised Ewing's sarcoma. *J Bone Joint Surg [Br]* 1978;**60–B**:567–74.

Codman E A. Epiphyseal chondromatous giant cell tumours of the upper end of the humerus. *Surg Gynecol Obstet* 1931;**52**:543.

Jaffe H L, Lichtenstein L. Benign chondroblastoma of bone: a re-interpretation of the so-called calcifying or chondromatous giant cell tumour. *Am J Pathol* 1942;**18**:969.

Juvara M E. Reconstitution de la tige osseuse fémoro-tibiale, interrompue par la resection d'une des extremité osseuses, qui constitue l'articulation du genou par une greffe, provenant de dédoublement de l'extremité osseuse opposee. *Bull Mémoires Soc Nat Chir* 1929;**55**:541.

Marcove R C, Lyden J P, Huvos A G, Bullough P B. Giant-cell tumours treated by cryosurgery. A report of twenty-five cases. *J Bone Joint Surg [Am]* 1973;**55–A**:1633–44.

Merle D'Aubigne R. Personal communication, 1982.

Merle D'Aubigné R, Dejouany J P. Diaphyso-epiphyseal resection for bone tumour at the knee. With report of nine cases. *J Bone Joint Surg [Br]* 1958;**40–B**:385–95.

Murray R O, Jacobson H G. *The radiology of skeletal disorders.* 2nd edn. London; Edinburgh: Churchill-Livingstone, 1977.

Parrish F F. Allograft replacement of all or part of the end of a long bone following excision of a tumour. Report of twenty-one cases. *J Bone Joint Surg [Am]* 1973;**55–A**:1–22.

Pritchard D J, Dahlin D C, Dauphine D T, Taylor W F, Beabout J W. Ewing's sarcoma. A clinico-pathological and statistical analysis of patients surviving five years or longer. *J Bone Joint Surg [Am]* 1975;**57–A**:10–16.

Shimkin M B. Cancer research. In: *Cancer, diagnosis, treatment and prognosis.* Ackermann L V, del Regato J A. eds. St. Louis: C V Mosby Co, 1970;28.

Sim F H, Chao E Y S. Prosthetic replacement of the knee and a large segment of the femur or tibia. *J Bone Joint Surg [Am]* 1979;**61–A**:887–92.

Simon M A, Kirchner P T. Scintigraphic evaluation of primary bone tumours. Comparison of technetium 99m phosphate and gallium citrate imaging. *J Bone Joint Surg [Am]* 1980; **62–A**:758–64.

Smillie I S. *Diseases of the knee joint.* Vol 14. Edinburgh: Churchill Livingstone, 1980;469.

Sweetnam R. Amputation in osteosarcoma. Disarticulation of the hip or high thigh amputation for lower femoral grafts. *J Bone Joint Surg [Br]* 1973;**55–B**:189–92.

Tormeno B, Istria R, Merle D'Aubigne R. La resection-arthrodese du genou pour tumeur. *Rev Chir Orthop* 1978;**64**:323.

Volkov M. Allotransplantation of joints. *J Bone Joint Surg [Br]* 1970;**52–B**:49–53.

Wilson J N, Lettin A W F, Scales J T. Twenty years of evolution of the Stanmore hinged total knee replacement. *Conference on Total Knee Replacement.* London: Institution of Mechanical Engineers, 1974; 61.

Woutters H W. Tumeur a cellules geantes de l'extremité distal du fémur avec fracture intra-articulare de genou. *Rev Chir Orthop Reparatr L'Appareil Moteur,* 1974;**60:Suppl 11**:316.

Index